The International Review of Child Neurology

FETAL NEUROLOGY

The International Review of Child Neurology

The International Review of Child Neurology

Fetal Neurology

Editors

Alan Hill, M.D., Ph.D., F.R.C.P. (C)

Professor and Head
Division of Neurology
Department of Paediatrics
University of British Columbia
British Columbia's Children's Hospital
Vancouver, British Columbia, Canada

Joseph J. Volpe, M.D.

A. Ernest and Jane G. Stein
Professor of Developmental Neurology
Professor of Pediatrics, Neurology,
and Biological Chemistry
Director, Division of Pediatric Neurology
Washington University School of Medicine
St. Louis, Missouri

Raven Press 🦫 New York

Raven Press, 1185 Avenue of the Americas, New York, New York 10036

Made in the United States of America

Library of Congress Cataloging-in-Publication Data
Fetal neurology.

    (The International review of child neurology)
    Includes bibliographies and index.
    1. Fetus—Diseases—Diagnosis. 2. Nervous system—Diseases—
Diagnosis. 3. Fetus—Physiology. 4. Pediatric neurology. I. Hill, Alan,
M.D. II. Volpe, Joseph J. III. Series. [DNLM: 1. Fetal Diseases.
2. Fetus—physiology. 3. Nervous System Diseases. WQ 210.5F4197]
RG627.F48   1989   618.3'268   88-42851
ISBN 0-88167-469-9

9 8 7 6 5 4 3 2 1

Preface

In the past decade or so, the neurology of the newborn has provoked so much interest that it seems reasonable to consider this area of neurology a discipline in its own right. However, those of us who have devoted most of our efforts to the study of the newborn have become increasingly aware of the importance of the intrauterine period in the determination of the nature and severity of neonatal neurological disease. Fortunately, other investigators such as those in obstetrics, perinatology, radiology, and developmental neurology have directed their special skills toward study of the fetus. Thus, because of the singular need to understand the nervous system of the fetus and because of the growing body of interesting information gleaned by recent studies of the fetus, we elected to devote this book to "fetal neurology."

We have divided the text into the broad categories of antepartum fetal assessment, intrapartum fetal assessment, and certain major, specific fetal conditions. Our contributors are experts in their fields, and at the end of each chapter we have added commentaries that we hope will put the work in perspective for the reader with a more general interest in neurology.

Concerning antepartum fetal assessment, recent studies of well-known means of evaluation, such as the fetal biophysical score, the nonstress test, and the contraction stress test, are presented. In addition, this section includes fascinating new insights into fetal behavioral states and movement, including eye movement. Finally, the application of Doppler ultrasonic methodology to assessment of fetal and placental blood flow is described, and the possibility is raised that perturbations of fetal circulation that are important in the genesis of brain injury can be detected and perhaps eventually prevented.

Concerning intrapartum fetal assessment, the importance of electronic fetal monitoring and assessment of fetal acid-base status is demonstrated. Although it is currently fashionable to de-emphasize the importance of intrapartum events in the genesis of neonatal brain injury, an overwhelming clinical experience together with studies in subhuman primates make it undeniably clear that brain injury does occur during the intrapartum period. It seems apparent that novel means of detecting the timing of such injury and of preventing the injury must be found.

Concerning certain major, specific fetal conditions, we chose to emphasize two common and challenging clinical problems, that is, fetal hydrocephalus and myelomeningocele. Additionally, we indulged ourselves somewhat with futuristic, although provocative discussions of fetal neurosurgery and the influence of the central nervous system on normal and abnormal muscle development.

We hope that this book provides an introduction for the neurologist to the time in the life of the patient that is often the most critical and invariably the most mysterious. Fetal neurology, although still a somewhat amorphous area of study, should evolve in the next decade into a new discipline in child neurology.

Alan Hill
Joseph J. Volpe

Foreword

The International Review of Child Neurology series is the official publication of the International Child Neurology Association (I.C.N.A.). This is the fifth volume in the series and broadens the horizons of child neurology into the area of fetal disorders.

When I.C.N.A. decided to launch the series it appointed Dr. John Stobo Prichard from the Hospital for Sick Children, Toronto, as its Senior Editor. He had been instrumental in the conception of the idea and its selling to I.C.N.A. Under his guidance the series had a successful beginning and, due to his enthusiasm, continued to thrive during his term as Senior Editor, during which he produced a total of four volumes.

Regrettably, Dr. Prichard passed away in 1986. We are sure that he will be long remembered for his contributions to the Department of Neurology at the Hospital for Sick Children and to the world of child neurology. He was one of the founding parents of I.C.N.A. and was responsible for the First International Child Neurology Congress held in Toronto in 1976. The International Review of Child Neurology will certainly be regarded as one of his major achievements.

There is no doubt that he would have welcomed the publication of this book on the neurology of the fetus as an appropriate and innovative expansion of his series.

P.G. Procopis

Acknowledgments

We wish to thank the editors of the International Review of Child Neurology Series, especially the late Dr. John Stobo Pritchard who initially invited us to contribute this volume. Drs. Isabelle Rapin, Peter Procopis, Joseph French, and William J. Logan have been helpful in the ongoing preparation of the manuscript. We acknowledge also the assistance of Dr. Alfred Brann, Jr., who reviewed the manuscript and made many helpful suggestions. Dr. Elke H. Roland assisted in many ways with helpful suggestions and with organization of the references. Finally, we appreciate the dedicated secretarial assistance of Karen Mewett.

Contents

II. Intrapartum Fetal Assessment

III. Major Specific Fetal Conditions

Contributors

Jason C. Birnholz
Department of Diagnostic Radiology
and Nuclear Medicine
Rush-Presbyterian–St. Luke's
Medical Center
Chicago, Illinois 60612

Harbinder S. Brar
Department of Obstetrics and Gynecology
Division of Maternal Fetal Medicine
University of Southern California
School of Medicine
Women's Hospital
Los Angeles County USC Medical Center
Los Angeles, California 90033

Frank A. Chervenak
Department of Obstetrics and Gynecology
The New York Hospital–Cornell
Medical Center
New York, New York 10021

Dermot E. FitzGerald
Angiology Research Group
Vascular Medicine Laboratory
St. Mary's Hospital
Dublin 20, Ireland

Alan Hill
Division of Neurology
Department of Paediatrics
University of British Columbia
British Columbia's Children's Hospital
Vancouver, British Columbia,
*   Canada V6H 3V4*

Glenn Isaacson
Department of Obstetrics and Gynecology
The New York Hospital–Cornell
*   Medical Center*
New York, New York 10021

Pierre Jacob
University of Ottawa Faculty of Medicine
The Children's Hospital
*   of Eastern Ontario*
Ottawa, Ontario, Canada K1H 8L1

J.A. Low
Department of Obstetrics and Gynecology
Queen's University
Kingston, Ontario, Canada K7L 3N6

Kim H. Manwaring
Division of Pediatric Neurosurgery
Phoenix Children's Hospital
Phoenix, Arizona 85006

Jeffrey P. Phelan
Department of Obstetrics and Gynecology
University of Southern California
*   School of Medicine*
Women's Hospital
Los Angeles, California 90033

Lawrence D. Platt
Department of Obstetrics and Gynecology
Division of Maternal Fetal Medicine
University of Southern California
*   School of Medicine*
Women's Hospital
Los Angeles County USC Medical Center
Los Angeles, California 90033

Heinz F.R. Prechtl
Department of Developmental Neurology
University Hospital
9713 E.Z. Groningen, The Netherlands

William F. Rayburn
Division of Maternal-Fetal Medicine
University of Nebraska
  College of Medicine
Omaha, Nebraska 68105

Harvey B. Sarnat
University of Calgary
Faculty of Medicine
Alberta Children's Hospital
Calgary, Alberta, Canada T2T 5C7

Barry S. Schifrin
AMI-Tarzana Regional Medical Center
Tarzana, California 91356

Carl V. Smith
Department of Obstetrics and Gynecology
University of Southern California
  School of Medicine
Women's Hospital
Los Angeles, California 90033

Bernard T. Stuart
Coombe Lying-in Hospital
Dublin 8, Ireland

Joseph J. Volpe
Division of Pediatric Neurology
Washington University
  School of Medicine
St. Louis, Missouri 63110

The International Review of Child Neurology

FETAL NEUROLOGY

Fetal Neurology, edited by
A. Hill and J.J. Volpe.
Raven Press, New York © 1989.

1

Fetal Behavior

Heinz F. R. Prechtl

*Department of Developmental Neurology, University Hospital,
9713 E.Z. Groningen, The Netherlands*

WHAT IS FETAL BEHAVIOR?

The term *behavior* is used in this context in the restricted sense of ''overt behavior.'' The connotation covers only observable movements of the fetus and so-called behavioral states and excludes speculations about subjective experience, feelings, intentions, emotions, and mood of the fetus. Such speculations lack scientific basis despite claims by prenatal psychologists.

Fetal movements and behavioral states should be studied in the conceptual context of developmental neurology. Thus, the recognition both of age-specific functional repertoires of the nervous system and of ontogenetic adaptations are relevant for fetal studies. The advantage of this approach is that the fetus can be studied in terms similar to those in which preterm and full-term infant behavior has been previously investigated. Such an approach facilitates homogeneity of terminology and provides an opportunity to compare prenatal with postnatal neural activity that spans the transition from intrauterine to extrauterine life. In fact, we have demonstrated a high degree of continuity of neural functions before and after birth (34). However, this does not ignore a few distinct changes after birth that provide functional adaptions to the extrauterine environment.

NEW METHODS

The study of fetal behavior has received a new impetus from the development of advanced ultrasound techniques that permit prolonged and repeated observations of the undisturbed fetus. This technique has great advantages over mechanical or electromagnetic recordings of fetal activity through the abdominal wall that do not allow the recognition of specific movement patterns. The subjective counting of movements by the expectant mother is even more limited and has a major degree of unreliability.

1

Real-time ultrasound equipment with multiple transducers in a linear array is the most suitable apparatus for investigation of fetal movements, provided the resolution and dynamics are sufficiently high. However, a problem relates to the size of the transducers. The large type (~12 cm length) provides excellent total viewing of the fetus in a longitudinal mid- or parasagittal plane during the first half of pregnancy. During the second half of pregnancy, the fetus grows beyond the range of available transducers and can be only partially viewed. A lack of larger transducers to date has prevented detailed studies of the older fetus. The simultaneous use of two transducers in a longitudinal alignment represents a partial solution to the problem.

HOW DOES THE FETUS MOVE?

A scientific interest in fetal movements has existed for 100 years. However, only recently has an answer been found to the questions concerning how the fetus moves and the timetable followed by emerging movement patterns. The noninvasive and apparently safe nature of ultrasound investigations (46) has enabled observations of the comprehensive motor repertoire in healthy and undisturbed fetuses in their natural environment. Previously our knowledge of fetal neural functions had been based on incidental observations of aborted fetuses and on the systematic studies of Minkowski (23), Hooker (13), and Humphrey (15) on exteriorized fetuses. Because of the dominance of the reflex theory at that time, these studies concentrated on responses to externally applied sensory stimulation. Although these investigations demonstrate the capacity of the fetal nervous system to respond to artificial stimuli, they tell little of the endogenously generated motility of the healthy fetus. Moreover, comparison of the cinefilm recordings made by Hooker (14) with the pictures obtained by ultrasound clearly indicate that the exteriorized fetuses were in a terminal condition and moved abnormally.

With the advent of ultrasound observations of spontaneous movements of the fetus in the undisturbed intrauterine environment, the problem of classification of these motor patterns has arisen. The most obvious and elementary distinction between movements is a classification based on their amplitude and speed, i.e., small versus large and slow versus fast, involving the whole body or the limbs only. Although this type of classification has been in use since Reinold's pioneer work (41,42), it soon became apparent that the complexity of movements by far exceeds the limited discrimination power of such categories. This became especially true as the resolution quality of real-time ultrasound equipment improved. More recent observations therefore have been related to previous neurological studies of the fetus (3–14) or infant (16–22). A shortcoming common to all earlier ultrasound investigations of fetal movement patterns and their developmental course relates to the relatively short duration of the observations (usually only a few minutes), the cross-sectional approach instead of a longitudinal follow-up and, last, but not least, the on-line observation without the possibility of repeated observation via a replay of a video tape recording.

A more systematic approach has been taken up in Groningen, where fetal studies have been carried out within the conceptual context of developmental neurology (5–9). These investigations were preceded by a longitudinal study of strictly selected low-risk preterm infants "because they are the only group whose behaviour can be compared, with any meaning, with the recorded behaviour of the intrauterine fetus during undisturbed pregnancies" (36). The design of the fetal investigations followed, to a large extent, the same line as this preterm research. Repeated observations of fetuses of carefully selected low-risk pregnancies were carried out longitudinally. They lasted 1 hr each and, during the last trimester, 2 hr. All sessions were recorded on videotape for off-line analysis. It was also expected that the existing classification of motor patterns of preterm infants would help to recognize at least some of the fetal movements that might have a similar appearance. Nevertheless, it came as a surprise that the total repertoire of fetal movements consists exclusively of motor patterns that also can be observed postnatally. It must be added, however, that the newborn's behavioral repertoire rapidly expands with patterns thus far never observed in the fetus (e.g., the Moro response). However, the striking similarity between fetal movements and postnatal motor patterns greatly facilitates a consistent and comprehensive descriptive classification and terminology. In the following, a short definition of the various types of fetal movements will be given (35).

Startles are quick, generalized movements that always start in the limbs and often spread to the trunk and neck. The duration of a startle is 1 sec or less. Usually they occur singly but sometimes they may be repetitive. They can be superimposed incidentally on a general movement.

General movements are also gross movements, but they are slow and involve the whole body. They may last from a few seconds to a minute. A peculiarity of these movements is the indeterminate sequence of arm, leg, neck, and trunk movement. They wax and wane in intensity, force, and speed. Despite this variability, they must be considered as a distinct pattern and easy to recognize if they occur again.

Hiccups are phasic contractions of the diaphragm, often repetitive at regular intervals. A bout of hiccups may last as long as several minutes. In contrast to the startle, the movement always starts in the trunk but may be followed by involvement of the limbs.

Fetal breathing movements are usually paradoxical. Every contraction of the diaphragm (which after birth leads to an inspiration) causes an inward movement of the thorax and a simultaneous movement of the abdomen outward. The sequence of "breaths" can be either regular or irregular. No amniotic fluid enters the lungs during breathing movements. Isolated breaths may resemble a sigh.

Isolated arm or leg movements may occur without other parts moving. The speed and amplitude of the movement may vary.

Twitches are quick extensions or flexions of a limb or the neck. They are never generalized and are not repetitive.

Clonic movements are repetitive, tremulous movements of one or more limbs at a rate of approximately three per second. There are rarely more than three to four beats in normal fetuses.

Isolated hand movements occur when the fingers flex or extend together repetitively or in isolation. Some hand postures may resemble hand gestures seen in later life. The hand may also rotate outward or inward (supination or pronation).

Hand-face contact is made when the hand accidentally touches the face either by an arm movement in the direction of the face or by a head movement in the direction of the hand. Hand-mouth contact occurs, but it is often difficult to judge precisely where the hand makes contact.

Retroflexion of the head is the backward bending of the head, varying in speed from slow to jerky. The head may remain in a retroflexed position from 1 sec to 1 min, often accompanied by an overextension of the spine.

Lateral rotation of the head occurs when the head is rotated from the midline to a lateral position or vice versa. This movement occurs in isolation. The speed is usually slow and the amplitude may vary.

Rhythmical side-to-side movements of the head are slow and may cover a range of 180°. As in postnatal rooting, the regularity is not accurate.

Anteflexion of the head is the forward bending of the head, which is usually slow but always consists of a lift-off from the surface on which the fetus is resting.

Opening of the mouth occurs in isolation, and the amplitude and speed may vary. Sometimes tongue protrusion is observed.

Yawn is a slow opening of the mouth, followed by maintenance of the position for several seconds and then by quick closure.

Rhythmical mouthing is a small and rhythmical quiver of the jaws without opening of the mouth, occurring in bursts of 5 to 10 movements with a rate of approximately four or five per second.

Sucking is a burst of rhythmical jaw movements with a rate of about one per second and of varying length, sometimes followed by swallowing, which indicates that the fetus is drinking amniotic fluid.

Stretch is a complex motor pattern consisting of overextension of the spine, retroflexion of the head, abduction, external rotation, and elevation of the arms. The movement lasts several seconds and occurs singly.

Rotation of the fetus may occur along the longitudinal axis or the transverse axis of the fetal body. These movements are always forceful. Alternating leg movements, when the feet are contacting the uterine wall, may result in a somersault over the head. Rotation around the sagittal axis is initiated by either rotation of the head or of the hip.

Eye movements can be distinguished as slow, rapid, and repetitive (nystagmoid). The displacement of the eyeball can be seen as a flicker of the echo behind the orbit or, more clearly, as shifts in the position of the echoes of the lenses.

WHEN DO THE DIFFERENT MOVEMENT PATTERNS APPEAR?

By analogy with the age-related gradual unfolding of the postnatal motor repertoire, a timetable of fetal motor patterns has been obtained, based on their emergence in the 12 individuals observed longitudinally (5). Up to the 7th week (postmenstrual age) when the crown-rump length is approximately 18 mm, the fetus remains immobile. The first discernible movements appear at about approximately 7½ weeks and consist of slow flexion and extension of the vertebral column with passive displacement of arms and legs. A few days later these movements are replaced by the first complex movements, e.g., general movements and startles, involving trunk, head, and limbs. Again only a few days later, isolated limb movements are observed. As can be seen in Fig. 1, the repertoire expands rapidly from 10 weeks onward. The width of the scatter formed by the different individuals is approximately 1½ weeks for frequently occurring movement patterns and much larger for rare movements. In the latter case, the movements are obviously missed during the 1-hr observation at earlier ages. Compared with previously published timetables (3,16), the ages of first appearance are considerably younger in our study. This is most probably owing to the relatively short duration of observations made by the earlier authors.

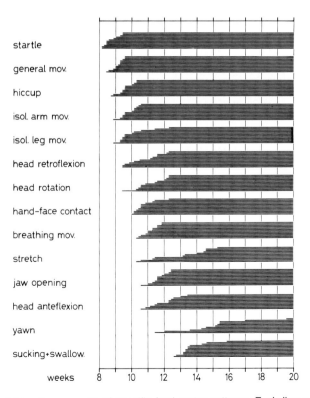

FIG. 1. Timetable of emergence of specific fetal motor patterns. Each line represents one fetus from a weekly follow-up study. Age in weeks and days; N = 12. (Data from ref. 5.)

QUANTITATIVE ASPECTS OF FETAL MOTILITY

Subjective reporting of fetal movements by the expectant mother and various kinds of objective recordings with mechanical, pressure, or electromagnetic devices have suggested that changes in the amount of movements may indicate neural dysfunction in the abnormal and compromised fetus. Usually these changes comprise a sudden decrease in activity or, sometimes, an excessive increase. Systematic quantitative assessment of fetal motility based on ultrasound observations is heretofore lacking, with the exception of the study by De Vries et al. (7), which included only the first half of pregnancy. For the second half of gestation, data are still scarce because of the aforementioned shortcomings of instrumentation. Only for breathing movements (32) and for gross body movements (without further specification) (31) are data available regarding the last 10 weeks of pregnancy.

During the first half of pregnancy, when a complete view of the fetus is still possible, the complete repertoire of distinct movements that occur during each of the 1-hr observations can be recorded. The result is an actogram (an example is given in Fig. 2). Such actograms, recorded with the aid of an event recorder during videotape replay, indicate the incidence and the temporal sequence of specific movement patterns. A data base obtained in this way allows analysis of the amount of specified motility per recording. It also permits analysis of the developmental course over the longitudinal recordings. Of great interest was the individual consistency and the differences between individuals. Only such normative data can provide a sound basis for a meaningful assessment of the compromised fetus and an answer to the question of whether quantitative measurements of motility are a sensitive discriminator between the normally or abnormally functioning fetal nervous system.

Fetal motility is not a homogeneous phenomenon but is based on activities of different movement generators. This leads to complex pictures as seen in the actograms. If the amount of specific movement patterns is considered per individual, it becomes clear that motility is not equally abundant or scarce in all components but that one specific movement pattern may occur relatively frequently whereas others are relatively rare. When the absolute incidences of all movement types are ranked, a consistent pattern emerges that changes only slightly with age (8). In contrast to this stability, the week-to-week variations of absolute measures per movement type vary considerably. This is a common finding in all kinds of longitudinal behavioral observations. It was, for example, also found in the motor activity in low-risk preterm infants (36). The mechanism that explains this phenomenon remains obscure. Because the observations were always carried out at the same time of the day, diurnal variations can be excluded as the cause of this variability. Despite these overall fluctuations in weekly values of the motor output, considerable interindividual differences exist in the degree of these fluctuations. Consistently stable fetuses turned out to be the exception rather than the rule, but they do exist. This fact renders improbable the possibility that the 1-hr recordings

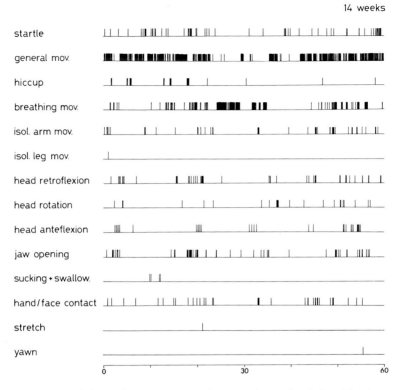

FIG. 2. Actogram of the various movements, from event recorder during 1-hr observation from repeated videotape replays.

are too short to be a representative sample. This conclusion is at least true for the younger ages when rest-activity cycles and behavioral states do not yet play a role.

The developmental course of the different movement patterns shows clear differences. For example, general movements increase in incidence from 8 to 10 weeks, then reach a plateau at 10% to 15% of the recording time, and remain at this level for the first two trimesters. Another type of developmental course is followed by the isolated arm movements, breathing movements, rotation of the head, and sucking, all of which gradually increase in incidence over the first half of pregnancy. Still different is the development of startles, which increase rapidly from 8 to 9 weeks, followed by a gradual decline. These differences in developmental trends explain the age-related shifts in the rank order of relative frequencies of occurrence, discussed previously, because there are individuals who move relatively frequently and others who move less, as well as fluctuations in the amount of activity within individuals. Consequently, a large scatter occurs when a larger number of individuals is plotted. That the scatter within individuals is smaller than within an ensemble of individuals is trivial but is frequently reported in the obstetrical literature. In any case, the large scatter in the quantitative movement data of a carefully selected low-risk group (7,8) makes quantitative assessment a less sensitive indicator of conditions that compromise the nervous system. Only extreme cases will exceed the wide normal ranges and will appear as clearly abnormal.

THE FETUS WITH NEURAL MALFORMATIONS

Although Preyer (40) described abnormal motor behavior in anencephalic fetuses and reported excessive activity occurring in bursts as a characteristic phenomenon, it was 100 years before a detailed description of movements in anatomically verified anencephalic fetuses was published (51). Although otherwise stated in the neuropediatric literature (19), their motor behavior is grossly disturbed. Even if the morphological organization of the spinal cord is intact, the coordination and the temporal sequence of the motor activity appeared to be abnormal. The clearest abnormality concerned the quality of the individual movements and especially that of general movements. In all such fetuses, the movements were forceful, jerky in character, and of large amplitude and caused large positional shifts in the uterus. They started abruptly, and during the movement, the same force and amplitude continued until the movement suddenly stopped. These qualities are in contrast to the fluent appearance and the waxing and waning of these movements in normal fetuses (51). This abnormality in anencephalic fetuses indicates a strong organizing influence of supraspinal structures on normal fetal activity. In a case with only low thoracic and lumbosacral spinal cord present, active displacement of an arm has been seen, although only ectopic nests of geometrically disorganized motor neurons were found in the paravertebral cervical region. These observations considerably aid the understanding of the generation of normal motor patterns because they show how little neural structure is necessary to generate movements, even if their quality is staggering and lacks normal features. Electron microscopy of the cervical spinal cord of normal fetuses (28) revealed remarkably few motor neurons with limited synaptic innervation at an age when the fetus moves with different distinct motor patterns (i.e., at 9–12 weeks). The conclusion can therefore be reached that early fetal motility is endogenously generated by a minimal but ordered neural structure and with minimal sensory input. Despite this immaturity of the nervous system's structure, the generated motor patterns appear coordinated and clearly distinguishable. Results from electrical recordings of neural activity in tissue cultures of the nervous system (11,45) corroborate these conclusions. As soon as a minimal differentiation of connectivity is reached, organized activity in burst-pause patterns occurs.

THE COMPROMISED FETUS

In a large number of complications of pregnancy, the question arises as to whether the integrity of the fetal nervous system is at risk or has already been impaired. Fetal well-being is usually monitored by fetal heart rate recordings or quantification of (subjectively or objectively) recorded fetal motility. It is best to monitor a combination of both of these phenomena in a "nonstress test," i.e., heart rate accelerations in response to fetal movements. A more comprehensive scoring system for monitoring of high-risk pregnancies has been suggested by Manning et al. (20,21) and has been called the biophysical profile. It includes the observation of fetal breathing movements, body movements, and "fetal tone" during a 30-min ultrasound recording. One can argue that the criteria for "movements" and "tone" could easily be refined in view of the present state of the art. Because the number of movements per unit time is not a sensitive criterion, it is not advisable to include this measure among the criteria. A much better characteristic of suboptimal neurological functioning is the change in quality of distinct movement patterns, e.g., the quality of general movements or of startles. This notion stems from investigations of preterm infants (37).

A comparison of a low-risk group and a neurologically impaired group of preterm infants, in a longitudinal study (2-hr observations, repeated weekly) of spontaneous motility, revealed only differences in the number of clonic movements. All other types of motor patterns failed to discriminate between the two groups (37). A continuation of these studies, including video recordings of preterm infants, demonstrated another abnormality of motor pattern of impaired preterm infants. The latter move monotonously, without subtle fluctuations in speed, amplitude, and force, e.g., in general movements or isolated arm movements. Although such subtle changes of the pattern can easily be recognized, especially when observed on videotape replay, they are difficult to measure exactly and to describe in terms other than fluency, variability, and smoothness. Touwen (48) has previously demonstrated this aspect of impaired neural functions in children, referring to the stereotypical aspects of abnormal postures and responses. Even if difficult to measure objectively, our visual "gestalt perception" is a powerful and sensitive instrument that has enabled us to grasp the multifaceted complexity of such phenomena. It is fashionable nowadays to underestimate the importance of such qualitative observations. However, it is becoming more and more evident that qualitative changes in motor patterns precede quantitative changes when the integrity of the nervous system is impaired. The validity of such subjective judgments, made with the unaided eye, must be tested. Only a high degree of intersubjectivity between different observers guarantees objectivity of the conclusions. Results of interpretations made by independent observers from the same videotapes of both normal and abnormal preterm infants have given unexpectedly high and reproducible interobserver agreements.

When the same technique was applied to fetuses with growth retardation (1), eight observers (89%) came to the same conclusion when they had to discriminate between normally and abnormally moving fetuses. The degree of familiarity with obstetric ultrasound examinations did not appear to play a role.

In 10 growth-retarded fetuses, varying in age from 20 to 35 weeks gestation, Bekedam et al. (1) noted "a general monotony of all movement patterns" in all but one. The movements were slow, lacked power and amplitude, and were characterized by a striking reduction in variability of intensity and speed of each movement, such that the normal waxing and waning of the movement disappeared. Although parameters such as speed, power, and amplitude were reduced, it must be emphasized that the overall monotony was the most impressive feature. This feature was also observed in the isolated movements. Subtle movements of the arm and hand of varied speed and intensity were seen only in normal fetuses. Another example of abnormal quality involved head movements, both isolated or as components of general movements. They were performed slowly with a small amplitude in the growth-retarded fetus, as if the movements were not fully executed. Although this pattern was characteristic for the group as a whole (apart from one case), interindividual differences in performance existed.

Although statistically significant differences between the growth-retarded fetuses and a matched control group were found for various movement types, such quantitative differences are of limited practical importance. The considerable overlap between the individual values of the two groups makes such quantification a poor discriminator.

Another example describing qualitative changes of fetal movement patterns observed by ultrasound is the study by Boue et al. (4) of fetuses with chromosomal anomalies. Without distinguishing between specific motor patterns as in the studies previously discussed, these investigators describe grossly abnormal motility in cases with trisomy 21 and 18 and monosomy 5p (cri du chat syndrome) at fetal ages of approximately 19 weeks of gestation.

FETAL BEHAVIORAL STATES

Behavioral states are temporarily stable conditions of neural and autonomic functions known as sleep and wakefulness. They are characterized by a distinct behavior of certain variables in concert. Observation or recording of such variables [e.g., eye movements, heart rate pattern, breathing pattern, electroencephalograph (EEG) pattern, motility] provide a method for monitoring behavioral states over long periods. There exist extensive studies in the full-term neonate, and several attempts have been made to define states in the preterm infant (29,47). In the healthy full-term newborn, the coordination between the variables is such that transitions from one state to another do not last longer than 2 to 3 min (i.e., all variables have changed their parameters to those characteristic for the new state) (30,44). It is this phenomenon of *alignment* between the variables at the transitions that develops at approximately 36 to 38 weeks conceptional age in the preterm infant. Before this age, states are "poorly organized" (29) as the separate variables fluctuate less consistently than later. On the other hand, there are periods of congruency between state variables that fit the state definition but that do not start and end simultaneously. The possibility of coincidence by chance would exist even if the separate variables oscillated completely independently from each other. Such an extreme condition does not usually seem to be the case as, from about 30 to 32 weeks onward, a certain bias in the relationship between particular state variables may exist (36).

Concerning the ontogeny of behavioral states in the fetus, Nijhuis et al. (25,26) were able to show in multiparous women that fetuses of 36 and 38 weeks gestation had developed behavioral states, the degree of organization of which was comparable to the states in full-term neonates. Of course, the selection of state criteria had to be adapted to the particular situation *in utero,* and these criteria differ in part from those employed in neonates. Three independent variables were chosen, i.e., fetal heart rate pattern (excluding accelerations during movements), eye movements present or absent, and gross body movements present or absent. An important step was achieved by the differentiation between "coincidence" and "true behavioral state." Coincidence was defined as any period in which the parameters of variables met the criteria of the particular state, although without the simultaneous changes during transitions (Fig. 3). With this distinction, it became much easier to focus on the ontogenetic events in the emergence of true behavioral states. In this context, the main questions are: what is the developmental course of the various types of coincidences (Fig. 4)?, when do synchronized transitions occur?, and are there age differences between the different kinds of transitions (between certain states)? A study by Van Vliet et al. (49) provides data for a group of fetuses of low-risk nulliparous women. There are certain minor differences from the previously studied multipara group but the increase between 32 and 40 weeks in the percentage of coincidences, mimicking state 1, was similar to that in the multipara group. Surprisingly, before 36 to 38 weeks, there was no prevalence in the synchronization of a certain type of transition. The occurrence of well-aligned transitions is inconsistent within the same individual fetus and seemingly follows no particular rule. Future research should concentrate on these aspects rather than debate the existence of states before 36 weeks without convincing data. However, it is clear that the choice of state variables is crucial. Single variables (e.g., fetal heart rate or eye movements) are insufficient to identify states and therefore are misleading.

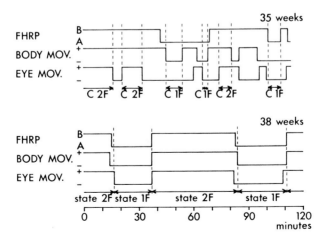

FIG. 3. Profiles of state variables at 35 and 38 weeks. **Top:** Independent fluctuations of the three variables with incidental meeting of the criteria for coincidence. **Bottom:** Same fetus with organized state. Synchrony of transitions. FHRP, fetal heart rate pattern. (From ref. 25.)

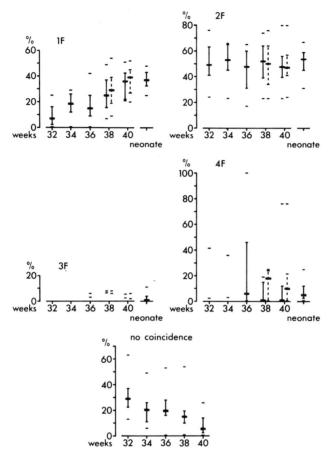

FIG. 4. Quantitative data of percentages of coincidence (*solid lines*) and states (*dashed lines*) from 32 to 40 weeks, and states in newborns for comparison. Given are medians, quartiles, and total ranges. (Data for fetuses from refs. 26 and 50; newborn data from ref. 33.)

It has become evident from newborn studies of the input-output relation to stimulation with different modalities (38) that behavioral states are not merely convenient descriptive categories of complex physiological regulations but capture specific modes of neural functions (33). The response intensity to one particular kind of stimuli not only changes with different behavioral states but different stimulus modalities behave differently in the same states. These regulatory properties of behavioral states are also to be expected in the fetus.

Behavioral States in the Compromised Fetus

Attention has been given to the possibility of abnormal development of behavioral states in research regarding fetuses with intrauterine growth retardation

(49,50) and in fetuses of mothers with type I diabetes (24). Studies in the full-term neonate with neurological impairment demonstrate that behavioral states may dissociate and fluctuations of the state variables may become independent (39). In the longitudinal study of eight growth-retarded fetuses from 32 to 40 weeks of gestation, only three showed well-organized states during the 2-hr continuous monitoring at 40 weeks of gestation. From 28 cases in the parallel low-risk control group, only one failed to demonstrate normal development of states. In contrast to the delay in maturation of states in the growth-retarded fetuses, values of the coincidence measures were undisturbed. What was obviously deviant in these fetuses was the *inability to synchronize the variables* at the transitions. This observation emphasizes the importance of discriminating between the coincidence and the true behavioral state with synchronized state transitions. The abnormalities in the development of behavioral states in growth-retarded fetuses would have been overlooked without this distinction.

Fetuses of insulin-dependent diabetic mothers had similar deviations of the normal development of behavioral states (24). Only three of eight fetuses studied at 38 weeks gestation had normal behavioral states, and these were fetuses of multiparous women. There was a clear delay in the maturation of states in the infants of nulliparous women despite careful metabolic control.

Thus, the compromised fetus may show abnormalities in the development of behavioral states. However, these signs are not specific.

FETAL RESPONSES TO STIMULATION

A high rate of endogenously generated movements is common to all stimulation experiments of the fetus. Only if experiments with stimuli are carefully balanced with experiments with sham stimulations and with a sufficiently long control period without stimulation is it possible to demonstrate responses with certainty. In addition, in fetuses of 36 weeks and older, behavioral states have to be taken into account, as responses are state dependent, i.e., their occurrence is restricted to particular behavioral states, depending on the sensory modality. The relationship between the various behavioral states and the responsiveness to stimuli of different modalities has been extensively investigated in newborn infants. There is every reason to expect a similar relationship in the near-term fetus.

Motor responses to tactile stimulation of various areas of skin are known from studies of the exteriorized fetus (15). Anecdotal observations are reported in the literature on "avoidance responses" to accidental touches of the fetus with the needle during amniocentesis.

Evidence that the near-term fetus can hear has been stated for many years but only recently have systematic and well-controlled studies shown a state dependence, similar to those in the newborn infant. Schmidt et al. (43) reported practically no responses during state 1F to a 2,000-Hz sine wave or to sawtooth-modulated sine waves of 120 dB, inconsistent responses during state 2F, and regular responses during state 3F and 4F (wakefulness). In an even more extensive study, Lecanuet et al. (17) confirmed these findings. The response decrement owing to repeated stimuli was the strongest in state 1F and less during state 2F. Moreover, the stimulus intensity was shown to play a role. In both studies, attention was paid to avoid mechanical vibratory stimulation during the sound stimulations.

Vibration is obviously the most potent stimulus with which to elicit changes in fetal movements and heart rate. Birnholz and Benacerraf (2) have employed a so-called electrolarynx firmly applied to the maternal abdomen such that it overlies a fetal ear. The output is approximately 110 dB in a frequency range of 250 to 850 Hz, and it produces a vibroacoustic stimulus. The fetal response consists of an eye blink and a startle reaction, such as head aversion, arm movements, and leg extension.

Recently, this vibroacoustic stimulation has been suggested as a test for fetal well-being during periods of low heart rate reactivity and low motor activity. When the stimulus is applied to a normal fetus during behavioral state 1F, the heart rate instantaneously increases by 30 to 50 beats per minute and usually remains at a high rate for 10 min or longer (27). A similar abrupt increase in fetal movements is observed and may last for an hour (12). Such long-lasting changes in fetal behavior can only be explained by an induced transition into another behavioral state, i.e., into state 4F. Under normal conditions without stimulation, such prolonged episodes of state 4F have never been observed. It may be concluded that the abrupt heart rate changes and the prolonged episodes of vigorous fetal activity are an abnormal response produced by these stimuli. Divon et al. (10) elicited consistent "fetal startle responses" with the electrolarynx. Because this reaction seems to be independent of the ongoing behavioral state, it may belong to the same category of responses as those caused by pain stimuli. In the neonate, the reactions to this latter modality were the only ones that were independent of state (18). It should be noted that pure sound stimulation does not lead to changes of fetal heart rate or to fetal movements longer than several seconds and, in addition, does not include changes in the behavioral state (43).

REFERENCES

1. Bekedam, D.J., Visser, G.H.A., DeVries, J.I.P., and Prechtl, H.F.R. (1985): Motor behaviour in the growth retarded fetus. *Early Hum. Dev.*, 12:155–166.
2. Birnholz, J.C., and Benacerraf, B.R. (1983): The development of human fetal hearing. *Science*, 222:516–518.
3. Birnholz, J.C., Stephens, J.C., and Faria, M. (1978): Fetal movement patterns: A possible means of defining neurologic developmental milestones *in utero*. *Am. J. Roentgenol.*, 130:537–540.
4. Boue, J., Vignal, P., Aubry, J.P., Aubry, J.C., and MacAleese, J. (1982): Ultrasound movement patterns of fetuses with chromosome anomalies. *Prenat. Diagn.*, 2:61–65.
5. DeVries, J.I.P., Visser, G.H.A., and Prechtl, H.F.R. (1982): The emergence of fetal behaviour. I. Qualitative aspects. *Early Hum. Dev.*, 7:301–322.
6. DeVries, J.I.P., Visser, G.H.A., and Prechtl, H.F.R. (1984): Fetal motility in the first half of pregnancy. In: *Continuity of Neural Functions from Prenatal to Postnatal Life: Clin. Dev. Med.*, edited by H.F.R. Prechtl, vol. 94, pp. 79–92. Blackwell, Oxford.
7. DeVries, J.I.P., Visser, G.H.A., and Prechtl, H.F.R. (1985): The emergence of fetal behaviour. II. Quantitative aspects. *Early Hum. Dev.*, 12:99–120.

8. DeVries, J.I.P., Visser, G.H.A., and Prechtl, H.F.R. (1988): The emergence of fetal behaviour. III. Individual differences and consistencies. *Early Hum. Dev.*, 16:85–103.

9. DeVries, J.I.P., Visser, G.H.A., and Prechtl, H.F.R. (1987): Diurnal and other variations in fetal movement and heart rate patterns at 20 to 22 weeks. *Early Hum. Dev.*, 15:333–348.

10. Divon, M.Y., Platt, L.D., Cantrell, C.J., Smith, C.V., Yeh, S.Y., and Paul, R.H. (1985): Evoked fetal startle response: A possible intrauterine neurological examination. *Am. J. Obstet. Gynecol.*, 153:454–456.

11. Droge, M.H., Gross, G.W., Hightower, M.H., and Czisny, L.E. (1986): Multielectrode analysis of coordinated, multisite, rhythmic bursting in cultured CNS monolayer networks. *J. Neurosci.*, 6:1583–1592.

12. Gelman, S.R., Wood, S., Spellacy, W.N., and Abrams, R.M. (1982): Fetal movements in response to sound stimulation. *Am. J. Obstet. Gynecol.*, 143:484–485.

13. Hooker, D. (1952): *The Prenatal Origin of Behaviour.* University of Kansas Press, Lawrence.

14. Hooker, D. (1952): Early human fetal activity. 16 mm film, Department of Anatomy, University of Pittsburgh.

15. Humphrey, T. (1978): Function of the nervous system during prenatal life. In: *Perinatal Physiology,* edited by U. Stave, pp. 651–683. Plenum, New York.

16. Ianniruberto, A., and Tajani, E. (1981): Ultrasonographic study of fetal movements. *Semin. Perinatol.*, 4:175–181.

17. Lecanuet, J.P., Granier-Deferre, C., Cohen, H., leHouezec, R., and Busnel, M.C. (1986): Fetal responses to acoustic stimulation depend on heart rate variability pattern, stimulus intensity and repetition. *Early Hum. Dev.*, 13:269–283.

18. Lenard, H.G., von Bernuth, H., and Prechtl, H.F.R. (1968): Reflexes and their relationships to behavioural state in the newborn. *Acta Paediatr. Scand.*, 3:177–185.

19. Lou, H.C. (1982): *Developmental Neurology.* Raven Press, New York.

20. Manning, F.A., Baskett, T.F., Morrison, I., and Lange, I. (1981): Fetal biophysical profile scoring—A prospective study in 1,184 high-risk patients. *Am. J. Obstet. Gynecol.*, 140:289–295.

21. Manning, F.A., Harman, C.R., Lange, I.R., and Morrison, I. (1986): Fetal assessment by biophysical profile scoring: 1985 update. *Eur. J. Obstet. Gynecol. Reprod. Biol.*, 21:331–339.

22. Milani-Comparetti, A., and Gidoni, E.A. (1967): Pattern analysis of motor development and its disorders. *Dev. Med. Child Neurol.*, 9:625–630.

23. Minkowski, M. (1928): Neurobiologische Studien am menschlichen Foetus. *Hand. Biol. Arbeitsmeth. Abt. v. Teil* 5B:511–618.

24. Mulder, E.J.H., Visser, G.H.A., Bekedam, D.J., and Prechtl, H.F.R. (1987): Emergence of behavioral states in fetuses of type-1-diabetic women. *Early Hum. Dev.*, 15:231–251.

25. Nijhuis, J.G., Martin, C.B., and Prechtl, H.F.R. (1984): Behavioural states of the human fetus. In: *Continuity of Neural Functions from Prenatal to Postnatal Life: Clin. Dev. Med.,* edited by H.F.R. Prechtl, vol. 94, pp. 65–78. Blackwell, Oxford.

26. Nijhuis, J.G., Prechtl, H.F.R., Martin, C.B., Jr., and Bots, R.S.G.M. (1982): Are there behavioural states in the human fetus? *Early Hum. Dev.*, 6:177–195.

27. Ohel, G., Birkenfeld, A., Rabinowitz, R., and Sadovsky, E. (1986): Fetal response to vibratory acoustic stimulation in periods of low heart reactivity and low activity. *Am. J. Obstet. Gynecol.*, 154:619–621.

28. Okada, N., and Kojima, T. (1984): Ontogeny of the central nervous system: Neurogenesis, fibre connection, synaptogenesis and myelination in the spinal cord. In: *Continuity of Neural Functions from Prenatal to Postnatal Life: Clin. Dev. Med.,* edited by H.F.R. Prechtl, vol. 94, pp. 79–92. Blackwell, Oxford.

29. Parmelee, A.H. (1975): Neurophysiological and behavioral organization of premature infants in the first months of life. *Biol. Psychiatry,* 10:501–512.

30. Parmalee, A.J., Jr., Wenner, W.H., Akiyama, Y., Schultz, M., and Stern, E. (1967): Sleep states in premature infants. *Dev. Med. Child Neurol.*, 9:70–77.

31. Patrick, J., Campbell, K., Carmichael, L., Natale, R., and Richardson, B. (1982): Patterns of gross fetal body movements over 24-hour observation intervals during the last 10 weeks of pregnancy. *Am. J. Obstet. Gynecol.*, 142:363–371.

32. Patrick, J., and Challis, J. (1980): Measurement of human fetal breathing movements in healthy pregnancies using a real-time scanner. *Semin. Perinatol.*, 4:275–286.

33. Prechtl, H.F.R. (1974): The behavioural states of the newborn infant (a review). *Brain Res.*, 76:1304–1311.

34. Prechtl, H.F.R. (ed.) (1984): *Continuity of Neural Functions from Prenatal to Postnatal Life: Clin. Dev. Med.,* vol. 94, p. 255. Blackwell, Oxford.
35. Prechtl, H.F.R. (1986): Prenatal motor development. In: *Motor Development in Children: Aspects of Coordination and Control,* edited by M.G. Wade, H.T.A. Whiting, pp. 53–64. Nijhoff, Dordrecht.
36. Prechtl, H.F.R., Fargel, J.W., Weinmann, H.M., and Bakker, H.H. (1979): Posture, motility and respiration in low-risk preterm infants. *Dev. Med. Child Neurol.,* 21:3–27.
37. Prechtl, H.F.R., and Nolte, R. (1984): Motor behaviour of preterm infants. In: *Continuity of Neural Functions from Prenatal to Postnatal Life: Clin. Dev. Med.,* edited by H.F.R. Prechtl, vol. 94, pp. 79–92. Blackwell, Oxford.
38. Prechtl, H.F.R., and O'Brien, M.J. (1982): Behavioural states of the full-term newborn. The emergence of a concept. In: *Psychobiology of the Newborn Infant,* edited by P. Stratton, pp. 53–73. John Wiley & Sons, Chichester.
39. Prechtl, H.F.R., Weinmann, H., and Akiyama, Y. (1969): Organization of physiological parameters in normal and neurologically abnormal infants: Comprehensive computer analysis of polygraphic data. *Neuropadiatrie,* 1:101–129.
40. Preyer, W. (1885): *Die spezielle Physiologie des Embryo.* Grieben, Leipzig.
41. Reinold, E. (1971): Fetale Bewegungen in der Frühgravidität. *Z. Geburtshilfe Gynäkologie* 174:220–225.
42. Reinold, E. (1976): Ultrasonics in early pregnancy. Diagnostic scanning and fetal motor activity. In: *Contributions to Gynecology and Obstetrics,* vol. 1, p. 148. S. Karger, Basel.
43. Schmidt, W., Boos, R., Gnirs, J., Auer, L., and Schulze, S. (1985): Fetal behavioural states and controlled sound stimulation. *Early Hum. Dev.,* 12:245–254.
44. Shirataki, S., and Prechtl, H.F.R. (1977): Sleep state transitions in newborn infants: Preliminary study. *Dev. Med. Child Neurol.,* 19:316–325.
45. Stafström, C.E., Johnston, D., Wehner, J.M., and Sheppard, J.R. (1980): Spontaneous neural activity in fetal brain reaggregate cultures. *Neuroscience,* 5:1681–1690.
46. Stark, C.R., Orleans, M., Haverkamp, A.D., and Murphy, J. (1984): Short and long-term risks after exposure to diagnostic ultrasound *in utero. Obstet. Gynecol.,* 63:194–201.
47. Stefanski, M., Schulze, K., Bateman, D., Kairam, R., Pedley, T.A., Masterson, J., and James, L.S. (1984): A scoring system for states of sleep and wakefulness in term and preterm infants. *Pediatr. Res.,* 18:58–63.
48. Touwen, B.C.L. (1978): Variability and stereotype in normal and deviant development. In: *Care of the Handicapped Child: Clin. Dev. Med.* edited by J. Apley, vol. 67, pp. 99–110.
49. VanVliet, M.A.T., Martin, C.B., Jr., Nijhuis, J.G., and Prechtl, H.F.R. (1985): Behavioural states in fetuses of nulliparous women. *Early Hum. Dev.,* 12:121–136.
50. VanVliet, M.A.T., Martin, C.B., Jr., Nijhuis, J.G., and Prechtl, H.F.R. (1985): Behavioural states in growth retarded human fetuses. *Early Hum. Dev.,* 12:183–198.
51. Visser, G.H.A., Laurini, R.N., DeVries, J.I.P., Bekedam, D.J., and Prechtl, J.F.R. (1985): Abnormal motor behaviour in anencephalic fetuses. *Early Hum. Dev.,* 12:173–182.

Fetal Neurology, edited by
A. Hill and J.J. Volpe.
Raven Press, New York © 1989.

2

Antepartum Fetal Monitoring: Fetal Movement

William F. Rayburn

Division of Maternal-Fetal Medicine, University of Nebraska College of Medicine, Omaha, Nebraska 68105

Evaluating fetal neurologic development presents considerable difficulties. Prior inferences about functional maturation have been derived from the examination of premature neonates and from direct observations of exteriorized fetal animal preparations. Present measures assess general well-being rather than direct cerebral function. Separate stages of neurologic organization can be defined only in concert with other parameters.

Recording fetal activity may serve as an indirect measure of central nervous system integrity and function. The coordination of fetal movement, which requires complex neurological control, is likely similar to that of the newborn infant. Techniques to assess fetal motion include real-time ultrasonography, maternal perception, pressure-sensitive electromechanical devices, and other such physiological devices.

Information gathered from such observations will be described in this chapter. Knowledge about types of fetal activity will be reviewed in relation to gestational age and in response to stimulation. Clinical applications from observed fetal motion will then be described.

MONITORING TECHNIQUES

Real-Time Ultrasonography

Real-time ultrasonography is a simple and reliable means for objectively recording fetal activity. Two-dimensional imaging is possible using phased or linear transducer arrays. An ultrasound transducer (usually 3.5 MHz) is placed on the recumbent mother's abdomen along the axis of the fetal abdomen. Resolution is sufficient to detect accurately propulsive movement of the trunk and lower extremities, respiratory movement, and hand-face contact.

Most observations occur during a short period (5–30 min), although specially designed experiments have been for up to 24 hr. For such prolonged periods, the ultrasound transducer should be held stationary by a device along the longitudinal axis of the fetal chest and abdominal wall. Isolated movements of fetal extremities may not be fully appreciated.

Maternal Peception

Perceived fetal motion by the compliant mother is the oldest and least expensive technique for monitoring fetal activity. Until recently, most clinical investigations have involved the description of fetal motion perceived by the mother or palpated by an observer. Several studies have suggested a positive relation between fetal motion perceived by the mother and that recorded by means of an electromagnetic device (48). Rayburn (39) found that 82% of all motion (nearly 100% if there was combined propulsive lower limb and trunk motion) viewed sonographically was perceived between 28 and 43 weeks gestation. The independent studies of Gettinger et al. (12), Rabinowitz et al. (38), and Hertogs et al. (17) also reported a significant positive correlation between the number of movements recorded by maternal perception and those viewed by real-time ultrasound scanning. The 95% confidence limits were wide, however (12).

Several methods for recording fetal activity have been described and are listed in Table 1. The mother should be asked to lie in a lateral recumbent position, pref-

TABLE 1. *Techniques for monitoring perceived fetal motion*

Principal investigator	Methods of recording	Evidence of fetal inactivity
Harper (16)	Three 1-hr periods, daily	Complete cessation
Leader (24)	30 min, four times daily	1 day of no movements or 2 successive days/week in which there were <10 movements/hr
Neldham (31)	One 2-hr period, three times weekly	≤3 movements/hr
O'Leary & Andrinopoulos (33)	Three half-hour periods, daily	0–5 movements/30 min for each of the 3 half-hour periods
Pearson (36)	12 hr (9:00 A.M.–9:00 P.M.), daily	<10 movements/12 hr
Rayburn (45)	≥1 hr (when convenient)	≤3 movements/hr for 2 consecutive hr
Sadovsky (49)	30 min to 1 hr, twice or three times daily	<2 movements/hr

erably in a quiet room, and concentrate on fetal activity. Perceived movement is to be routinely reported on a specially designed chart such as that used in our clinic (Fig. 1). The recording of perceived fetal motion during the second half of pregnancy is not dependent on a strict timetable.

Maternal compliance has been generally favorable in both outpatient and inpatient settings. This is especially true if that person appreciates the nature of the underlying antepartum complication, understands the charting instructions, and is able to see the same group of physicians regularly. An adequate explanation for keeping a movement chart should be provided, and the importance of recognizing a reduction in fetal activity should be stressed. The few persons who are incapable of recording fetal movement often improve their accuracy when taught using ultrasonography.

Electromechanical Devices

Fetal movement may alter the configuration of the maternal gravid abdomen. Electromechanical devices containing strain gauges of piezoelectric materials receive these forces and transform mechanical energy into electrical current. The tocodynamometer is an example of a simple strain gauge instrument (54). Two or more pressure transducers were placed on the maternal abdomen over different parts of the fetus to increase sensitivity. A rapid paper speed is necessary to better appreciate pressure changes caused by fetal movements. High frequency extremity motion and the respiratory movements of less than 1-sec duration may be distinguished from other fetal body motions lasting less than 1 sec.

Sadovsky and associates (50) have also described the use of highly sensitive piezoelectric material that conforms to the maternal abdomen. Energy transmitted from such activity produces an electric current that causes a deflection on the recorder. Although these electromechanical recording devices are available commercially, they are used primarily for investigation purposes because of cost containment. Like ultrasonography, these instruments are thought to be safe for human investigation because sound energy is either nonexistent or quite low.

Other

Granat and associates (15) reported the use of an integrative electromyogram (EMG) as a means for monitoring fetal activity. Recordings were derived from electrodes attached to the maternal abdominal circumference. The correlation between objective and subjective (maternal self-assessment) scores of fetal activity was generally confirmed. However, methods for monitoring fetal activity based on short-term recording are to be questioned.

Colley et al. (4) have recently reported on the use of a phonogram as a measure of fetal activity. A wide-band width sensor for total acoustic phonography may be used to detect fetal body and respiratory activities. The fetal phonogram offers a

NAME _Mary Beyers_

DATE _10/12/81_

FETAL MOVEMENT CHART

Instructions:

A daily diary of your baby's movements provides useful information. Please mark down any time the baby moves during at least one convenient hour each day. Try to count while lying on your left side, so that you get enough rest, and the circulation to the baby is improved. Should there be any concern, please notify the office. Otherwise, return this form when you return to the clinic or labor hall.

DAY	HOUR	COUNTINGS	TOTAL
Monday	9–10 am	Ɫ Ɫ Ɫ Ɫ Ɫ //	27
Tuesday	2–3 pm	Ɫ Ɫ Ɫ ////	19
Wednesday	10–11 am	Ɫ Ɫ Ɫ Ɫ Ɫ Ɫ //	32
Thursday	7–8 pm	Ɫ Ɫ Ɫ Ɫ ////	24
Friday	8–9 pm	Ɫ Ɫ Ɫ //	17
Saturday	4–5 pm	Ɫ Ɫ Ɫ Ɫ Ɫ Ɫ Ɫ /	36
Sunday	7–8 am	Ɫ Ɫ Ɫ Ɫ Ɫ /	26
Monday	10–11 pm	Ɫ Ɫ Ɫ Ɫ ////	24
Tuesday	7–8 pm	Ɫ Ɫ Ɫ Ɫ Ɫ Ɫ	30
Wednesday	9–10 am	Ɫ Ɫ Ɫ /	16
Thursday	2–3 pm	Ɫ Ɫ Ɫ Ɫ	20
Friday	7–8 pm	Ɫ Ɫ ///	13
Saturday	10–11 pm	Ɫ Ɫ Ɫ Ɫ Ɫ Ɫ ///	33
Sunday	4–5 pm	Ɫ Ɫ Ɫ Ɫ Ɫ //	27
Monday	7–8 pm	Ɫ Ɫ Ɫ Ɫ /	21
Tuesday	7–8 pm	Ɫ Ɫ Ɫ Ɫ Ɫ	25
Wednesday	8–9 pm	Ɫ Ɫ Ɫ ///	18
Thursday	3–4 pm	Ɫ Ɫ Ɫ Ɫ Ɫ Ɫ ////	34

FIG. 1. An example of a fetal movement chart with instructions. (From ref. 40.)

noninvasive method for assessing the fetus over long periods and at any place. Further work needs to be done on signal processing and discerning differences between normal and complicated pregnancies.

PHYSIOLOGY OF FETAL ACTIVITY

Types of Fetal Movement

Types of fetal movements reflect differing central nervous system activities, and specific muscle actions respond to different brain-received stimuli. The types of motion observed for each fetus were described by Birnholz et al. (1) in 1975 using continuous observations with real-time ultrasonography. Fetal motion had been previously characterized by Hooker (19) and Humphrey (20) with particular attention to extension of the head or limbs relative to the trunk, rotation or displacement of the torso, or individual phenomena related to specific limb, regional, or organ activity. Descriptions of specific movements are shown in Table 2.

The earliest fetal movements such as independent limb, trunk twitches, and isolated head motion are sporadic and have spastic or jerky qualities. These give way to more combined, sustained, and regular motions as integration progresses.

Types of fetal movements in late gestation have been separately described by Rayburn (39) and Patrick et al. (34) during continuous observations using real-time ultrasonic scanning. These include stretching or rolling, isolated movements

TABLE 2. *Types of fetal movements viewed ultrasonographically throughout gestation*

Twitch—Single gross episode of trunk flexion and head extension without separate or associated limb movement.

Independent limb—Asymmetrical or unilateral extensor movements of the arms or legs.

Isolated head—Extension, flexion, or rotation of the head without associated trunk or limb movements.

Combined/repetitive—Simultaneous or serial movements of the head or trunk and limbs that do not have a sudden, jerky, or "spastic" quality. Repeated head bobbing and the combination of head extension or rotation following contact between the hand and face are included in this category.

Quasi-startle—Sudden displacement of the entire body followed by a "relaxation" phase in which the body settles dependently within the amniotic fluid. This movement is initiated by a vigorous extensor movement of both hands or legs.

Limb-joint—Smooth sequential "locomotive" movements of an arm or leg, including flexion at the knee or elbow.

Hand-face—The hands contact and remain touching the face without extension (or other aversive movement) of the head. Hand apposition to the mouth and repetitive mandibular movement (probably thumb sucking) is included in this category.

Diaphragm—Vigorous diaphragmatic excursions, tending to occur suddenly and without temporal regularity (usually accompanied by excursions of the chest wall).

Respiratory—Periodic repetitive movements of the diaphragm with simultaneous chest wall excursions.

From ref. 1.

of extremities, and high frequency motion. The relation between visualized and perceived fetal movements is described in Table 3. Perceived fetal motion is primarily related to the strength of lower limb movement. Vigorous or sustained activities result from combined lower limb and trunk motion and are commonly referred to as "stretching," "kicks," and "roll-overs." These body movements are not significantly altered by fetal position or presentation, fetal sex, or twinning (40).

Simple respiratory movements are not perceived by the mother. An exception would be strong diaphramatic motions ("hiccoughs" that occur on one to four occasions per day and usually last 1–13 min). These gentle, regular, and rhythmic respiratory movements, occurring as frequently as every 2 sec, are usually easily distinguishable by the mother from fetal extremity movement or maternal aortic pulsations. Their significance is unclear, but "hiccoughs" are not thought to be a worrisome sign.

Gestational Age

The type of motion corresponds with the fetal developmental status. Ultrasonographic observations by Birnholz et al. (1) have been used to describe fetal movements as early as the first trimester. Several patterns can be recognized, and those described in Table 2 appear to correlate with gestational age (Fig. 2). Simple extremity motion visualized sporadically as early as the seventh gestational week has a jerky or spastic character. As integration proceeds, these movements give way to more complex activities that are more regular and sustained. Combined displacements of the limbs, torso, and head begin between the 12th and 16th week.

Fetal movements can be consistently perceived by the mother as early as the 16th week ("quickening"). By the 20th gestational week, fetal motor behavior involves a repertoire of basic motor patterns similar to those in the infant. These movements become strong and more frequent as they become more easily recognized.

Using real-time ultrasound during a 24-hr observation period, Natale et al. (29) have described the percentage of time in which the fetus is active. Visualized mo-

TABLE 3. *Classification of perceived gross fetal body motion*

Types of motion	Visualized movement	Movement perception	Duration	Strength
Simple or isolated	Trunk and extremity	"Kick, jab, startle"	Short (1–15 sec)	Strong
Rolling or stretching	Entire fetal body	"Rollover, stretch"	Sustained (3–30 sec)	Strong
High-frequency	Chest wall Isolated extremity	"Hiccough" "Flutter, weak kick"	Rapid (<1 sec)	Weak

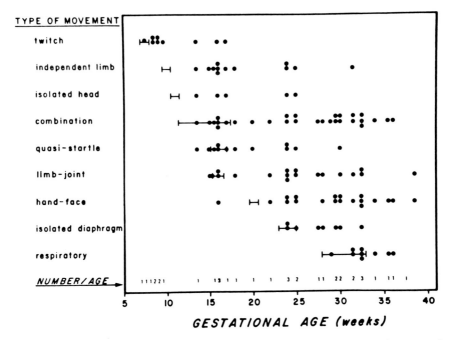

FIG. 2. Types of fetal movement and gestational age. Total number of pregnancies scanned at each gestational age is shown at baseline. (From ref. 1.)

tion involved approximately 14% of the time between 24 and 28 weeks gestation, and the number of visible gross body movements was 45 per hour. Both the percentage of time spent moving and the number of movements seen per hour increased in the late evening and early morning hours. The percentage of time spent moving and the number of movements per hour were greater than those reported in term fetuses.

Data reported in the literature (34,40) reveal that fetal activity is greatest between 28 and 32 weeks gestation. This may be attributable to a maximal intrauterine volume in relation to fetal size. A gradual decrease in the number of perceived fetal motions is expected to occur thereafter and may relate to the decreased amniotic fluid volume, increased fetal size, increased likelihood of placental insufficiency, and improved coordination of fetal movements. Despite this, the actual amount of perceived vigorous and sustained fetal motion should remain unchanged (40).

Fetal activity patterns during the third trimester have also been recently reported by Manning and associates (26). Fetal movements were not found to decrease significantly with gestational age. The mean frequency of fetal movement during a 20-min observation period involved 16.5 movements. This number of movements per hour would be expected to be less for pregnancies complicated by diabetes, hypertension, or Rh isoimmunization, in which fetal distress is more likely. The presence of at least one fetal movement per 20-min period was found to be a reassuring sign of a normal fetus as long as there were no acute changes.

Patrick et al. (34) also made 24-hr observations of gross fetal body movements using real-time ultrasonography between 30 and 39 weeks gestation. The transducer was positioned to permit continuous observation along a longitudinal cross section of the fetal chest and abdomen. All segments were viewed on a videomonitor and recorded. A summary of the data is shown in Table 4. The percentage of time spent moving was approximately 10%, and the number varied widely but was approximately 30 movements per hour. This is compatible with gross body movements perceived by the reliable mother as reported by Rayburn (40). The longest absence of gross body movements was 75 min.

Unless fetal distress is apparent, the mean value and pattern of fetal activity do not seem to decrease in the week before delivery (40). This observation dispels the common belief that a sudden decrease or loss of fetal activity is predictive of impending labor and supports the contention that fetal behavior may involve longer physiologic rest periods.

Time of Day

Each fetus has its own pattern of daily activity. The establishment of a normal range of fetal activity is often difficult because the number of movements per hour is highly variable (12,15). Perceived periods of fetal activity and inactivity appear to be unrelated to the time of day while the mother is awake or to a strict timetable between 24 and 44 weeks (40). Many mothers often report an increase in fetal

TABLE 4. *Summary of fetal movement observations during a 24-hr period between 30–39 weeks gestation using continuous ultrasonic scanning of the fetal abdomen and trunk*

Data	Gestational age (weeks)			
	30–31 (n = 9)	34–35 (n = 11)	38–39 (n = 11)	30–39 (n = 31)
% Time spent moving				
Mean (±SEM)	9.3 ± 0.9	9.8 ± 0.7	11.2 ± 0.9	10.2 ± 0.5
Daily range	5.1 – 13.6	5.0 – 13.7	6.8 – 16.3	5.0 – 16.3
Hourly range	0 – 29.7	0 – 50.1	0.4 – 38.5	0 – 50.1
No. movements/hr				
Mean	32.5 ± 2.2	28.1 ± 1.8	32.1 ± 2.1	30.8 ± 1.2
Daily range	22.3 – 43.5	16.5 – 37.5	24.0 – 45.4	16.5 – 45.4
Hourly range	0 – 86	0 – 71	3 – 130	0 – 130
Mean length of gross body movements (sec)	9.6 ± 0.3	11.6 ± 0.3	11.2 ± 0.3	10.8 ± 0.2
Longest absence of gross body movement (min)	60	75	50	75

From ref. 34.

activity during the evening hours or at bedtime. This may be attributable to the mother's activity during the day, which either prevents her from paying full attention to her fetus' activity or may cause the fetus to remain content or "quiet."

Ultrasonic imaging has allowed more precise measurement during the final trimester. Patrick and associates (34) have reported that the mean hourly number of visualized gross fetal body movements with ultrasound examination is greatest during the late night (between 2100 and 0100 hr). The hourly incidence of gross fetal body movements between 2100 and 0100 hr was 17%, which was significantly greater than 11% during the rest of the day. Roberts et al. (47) have reported gross fetal body movements to be present for a mean of 18% of the time, with a range over a 24-hr period with ultrasound visualization being between 11% and 26%. The incidence of fetal trunk movement was greatest in the late evening and least around midday. The mean number of movements calculated during a 30-min period was 29 (range 3–108).

Fetal Heart Rate Changes

The synchronous onset of fetal heart rate changes coincident with fetal body movement suggests a coordination of both functions. This control presumably resides in the brain, and cortical nerve cells associated with motor functions and cardiovascular response are located in close proximity. Navot and associates (30) evaluated the rate of fetal heart rate accelerations associated with fetal movements according to gestational ages in pregnancies with subsequent favorable outcomes. A continuous record of fetal heart rate changes was performed with a cardiotocograph in 242 patients. The ratio of heart rate accelerations with movements per total movement increments was found to increase with gestational age (Fig. 3). It is possible that the more premature fetus is unable to react to stimuli with accelerations of the heart rate because of neuromotor immaturity. Either the stimulus may not be perceived consistently by the fetus or the reaction by an acceleration in the heart rate may not occur or be negligible.

The association between fetal heart rate patterns and movements has been reported between 20 and 41 weeks gestation by Sorokin et al. (53) and Rabinowitz et al. (38). Fetal activity was detected by Sorokin et al. (53) using two tocodynamometers on the maternal abdomen, and the fetal heart rate was recorded using an abdominal electrocardiogram between 20 and 30 weeks. Their findings suggested that fetal heart rate criteria for evaluating well-being (accelerations: reassuring; decelerations: worrisome) are different in the very premature fetus than the term fetus. Fetal heart rate decelerations are common between 20 and 30 weeks but less common with advancing gestation. The frequencies of heart rate accelerations and acceleration/deceleration ratios increase with advancing gestation.

Fetal movements as felt by the pregnant woman and visualized by real-time ultrasonography were correlated with fetal heart rate accelerations by Rabinowitz et al. (38) in 52 normal and high risk pregnant women between 33 and 41 weeks. All movements seen on ultrasonic evaluation or felt by the mother were associated

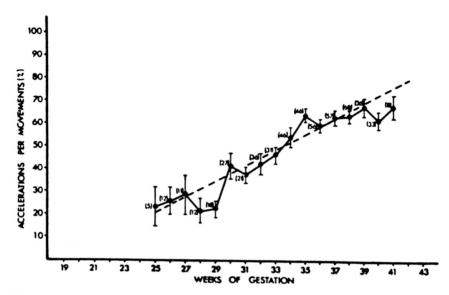

FIG. 3. Percentage of recorded fetal heart rate accelerations per total fetal movement in a 20-min period between 25–42 weeks gestation. Mean ± SE; numbers in parentheses are numbers of cases. Test of linearity, p < 0.05. (From ref. 30.)

with large or small fetal heart rate accelerations. The large accelerations (more than 15 bpm, lasting 15 sec or more) were associated with 78.6% of the fetal movements felt by the mother and 99.6% of propulsive fetal movements seen by real-time ultrasonography. In contrast, small accelerations were associated with 53% of perceived fetal movements and 82.4% of all visualized movements. Mothers felt 76% of fetal movement seen by ultrasonography. The conclusion from this investigation was that fetal movements could be verified by the existence of large fetal heart rate accelerations.

The influence of gross fetal body movements on the daily patterns of fetal heart rate near term was examined by Patrick and associates (35) in a study involving 12 healthy fetuses between 38 and 40 weeks gestation. During a 24-hr period of continuous observation, a combined fetal and maternal echocardiogram was obtained from three needle electrodes placed subcutaneously on the maternal abdominal wall. The fetuses had gross fetal body movements 12.0% ± 0.6% of the time (daily range, 8.3%–14.7%). The hourly fetal heart rate was increased by 18.1 ± 0.4 bpm during movements compared with times of no movement.

Extremes of Fetal Activity

A behavioral state is a term used to describe the pattern of breaking the controlled physiologic activity manifested by awake and sleep time. These states may be determined by the collection of many measurable physiologic variables such as gross body movements, heart rate and rhythm, electroencephalographic patterns, respiratory rate and rhythm, and eye movements. The fetal heart rate and body movements are the only variables which can be measured in an noninvasive manner before delivery.

Inactive

Analogues of behavioral states are present in the fetus and have cycling patterns. Using these two parameters, active and inactive (or quiet) fetal periods have been described recently by Dierker and associates (7). Groups of uncomplicated pregnancies were compared between 28 and 30 weeks and 38 and 40 weeks. A period of fetal movement with increased variability of the heart rate was classified as active, and one with absent movement and diminished heart beat was classified as quiet. Their results indicated significant differences in the number of active-quiet cycles per hour and the length of active intervals between the two gestational periods. The time spent in the active and quiet periods is longer in older fetuses. Active periods were described by these same investigators to average 40 min. Fetal inactivity of more than 1 hr was not thought to represent a physiologic rest period and may be associated with an increase of fetal jeopardy and distress. Decreased fetal movement may occur in response to hypoxia or other metabolic derangements.

Distinguishing between an abnormally low activity pattern and a physiologic rest period is important but difficult. Different definitions of fetal inactivity according to recorded maternal perception are described in Table 1. Half-hour periods of maternal self-recording have been recommended by several investigators for patient convenience. However, this appears to be less than the shortest of fetal rest-activity cycles. A 1-hr period or more of recording is therefore thought to be better for more objective and subjective scores of fetal activity.

Evidence for fetal inactivity has been defined clinically at our institution as three or fewer perceived fetal movements per hour for at least 2 consecutive hr. This lack of perceived propulsive motion occurs in 2.5% of all pregnancies and is twice as often in complicated than uncomplicated pregnancies (36,40). Using ultrasonic imaging between 30 and 39 weeks gestation, Patrick et al. (34) found the mean percentage of intervals with no gross movement to be less than 10% of a 2-min observation period, less than 5% for 30 min, and 2% for 40 min or more (Fig. 4).

Excess Activity

Another unusual behavioral state involves excess fetal activity. This pattern cannot be easily defined on a short-term basis. Rayburn (44) has defined evidence for long-term excess fetal activity as being an average of 40 or more perceived fetal motions per hour for at least a 14-day period. Such activity occurred in 5% of the general pregnancy population (Fig. 5). No association was found between excess fetal activity and premature labor, umbilical cord complications, or congenital

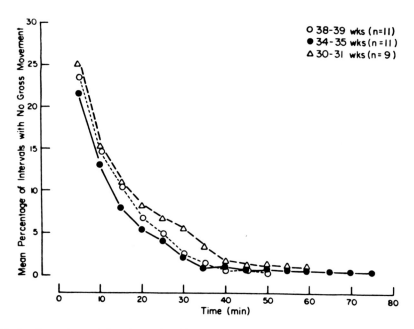

FIG. 4. Percentage of time intervals with no gross fetal body movements seen. (From ref. 34.)

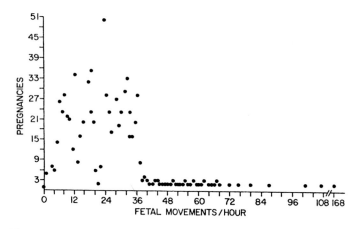

FIG. 5. Mean number of perceived fetal movements per hour among 1,156 pregnancies within the last trimester. (From ref. 44.)

anomalies. These fetuses remained vigorous during labor and did well following delivery. An examination of these infants during their first year revealed an unusual growth, developmental, or temperamental pattern compared with healthy infants with normal activity rates. Evidence for excess activity may represent an increased active/inactive behavioral state, although an explanation for why the fetus is apparently so active remains unclear.

RESPONSE TO STIMULATION

Uterine Compression or Contractions

Palpation or vigorous shaking of the uterine fundus during the second half of pregnancy does not always initiate fetal motion. Even forceful manipulation of the uterus and fetus will not cause an unarousable fetus to become active. This relation is also found in the newborn infant who is difficult to awaken from sleep.

Richardson et al. (46) have reported on the effects of external physical stimulation on the fetus near term. Seventeen healthy women between 36 and 42 weeks gestation underwent vigorous shaking of the uterus to assess any change in fetal behavior. Fluctuations in the fetal heart rate, heart rate variability, gross body movements, and breathing movements did not show any significant change after external stimulation.

The stress of uterine contractions on fetal activity has been studied separately by Nyholm et al. (32) and Carmichael et al. (3). Fetal motion was found to continue during labor and was a reliable indicator of fetal well-being. Although not absolute, the lack of fetal heart rate accelerations coincident with perceived fetal motion should arouse suspicion of fetal compromise. In contrast, an acceleration of fetal heart rate is reassuring of the present fetal health but is not complete assurance that distress will not appear later in labor. It may be concluded that the presence of gross fetal body movements before and during spontaneous labor at term is a consistent index of fetal well-being.

Sound Stimulation

Several investigators have claimed that a fetus responds to very loud sounds (greater than 500 cps) by increased activity and an associated increase in heart rate. A fetus who is difficult to arouse by sound stimulation may not necessarily be in jeopardy, and sound stimulation is not considered to be worthwhile for the clinical assessment of fetal well-being.

Leader et al. (25) has described the assessment of fetal neurologic integrity by assessing habituation, the response decrement that occurs when an organism is repeatedly stimulated. A standard Ronson electric toothbrush was used as a stimulus when placed on the maternal abdominal wall. Sound waves from this device were related to simultaneous fetal movements. Using three methods of assessment (electrocardiography, real-time ultrasonography, maternal perception), the fetal response to this vibration was studied in 40 normal human fetuses and compared with high risk pregnancies in which the fetus was at increased risk for neurologic damage. Highly significant differences were found in habituation patterns between the two groups. Failure to obtain a behavioral response to a stimulus was unusual in the normal fetus and was associated with a high incidence of abnormal fetal heart rate tracings and unfavorable fetal outcomes. Five infants found to have major central nervous system abnormalities (anencephaly, microcephaly) showed no response to stimulation. They died during labor and could not be tested further.

Other investigations have shown in animal studies that the failure to habituate to repeated stimuli has been found in decerebrate rats and those under the influence of barbiturates, amphetamines, and lysergic acid diethylamide (LSD) (5,6,23, 52,57). Impaired habituation has been reported in human fetuses and infants despite repeated stimuli in cases of traumatized newborn infants, hyperkinetic and autistic children, and infants with Down's syndrome or other brain damage (2,8,11,18,55,56).

Maternal Glucose Levels

Conflicting reports have related fetal activity with maternal glucose levels. Gross fetal body motion and heart rate accelerations are not thought to increase by a recent meal (34,43). Body movements may increase during the most rapid rise in maternal glucose levels following 25 to 100 g intravenous glucose challenge. This change is probably related more to an increase in respirations than to an increase in gross body movement. Sustained maternal hyperglycemia in the third trimester may be associated with a decrease in the number of fetal movements lasting more than 1 sec and an increase in inactivity during the first hour following intravenous glucose infusion. According to a recent study by Edelberg et al. (9), fetal movements and behavior return to baseline during the second and third hour following a glucose infusion to achieve maternal glucose levels of 120 mg/dl.

Cigarette Smoking and Medications

Maternal cigarette smoking may temporarily reduce fetal body motion and breathing (14). The depressant effect of nicotine on the central nervous system and increase in maternal carboxyhemoglobin levels or an unknown toxin may account for this decrease in movement.

Drugs that have sedating qualities such as alcohol, barbiturates, narcotics, methadone, or benzodiazepines are known to cross the placenta readily and may reduce the duration and number of fetal movements. Altered behavioral states are expected to reverse following clearance of the drug. Drugs taken in recommended doses to treat medical complications or preterm delivery are not thought to influence perceived fetal motion (34).

Maternal Exercise

Fetal movement may be influenced by maternal activity and position. Whether a change in maternal position will alter the frequency of gross fetal body motion is unclear, although Minors and Waterhouse (28) have reported that mothers record the most fetal movement while lying, less when sitting, and least when standing.

There has been no apparent relation between the mother's activity and changes in the daily rates of fetal movement according to Edwards and Edwards (10). Many women involved in such vigorous exercise as swimming or jogging will report a decrease in fetal movement shortly after these exercises. These fetuses should be expected to become active once the mother has rested unless there is an antepartum complication.

Other

The response of fetal activity to light stimulation has not been shown to be clinically useful. Preliminary reports have claimed that intense light on the gravid abdomen may increase fetal activity, but these studies require further confirmation (37).

Fetal activity may be increased in cases of acute maternal stress according to ultrasound visualization by Ianniruberto and Tajani (21). These movements may be numerous, disordered, and vigorous. Severe maternal stress or electric shock may be accompanied by inhibition of fetal body motion that is reversed with the correction of the stressful condition.

CLINICAL APPLICATION

Fetal activity monitoring is a surveillance technique that is helpful while managing certain complicated pregnancies. It serves as a signal for impending fetal jeopardy and possible death, although it is not a direct test of placental function. The maternal awareness of a loss or recent decrease in propulsive fetal motion has been traditionally regarded as a warning sign, especially when chronic uteroplacental insufficiency is suspected.

Stillbirth or Perinatal Asphyxia

Several reports have suggested the value of documenting fetal activity. Goodlin and Haesslein (13) have reported that 81% of inactive fetuses require resuscitation, which suggests prior compromise. Leader and associates (24) have found that 15% of their patients perceived fetal inactivity, and 45% of these had unfavorable neonatal outcomes. Sadovsky et al. (51) reported fetal inactivity to be a sensitive alarm signal of impending fetal death. This is particularly true when reduced activity is associated with conditions in which fetal distress is chronic rather than acute in nature. A recent 4-year experience by Rayburn et al. (40) revealed that approximately half of fetuses perceived to be inactive became either stillborn or did poorly during labor and immediately after delivery.

Not all antepartum stillbirths can be avoided using the monitoring of fetal motion. Many pregnant women have no apparent complication, and no obvious gross abnormalities are often observed in the neonate, placenta, or umbilical cord. These women often describe a sudden and unexplainable loss of perceived fetal motion before death is documented. Antepartum conditions listed in Table 5 compare prior fetal activity patterns and perinatal conditions associated with stillbirth. The cause of stillbirths following documented inactivity is most likely hypoxia. The usefulness of fetal movement monitoring is therefore greatest in high risk pregnancies, when chronic uteroplacental insufficiency is present. A decrease in the intensity and number of fetal movements is most likely to occur under these circumstances.

Reduced fetal motion alone is insufficient reason for delivery. Real-time ultra-

TABLE 5. *Events associated with stillbirth and prior fetal activity pattern*

Inactive fetus:
  Fetal abnormality
    Severe anemia
    Hydropic changes
    Severe growth retardation
    Major anomaly
  Placental abnormality
    Severe degenerative changes
    Abruptio placentae
  Umbilical cord complication
    Occult prolapse
    Nuchal cord
    Torsion near placental insertion
  Uterine rupture

Active fetus:
  Abruptio placentae (50–100%)
  Umbilical cord complication
    Prolapse
    Hematoma
    Nuchal cord
  Amniotic fluid
    Oligohydramnios
  Major fetal anomaly
  Uterine rupture

sound imaging is often performed to search for fetal trunk and lower extremity motion. Propulsive motions are reassuring and do not require further evaluation as long as the underlying complication remains stable. Ultrasound imaging is helpful in determining the mother's accuracy in perceiving certain types of fetal activity. Antepartum fetal heart rate testing is another alternative to search for compromise. A reactive pattern (adequate heart rate accelerations) is sufficient documentation of coincidental fetal motion. Fetal inactivity confirmed by ultrasound visualization or with fetal heart rate monitoring would require repeat fetal evaluation or delivery depending on gestational age and the underlying complications.

Congenital Malformations

Knowledge of an anomalous infant before labor would assist the physician in preparing the parents-to-be, managing the timing and method of delivery, and preparing for the immediate care of an infant whose deformity may be correctable. A cessation of fetal activity in the presence of oligohydramnios or polyhydramnios is strongly suggestive of a malformation. A lack of vigorous motion may relate to abnormalities of central nervous system pathways, muscular dysfunction, or mechanical restriction in lower extremity motion.

Most malformed infants are described as being active *in utero*. In a recent review of activity patterns of 58 malformed infants, Rayburn and Barr (41a) found that 42 (72%) were active and had patterns indistinguishable from those of unaffected infants. The remaining 28% were documented to be inactive, and all major malformations were visualized ultrasonographically before delivery. These involved hydrocephalus, nonimmune hydrops, bilateral renal agenesis, and bilateral hip dislocation. Perceived fetal inactivity with subsequent ultrasonic documentation may therefore be helpful in recognizing certain major malformations.

Fetuses with open neural tube defects are commonly active *in utero*. The spinal cord remains relatively intact until late gestation with sufficient quadriceps and iliopsoas muscle function for lower limb motion. When viewed ultrasonographically, fetuses with anencephaly or myelomeningoceles often have spastic positioning and limb motion that is characteristic of upper motor neuron lesions (51).

Fetal Growth Retardation

Several authors have reported a significant decrease in activity among fetuses found to have intrauterine growth retardation (22,27,41,42). A strong relation exists between these two findings and other signs of fetal distress, impending death, or major malformation. Despite these findings, most mildly growth-retarded fetuses have activity patterns that are clinically indistinguishable from those of more appropriately sized fetuses (7,27,41). It is usually only the severely growth-retarded infants (lower 5th percentile for expected birth weight) in which delayed fetal activity would be expected. An underlying medical, genetic, or chronic infectious complication is usually present under these conditions.

CONCLUSION

Monitoring fetal activity during pregnancy has provided much insight into the functional maturation of the developing nervous system. A progressive complexity in stimulus reactions suggests the possibility that several stages of neurologic organization may be defined in concert with other parameters of intrauterine development. Behavioral patterns *in utero* relate to subsequent motor development during infancy and later. Observation of the fetus is best performed using real-time ultrasound imaging. Monitoring fetal motion in high risk pregnancies had been shown to be clinically worthwhile in predicting impending fetal death or compromise when placental insufficiency is long-standing. The presence of perceived vigorous fetal activity is reassuring. Perceived inactivity would require a reassessment of any underlying antepartum complication and a more precise evaluation by antepartum fetal heart rate testing or real-time ultrasonography.

REFERENCES

1. Birnholz, J.C., Stephens, J.C., and Faria, M. (1978): A possible means of defining neurologic developmental milestones *in utero*. *Am. J. Roentgenol.,* 130:537–540.
2. Bronstein, A.I., Itina, N.A., and Kamenetsaia, A.G. (1968): The orienting reaction on newborn children. In: *Orienting Reflex and Exploratory Behaviour,* edited by L.G. Varonin, A.N. Leotiev, A.R. Luris, E.N. Sokolov, O.S. Vinogradova. Moscow Academy of Pedagogical Sciences of RSFSR.
3. Carmichael, L., Campbell, K., and Patrick, J. (1984): Fetal breathing, gross fetal body movements, and maternal and fetal heart rates before spontaneous labor at term. *Am. J. Obstet. Gynecol.,* 148:675–679.
4. Colley, N., Talbert, D.G., Abraham, N.G., et al. (1986): The fetal phonogram: A measure of fetal activity. *Lancet,* 1:931–935.
5. Davis, M., and Gendelman, P.M. (1977): Plasticity of the acoustic startle response in the acutely decerebrate rat. *J. Comp. Physiol. Psychol.,* 91:549–643.
6. Davis, M., Svensson, T.H., and Aghajanian, G.K. (1975): Effects of D- and L-amphetamine on habituation and sensitization of the acoustic startle response in rats. *Psychopharmacology,* 43:1–11.
7. Dierker, L.J., Pillay, S.K., Sorokin, Y., et al. (1982): Active and quiet periods in the preterm and term fetus. *Obstet. Gynecol.,* 60:65–70.
8. Dustman, R.E., and Callner, D.A. (1979): Cortical evoked responses and response decrement in non-retarded and Down's syndrome individuals. *Am. J. Ment. Defic.,* 83:391–397.
9. Edelberg, S., Dierker, L., Kalhan, S., et al. (1985): Maternal hyperglycemia and fetal movement. Annual Meeting of the Society of Perinatal Obstetricians, Las Vegas, Nevada.
10. Edwards, D.A., and Edwards, J.S. (1970): Fetal movement: Developmental and time course. *Science,* 169:95–97.
11. Eisenberg, R., Coursin, D.B., and Rupp, N.R. (1966): Habituation to an acoustic pattern as an index of differences among human neonates. *J. Aud. Res.,* 6:239–248.
12. Gettinger, A., Roberts, A.B., and Campbell, S. (1978): Comparison between subjective and ultrasound assessments of fetal movement. *Br. Med. J.,* 2:88.
13. Goodlin, R.C., and Haesslein, H.C. (1977): When is it fetal distress? *Am. J. Obstet. Gynecol.,* 128:140.
14. Goodman, J.D., Visser, F.G.A., and Dawes, G.S. (1984): Effects of maternal cigarette smoking on fetal trunk movements, fetal breathing movements and the fetal heart rate. *Br. J. Obstet. Gynaecol.,* 91:657–661.
15. Granat, M., Lavie, P., Adar, D., et al. (1979): Short-term cycles in human fetal activity. *Am. J. Obstet. Gynecol.,* 134:696–701.

16. Harper, R.G., Greenberg, M., Farahani, G., et al. (1981): Fetal movement, biochemical and bio-physical parameters, and the outcome of pregnancy. *Am. J. Obstet. Gynecol.*, 141:39–42.

17. Hertogs, K., Roberts, A.B., Cooper, D., et al. (1979): Maternal perception of fetal motor activity. *Br. Med. J.*, 2:1183–1185.

18. Holloway, F.A., and Parsons, O.A. (1971): Habituation of the orienting response in brain damaged patients. *Psychophysiology*, 8:623–634.

19. Hooker, D. (1952): The prenatal origin of behavior. 18th Porter Lecture. Lawrence, University of Kansas Press.

20. Humphrey, T. (1964): Some correlations between the appearance of human fetal reflexes and the development of the nervous system. *Prog. Brain Res.*, 4:93–133.

21. Ianniruberto, A., and Tajani, E. (1981): Ultrasonic study of fetal movements. *Semin. Perinatol.*, 5:175–181.

22. Jarvis, G., and MacDonald, H. (1979): Fetal movements in small-for-dates babies. *J. Obstet. Gynaecol.*, 86:724–727.

23. Key, B.H. (1961): Effects of chlorpromazine and lysergic acid diethylamide on the role of habituation of the arousal response. *Nature*, 190:275–277.

24. Leader, I., Baillie, P., and Van Schalkwyk, D.H. (1981): Fetal movements and fetal outcome: A prospective study. *Obstet. Gynecol.*, 57:431–436.

25. Leader, L.R., Baillie, P., Martin, B., et al. (1982): Fetal habituation in high-risk pregnancies. *Br. J. Obstet. Gynaecol.*, 89:441–446.

26. Manning, F.A., Platt, I.D., and Sipos, I. (1979): Fetal movements in human pregnancies in the third trimester. *Obstet. Gynecol.*, 6:699–702.

27. Mathews, D.D. (1975): Maternal assessment of fetal activity in small-for-dates infants. *Obstet. Gynecol.*, 45:488–493.

28. Minors, D., and Waterhouse, J. (1979): The effect of maternal posture, meals, and time of day on fetal movements. *Br. J. Obstet. Gynaecol.*, 86:717–723.

29. Natale, R., Nasello-Paterson, C., and Turliuk, R. (1986): Fetal breathing and fetal body movements in the human fetus at 24 to 28 weeks gestation. 33rd Annual Meeting of the Soc. Gynecol. Invest., Toronto, Ont., Can.

30. Navot, D., Yaffe, H., and Sadovsky, E. (1984): The ratio of fetal heart rate accelerations to fetal movement according to gestational age. *Am. J. Obstet. Gynecol.*, 149:92–94.

31. Neldham, S. (1980): Fetal movements as an indicator of fetal well-being. *Lancet*, 1:1222–1224.

32. Nyholm, H.C., Hansen, T., and Neldham, S. (1983): Fetal activity acceleration during early labor. *Acta Obstet. Gynecol. Scand.*, 62:131–133.

33. O'Leary, J.A., and Andrinopoulos, G.C. (1981): Correlation of daily fetal movements and the nonstress test as tools for assessment of fetal welfare. *Am. J. Obstet. Gynecol.*, 139:107–108.

34. Patrick, J., Campbell, K., Carmichael, L., et al. (1982): Patterns of gross fetal body movements over 24-hour observation intervals during the last 10 weeks of pregnancy. *Am. J. Obstet. Gynecol.*, 142:363–371.

35. Patrick, J., Campbell, K., Carmichael, L., et al. (1982): Influence of maternal heart rate and gross fetal body movements on the daily pattern of fetal heart rate near term. *Am. J. Obstet. Gynecol.*, 144:533–538.

36. Pearson, J.F., and Weaver, J.B. (1976): Fetal activity and fetal well-being: An evaluation. *Br. Med. J.*, 1:1305–1307.

37. Polishuk, W.Z., Laufer, N., and Sadovsky, E. (1975): Fetal reaction to external light. *Harefuah*, 89:395–396.

38. Rabinowitz, R., Persitz, E., and Sadovsky, E. (1983): The relation between fetal heart rate accelerations and fetal movements. *Obstet. Gynecol.*, 61:16–18.

39. Rayburn, W.F. (1980): Clinical significance of maternal perceptible fetal motion. *Am. J. Obstet. Gynecol.*, 138:210–212.

40. Rayburn, W.F. (1982): Clinical applications of monitoring fetal activity. *Am. J. Obstet. Gynecol.*, 144:967–980.

41. Rayburn, W.F. (1982): Fetal activity patterns in hypertensive pregnancies. *Clin. Exp. Hypertens.*, 1:119–126.

41a. Rayburn, W.F., and Barr, M. (1985): The malformed fetus: Diagnosis and pregnancy management. *Obstet. Gynecol. Annu.*, 14:112–126.

42. Rayburn, W.F., Motley, M.E., Stempel, L.E., et al. (1982): Antepartum prediction of the postmature infant. *Obstet. Gynecol.*, 60:148–153.

43. Rayburn, W.F., Motley, M.E., and Zuspan, F.P. (1982): Conditions affecting nonstress tests. *Obstet. Gynecol.,* 59:490–493.

44. Rayburn, W.F., Rayburn, P.R., and Gabel, L.L. (1983): Excess fetal activity: Another worrisome sign? *South. Med. J.,* 76:163.

45. Rayburn, W.F., Zuspan, F.P., Motley, M.E., et al. (1980): An alternative to antepartum fetal heart rate testing. *Am. J. Obstet. Gynecol.,* 138:223–226.

46. Richardson, B., Campbell, K., Carmichael, L., et al. (1981): Effects of external physical stimulation on fetuses near term. *Am. J. Obstet. Gynecol.,* 139:344–352.

47. Roberts, A.B., Little, D., Cooper, D., et al. (1979): Normal patterns of fetal activity in the third trimester. *Br. J. Obstet. Gynaecol.,* 86:4–9.

48. Sadovsky, E., Mahler, Y., Polishuk, W.Z., et al. (1973): Correlation between electromagnetic recording and maternal assessment of fetal movement. *Lancet,* 1:1141–1143.

49. Sadovsky, E., and Polishuk, W.Z. (1977): Fetal movements *in utero. Obstet. Gynecol.,* 50:49–55.

50. Sadovsky, E., Polishuk, W.Z., Yaffe, H., et al. (1977): Fetal movements recorder: Use and indications. *Int. J. Gynaecol. Obstet.,* 15:20–24.

51. Sadovsky, E., Yaffe, H., and Polishuk, W.Z. (1974): Fetal movement monitoring in normal and pathologic pregnancy. *Int. J. Gynaecol. Obstet.,* 12:75–79.

52. Sagvolden, T., and Webster, K. (1974): Habituation of the startle reflex in rats with septal lesions. *Behav. Biol.,* 12:413–418.

53. Sorokin, Y., Dierker, L.J., Pillay, S.K., et al. (1982): The association between fetal heart rate patterns and fetal movements in pregnancies between 20 and 30 weeks of gestation. *Am. J. Obstet. Gynecol.,* 143:243–249.

54. Sorokin, Y., Pillay, D., Dierker, L.J., et al. (1981): A comparison between maternal, tocodynamometric, and real-time ultrasonographic assessment of fetal movement. *Am. J. Obstet. Gynecol.,* 140:456–460.

55. Thompson, R.F., and Spencer, W.A. (1966): Habituation: A model for the study of neuronal substrates of behaviour. *Psychol. Rev.,* 73:16–43.

56. Tizard, B. (1968): Habituation of EEG and skin potential changes in normal and severely subnormal children. *Am. J. Ment. Defic.,* 73:34–40.

57. Webster, W. (1969): Auditory habituation and barbiturate induced neurological activity. *Science,* 164:970–971.

Fetal Neurology, edited by
A. Hill and J.J. Volpe.
Raven Press, New York © 1989.

Commentary on Chapters 1 and 2

*Alan Hill and **Joseph J. Volpe

*Division of Neurology, Department of Paediatrics, University of British Columbia,
British Columbia's Children's Hospital, Vancouver, British Columbia, Canada V6H 3V4;
and **Division of Pediatric Neurology, Washington University School of Medicine,
St. Louis, Missouri 63110*

These two chapters are concerned with fetal motility and related activities and provide a fascinating complement to each other because the authors are from two quite different disciplines. Prechtl provides the perspective of an investigator with a long and illustrious interest in the development of human behavior, and Rayburn provides the perspective of a specialist in perinatal medicine with a particular interest in the clinical applicability of this new area of research. In Prechtl's chapter, the importance of the quality of movement in clinical assessment is a critical point, soundly made, and in Rayburn's chapter, the anatomic and physiologic substrates of such linkages as fetal heart rate and motility are addressed. Both chapters provide us with the exciting sense that a neurological examination of the fetus is on the horizon and that our striking deficiencies of understanding of the status of the nervous system in our fetal patients will lessen dramatically in the next decade.

Careful evaluation of the quantity and quality of movement represents an integral component of the neurological examination at all ages. This fundamental principle of neurological evaluation has been extended recently to include the assessment of fetal movement as a "fetal neurological examination."

Several techniques permit the monitoring of fetal movements. The oldest, most convenient and widely used method is the systematic recording of activity perceived by the mother. Electromechanical devices are used primarily as investigative tools at the present time. However, recent advances in the resolution capability of modern ultrasonography, particularly when combined with video recordings, now are affording the most detailed longitudinal evaluations of fetal movement available to date.

Real-time ultrasonography may detect the presence of fetal movement as early as the second month of gestation. Serial and prolonged examinations with this presumably innocuous technique are capable of demonstrating distinct maturational changes in movement of the developing fetus. The time of appearance of specific spontaneous movement patterns and reflex activity following stimuli are remarkably constant (1). Thus, the relationship of the patterns of movement to gestational age in healthy fetuses may be used as an index of fetal well-being. In this context, preliminary observations suggest that in the abnormal fetus, changes in the quality of movement precede changes in the quantity of movement and therefore may be a more sensitive indicator of abnormalities (2). This notion is supported by reports of abnormal quality of movements in fetuses with anencephaly, chromosome abnormalities, and growth retardation. Furthermore, a decrease in quantity of spontaneous fetal activity may be valuable for the diagnosis of congenital neuromuscular disease. Similarly, in infants with other types of cerebral injury, e.g., hypoxic-ischemic injury and congenital infections, the abnormal modifying influence of injured cerebral structures may produce recognizable abnormal patterns of fetal movement.

Detailed analysis of fetal behavior by real-time ultrasonography, including assessment of body movements, ocular movements, posture, breathing, and heart rate, has led to the identification of four distinct behavioral states in the fetus by 38 weeks of gestation (4,5). The inability to synchronize several behavioral variables during transitions between these different behavioral states has been demonstrated to be associated with fetal compromise. Such observations may be refined further by assessment of the habituation response of the fetus to vibrotactile or acoustic stimuli (3). However, the evaluation of fetal response to mechanical stimulation through the maternal abdominal wall is complicated by the fact that it is difficult to prove that a particular movement following a stimulus is a direct result of the stimulus and does not merely represent a spontaneous movement occurring coincidentally at that time, especially in view of the high baseline rate of spontaneous fetal activity.

A combination of fetal movement with fetal breathing, fetal heart rate reactivity, and amniotic fluid volume are included in the ''fetal biophysical score.'' This refined method of antepartum assessment is discussed in greater detail in a later chapter.

Comparison of longitudinal observations of fetal behavior with the well-established patterns of postnatal behavior in low-risk premature infants has demonstrated striking similarities between fetal and preterm infant behavior at the same conceptional age. Thus, movement patterns observed in the fetus may be observed after birth, with the addition of certain specific movements that represent an apparent adaptation to the extrauterine environment, e.g., Moro reflex. Thus, the terminology used to describe movement patterns in the newborn may be applied also to fetal movements (6,7). The reduced effect of gravity *in utero* may cause certain fetal movements to appear more fluent than the equivalent movements observed postnatally (e.g., the sudden relaxation of the body causes a more gradual drop of an elevated limb. Similarly, anteflexion of the head or rotation of the body, which is normally observed at 3 to 4 months post-term, may be observed in the intrauterine environment because of the buoyancy effect of amniotic fluid) (2).

Although assessment of spontaneous movements of the human fetus is gaining increasing importance as a diagnostic index of fetal well-being, the underlying morphological substrate of these movements and their functional significance during prenatal life are understood less clearly. This relates in part to the limited knowledge of the ultrastructure of the central nervous system and muscles in the fetus, particularly regarding synapse and motor end-plate formation. Indeed, the last trimester is the maturational time of onset of such events as synaptogenesis and elaboration of axonal and dendritic ramifications, events still to be defined quantitatively in human brain regions. Thus, future research directed toward the correlation of fetal movements with neurological outcome should provide important data regarding maturation of neural and muscular structures in the human fetus.

REFERENCES

1. Birnholz, J.C., Stephens, J.C., and Faria, M. (1978): Fetal movement patterns: A possible means of defining neurologic developmental milestones *in utero*. *Am. J. Roentgenol.*, 130:537–540.
2. DeVries, J.I.P., Visser, G.H.A., and Prechtl, H.F.R. (1982): The emergence of fetal behaviour. I. Qualitative aspects. *Early Hum. Dev.*, 7:301–322.
3. Gelman, S.R., Wood, S., Spellacy, W.N., Abrams, R.M. (1982): Fetal movements in response to sound stimulation. *Am. J. Obstet. Gynecol.*, 143:484–485.
4. Nijhuis, J.G., Martin, C.B., and Prechtl, H.F.R. (1984): Behavioural states of the human fetus. In: *Continuity of Neural Functions from Prenatal to Postnatal Life: Clin Dev Med*, edited by H.F.R. Prechtl, vol. 94, pp. 65–78. Blackwell, Oxford.
5. Nijhuis, J.G., Prechtl, H.F.R., Martin, C.B., and Bots, R.S.G.M. (1982): Are there behavioural states in the human fetus? *Early Hum. Dev.*, 6:177–195.
6. Prechtl, H.F.R., Fargel, J.W., Weinmann, H.M., Bakker, H.H. (1979): Posture, motility and respiration in low-risk, preterm infants. *Dev. Med. Child Neurol.*, 21:3–27.
7. Prechtl, H.F.R., and Nolte, R. (1984): Motor behaviour of preterm infants. In: *Continuity of Neural Functions from Prenatal to Postnatal Life: Clin Dev Med*, edited by H.F.R. Prechtl, vol. 94, pp. 79–92. Blackwell, Oxford.

Fetal Neurology, edited by
A. Hill and J.J. Volpe.
Raven Press, New York © 1989.

3

Ultrasonic Fetal Neuro-ophthalmology

Jason C. Birnholz

Department of Diagnostic Radiology and Nuclear Medicine, Rush-Presbyterian–St. Luke's Medical Center, Chicago, Illinois 60612

Recent advancements in ultrasound scanning have enabled visualization of the anatomic structure of the eye as well as eye movements in the fetus (5). Occasionally, evaluation of the fetal eye is of interest because of a family history of a specific genetic/ophthalmic disorder. More commonly, specific ocular and facial abnormalities on initial ultrasound scans may suggest a particular syndrome or malformation. Because parts of the eye, such as the optic nerve, are direct embryologic derivatives of the forebrain, evaluation of the fetal eye may provide an indirect but technically facile method for monitoring development of the central nervous system. This chapter will review the current applications of ultrasonic fetal ophthalmology and will suggest directions for future research.

TECHNICAL BACKGROUND

The general principles of ultrasound imaging are well known. Recent technical advances have improved image quality and permit detailed examinations, including evaluation of the fetal eye. The instrument that we prefer utilizes an 80 (or more) wave length aperture, as well as a multielement array with dynamic focusing on both transit and receive portions of the cycle. Uniform field insonation and side lobe suppression result in such improved spatial resolution so that the basic Rayleigh limit for diffraction-limited methods is approached more closely than with earlier devices. In addition, speckle reduction via frame averaging provides a "clean" image with optimal contrast resolution.

At higher frequencies, the principal limitation on spatial resolution results from display inadequacies, rather than acoustic pulse features or signal processing. A useful calculation in this regard is the ratio of display screen pixels per tissue millimeter. The most recent equipment may provide 1,024 pixel by 500 (TV) line display and incorporates options for magnification imaging. In this mode, the tissue region is interrogated solely and the full display surface is "concentrated" on a limited area. Magnification technique provides an additional advantage by achieving high sampling rates over a small area, which permits visual recognition of subtle or otherwise imperceptible tissue movement.

The analysis of frequency shifts of reflected pulses provides information about the velocity of the target along the direction of the sonic beam. This has been termed *the Doppler shift phenomenon.* The conventional Doppler recording generally samples a unidirectional or "ice pick" movement component only. However, Doppler shifts may be determined for an entire imaging field, provided that some loss in sensitivity or sampling rate is accepted. Velocities may be overlayed on the original monochrome image as a series of colors by a method referred to as "color flow mapping." Doppler shifts of 3 to 7 MHz acoustic pulses, which correspond to the relatively rapid movement of blood within vessels, are not optimal for the display of fetal eye movements. Moving target indicator (MTI) techniques, which display differences between image frames and may be implemented in off-line computer graphics terminals, have not been applied in this area.

The fetal eye is a "high contrast" target of fluid bounded by an elastic, multilayered boundary, a combination that is optimal for ultrasound imaging. Consequently, the technical issues associated with antenatal study of the eye are principally related to scan plane selection. In approximately 85% of cases, the eye may be visualized via bone-free portals, located anterior or lateral to the face, i.e., through the nonattenuating layer of amniotic fluid. Coronal views are obtained by positioning the probe above the brow (Fig. 1) or lateral to the face (Fig. 2). This plane is useful for studying orbitofacial topography, as well as for specifically visualizing the lens, anterior chamber structures, and lids (Figs. 3 and 4).

Positioning the probe in the front of the eyes, in a plane parallel to the base of the cranium (i.e., scan plane along the intraorbital line), permits measurement of orbital separation (Fig. 5) and simultaneous visualization of both lenses. The vitreous and hyaloid artery (see below) may be studied by sweeping through the volume of the eye in either basal or sagittal plane orientations (Fig. 6). Similarly, these planes may also be used for visualization of the apical fat pad, the extraocular muscles, and the optic nerve with its associated vessels. Inasmuch as these scanning positions are directed "into" the ophthalmic artery, their scanning angle would appear to be optimal for Doppler recording of the arterial wave form (Fig. 7), although this method of data collection has not been applied to date.

STRUCTURAL DEVELOPMENT

The bony orbital margins may be visualized clearly by the beginning of the 9th week after conception (Fig. 8). Severe holoprosencephaly may be diagnosed at that time either on the basis of the abnormal intracranial appearance or from orbitofacial abnormalities (i.e., cebocephaly, hypotelorism) that are present in the ma-

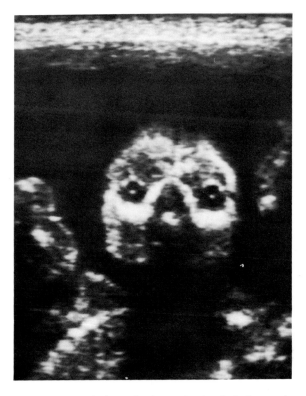

FIG. 1. The probe is positioned above the brow showing both lenses. Large scale markers = 10 mm distance.

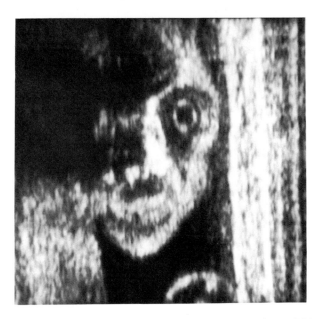

FIG. 2. The lateral coronal view shows half the face. The scan plane of this view passes through the lens of the left eye.

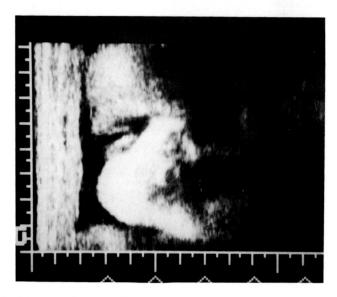

FIG. 3. The lids are partly open in this lateral coronal view of a well-nourished third-trimester fetus. This is an anterior scan plane.

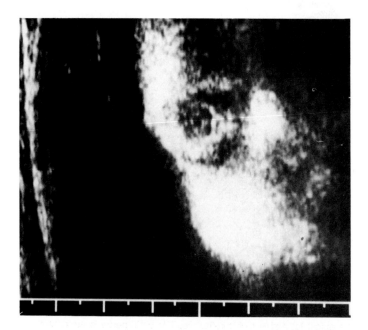

FIG. 4. The central 2.5-mm circle is the pupil. This scan plane passes through the iris.

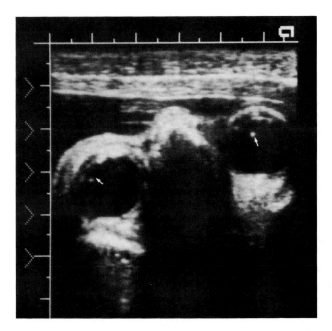

FIG. 5. This is a base plane view through both globes. The arrows point to the posterior capsule of the lens and show the central axis of each eye. The minute dimple of the retinal surface of the left eye (10 o'clock arrow position) is the optic disk.

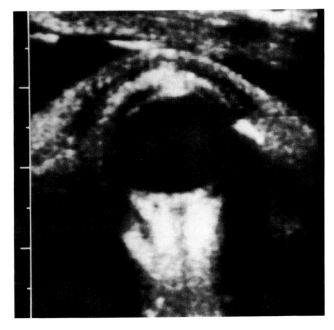

FIG. 6. The apical fat pad is highly reflective. The optic nerve is the central, less reflective structure.

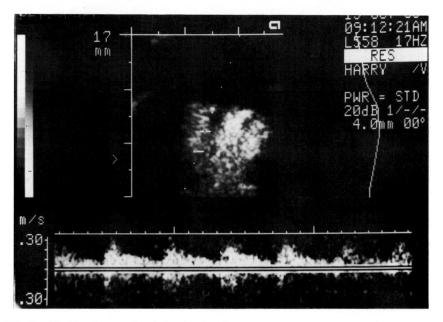

FIG. 7. The Doppler sample window is placed next to the optic nerve including the ophthalmic artery. The waveform plots flow velocity versus time.

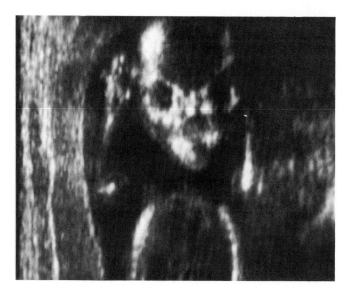

FIG. 8. The bony orbits are well defined before the end of the first trimester and may be studied then or subsequently.

jority of cases (9). Abnormal configurations of the orbits caused by skeletal dysplasias, e.g., osteogenesis imperfecta, hypophosphatasia, and fibrous dysplasia may not be evident until later in pregnancy. Nasofrontal encephaloceles may be recognized early in gestation (Fig. 9). Amniotic band deformations may have a variable time of onset (22).

The ocular globe may be visualized after approximately 14 weeks postconceptual age. At this time, the lens appears cupshaped. A bright, linear reflection, which represents the hyaloid artery, extends from the posterior chorioretinal boundary and inserts eccentrically into the posterior surface of the lens (Fig. 10) (6,27). This vessel, which is part of the carotid system developmentally, is a continuation of the ophthalmic artery and ramifies greatly throughout the vitreous and along the lens surface in the first trimester. The vitreal elements of the vessel regress early, whereas the main arterial trunk, which has a tight endothelial investment, maintains its linear reflectivity until 20 weeks after conception when it becomes segmented or "beaded" in appearance. The vessel subsequently regresses (i.e., becomes invisible by ultrasound) during a 2-week period, beginning at the retinal end. Residual fragments seen just behind the lens in the early third trimester correspond to the later ophthalmoscopic finding, termed *the Mittendorf spot*. Regression of the central and proximal parts of the artery is completed by the time the fused lids separate. However, the mechanism involved is presumably different from the hypothesis that desmosomal lid bridges are lysed by lipids that are secreted from maturing Meibomian glands (1). Occasionally the hyaloid artery may persist into childhood as a "normal" variant (21). In our experience, regression is usually completed by 24 weeks postconceptual age, and there appears to be an increased incidence of aneuoploidy, specifically Down's syndrome, in those cases in whom "beading" is delayed beyond 28 weeks. Following regression of the hyaloid artery, the vitreous appears anechoic with ultrasound imaging because the canal of the Cloquet and other anatomic channels within the vitreous are invisible with this technique.

Abnormalities of the anterior chamber have been observed in the fetal alcohol syndrome (23) and with acute maternal cocaine use (16). Coloboma may occur as an isolated finding or may be associated with several syndromes. Although it is possible to visualize the iris (see below) and aqueous humor by ultrasound, these anatomic structures are not generally included in a primary dysmorphology survey because their visualization depends greatly on uncontrolled physical variables, such as their size and depth, fetal position, and amniotic fluid volume. Lid appearance may be helpful later in the third trimester, specifically for the detection of epicanthal folds (Fig. 11) or an anti-Mongoloid slant of the eyes. However, it must be remembered that epicanthal folds are not a feature of abortuses with trisomy 21 during the second trimester (31). The lens may be visualized during the second and third trimesters because of the high reflectivity of the corneoscleral limbus. I have not observed congenital cataracts *in utero*, although they might be expected to be visible by ultrasound technique. However, corneal clouding should not affect sound transmission or reflection in the low megahertz range.

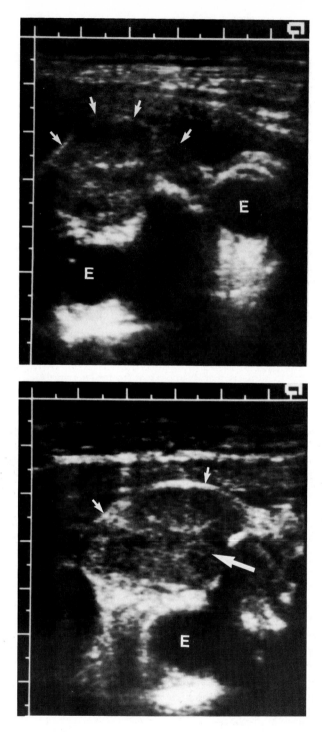

FIG. 9. There is a soft tissue mass (*arrows*) protruding beyond the left eye in this base view (**top**). The eyes are centrally marked with "E." A large bony defect (*large arrow*) is seen in the magnification view (**bottom**) of the left side. The eye is itself normal.

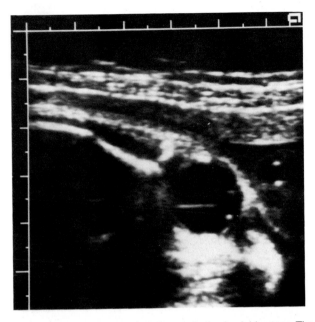

FIG. 10. The linear reflector traversing the vitreous is the hyaloid artery. The lens is positioned at 3 o'clock.

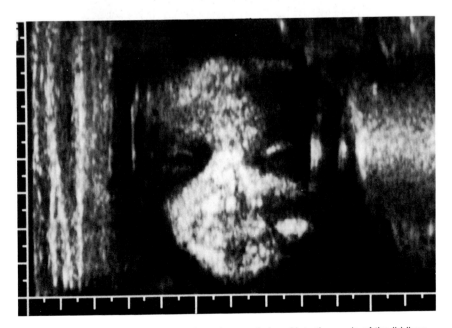

FIG. 11. Both lids are seen in this lateral coronal view. Note the angle of the lid lines.

Although the fetal eye is not precisely spherical (26), for practical purposes it may be assumed that the average transvitreous diameter is a representative measure of its size. Such measurements, as a function of gestational age, provide an *in vivo* standard for volumetric growth of the eye, and these measurements correspond to those previously obtained at postmortem examination of excised reexpanded specimens (26,32).

The association between microphthalmia and "mental retardation" (35) was recognized before present diagnostic methods were developed to classify these patients according to their intracranial anatomy, metabolic features, or genetic pedigree. Microphthalmia, which is recognizable *in utero* by ultrasound, often implies significant cerebral growth deficit such as may be observed in trisomy 13, trisomy 18, holoprosencephaly, microcephaly, and severe hydrocephalus.

The rate of volume growth of the fetal eye is not linear. There appear to be spurts or accelerations of growth that alternate with plateaus and this nonlineauts of growth resembles the discontinuous pattern of growth of the brain itself (10). At the present time, it is not clear to what extent the apparent variation in timing of these phases is due to inaccurate calculation of gestational age rather than true biological variation. However, it is possible to distinguish delayed growth from progressively diminishing or retarded growth. Delayed regression of the hyaloid artery, which has been discussed previously, is often associated with delay in cerebral sulcation during the third trimester. We have studied cerebral mantle thickness, calculated from the ventricular margin to cerebral surface at the level of the central sulcus, during the second trimester (J.C. Birnholz, *unpublished observations*). During this time period, a triphasic pattern of growth may be observed with, first, increasing growth in width between 14 and 16½ weeks, followed by a relative plateau during the next 2 weeks, and then a great increase in thickness during the following 3 weeks. These phases appear to correspond to primary neuronal proliferation, followed by the first phase of neuronal migration and, finally, by glial proliferation (33). We have observed three cases of trisomy 21 and one of triploidy that demonstrated delayed cortical growth during the second trimester with subsequent "normalization" of cerebral mantle thickness by the beginning of the third trimester. The ocular volumes in those cases demonstrated a similar delayed pattern of growth.

FUNCTIONAL DEVELOPMENT

Functionally, the eye, the visual cortex, and the intervening pathways operate as a unit. At the present time, there is no noninvasive method to test "vision" in the fetus. However, we have demonstrated that simple responses to light may be elicited in the fetus during the third trimester (5). These investigations were conducted following auditory stimulation, when lids were observed to open spontaneously, suggesting a behavioral state (28) of "arousal" or "alertness." A bright light source (without heat), placed in direct contact with the skin of the maternal abdomen immediately overlying a fetal eye, was switched on when the lids were open. Almost immediate closing of the eyes was observed (17). In one instance, when the light source was placed in a more peripheral location, an orienting response that resembled the head-turning response toward diffuse light present in the normal newborn infant (11) was observed. Slender mothers who were either Caucasian or had relatively little melanin pigmentation were selected for these preliminary studies. Obviously, light level within the uterus represents an uncontrolled parameter that will vary from case to case. This fact most probably precludes the development of a reliable prenatal test based on these observations. An additional problem is the issue of spectral filtering of light, which results in a stimulus that is both dim and red. Thus, the assumption that the baseline intra-amniotic environment is uniformly dark is probably false. There are anecdotal descriptions of maternal sensations of altered fetal movement during sunlight exposure, e.g., sunbathing. Conversely, there is no evidence that prenatal light stimulation is essential for development of vision in humans. However, postnatal visual experience influences both sensory and morphologic growth and morphologic visual growth patterns, including induction of myopia (12) and amblyopia (36).

Despite the formidable technical difficulties, studies of visual responsiveness in the fetus may provide clinically relevant information about the functional state of the central nervous system, analogous to the information provided by evoked response testing to auditory stimuli (15). For example, visual pattern fixation in newborn infants has been demonstrated to have predictive neurologic value (24). Because ultrasound guided amniocentesis has become an essentially risk-free procedure, it should be possible to insert fiberoptic instruments into the amniotic space to standardize stimulation if preliminary studies in this field appear encouraging. Any experimental design must take into consideration that the newborn infant has a fixed accommodation distance (median 19 cm) (14) until 2 to 4 months of age.

Light sensitivity is a basic visual perceptual capability, similar to contrast and color discrimination, form and pattern perception, and motion detection. To date, ultrasound studies of fetal vision have generally used a motor endpoint to assess visual sensation. However, it must be remembered that vision also relies greatly on associative pathways, which become operative much later during development than does receptor function.

DEVELOPMENTAL DYNAMICS

Ultrasonic studies of ocular dynamics have principally involved recording the presence or absence of globe movements (3). The lens is viewed in a (lateral) coronal plane so that ocular movement can be tracked in any of its possible directions. Movements may be distinguished by their velocity (i.e., slow, fast), as well as by their angular deviation from a resting or previous lens position or by their sequential properties (i.e., isolated, two or three conjoint movements, or longer saccades). As previously discussed, the sampling of data will depend on the frame rate and field size of the imaging system. Ocular dynamics may be characterized by time statistics, including incidence, transition probabilities, and observed periodicities.

The normal developmental sequence of eye movements has not been quantitated for any specifically defined, sufficiently large fetal population. Individual lens movements of slow velocity and large amplitude may be seen between 12 and 14 weeks conceptual age. These appear to occur infrequently and randomly. More rapid eye movements emerge by 20 weeks postconceptual age. Conjugate, rapid eye movements (REM) develop subsequently at the beginning of the third trimester and increase in frequency and duration until approximately 32 weeks postconceptual age. After this gestational age, phases of deep sleep with relative ocular immobility are observed with increasing frequency. Early in gestation, eye movements occur randomly in any (or all) directions with slow return to central resting position. Later, the eyes may remain deviated following a movement, and transverse-lateral excursions tend to predominate. Later in the third trimester, slow eye movements, often with lateral or medial "fixation" and with open lids, become interspersed with REMs of increasing frequency, possibly representing an "alert" state.

The anatomic loci initiating various types of eye movements as well as their control circuits remain to be elucidated. It may be assumed that most of the ocular activity observed prenatally originates from subcortical levels. In this context, observations in newborn kittens are of interest, which demonstrate that organized eye movements occur spontaneously and may be elicited by direct stimulation of the superior colliculus, before visual signals themselves are capable of activating the colliculus (34).

Any discussion of fetal eye movements must include a notion of behavioral states (28), i.e., operating levels of the nervous system that are consistent, recognizable, recurrent, and which eventually become periodic. In general, state differentiation in the fetus occurs before the final month of pregnancy, although the precise timing of the transition from only transient combinations to stable patterns (that may be classified as particular "states") has not been identified. Rapid eye movements are recognized as the principal component of active sleep. In our studies of synchronization of movements of the larynx and diaphragm, we have observed fluttering excursions of the upper airway that modulate tracheal fluid flow (Fig. 12), coincident with REM activity, between 26 and 30 weeks post-conceptual age.

The principal clinical application for observation of REMs in the fetus is in the assessment of fetal hypoxemia. Physiologic compensatory mechanisms of the fetus are provoked by failing placental function. Increased venous return to the heart occurs by relaxation of the sphincter that normally limits blood flow through the ductus venosus (19). There is preferential maintenance of cerebral, myocardial, and adrenal circulations by increased vascular resistance systems. There is a decline in endogenous growth factor secretion from the gut. There is also energy conservation by a decrease in fetal heart rate of 8 to 10 beats/min and by decreased body movements in general and both diaphragm and eye movements in particular. Graded decrease in REMs with progressive hypoxemia has been demonstrated in fetal sheep (18), an effect that is presumably mediated via central suppression at

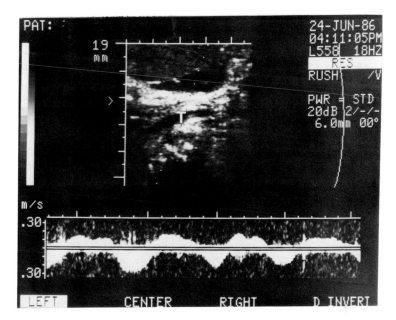

FIG. 12. The Doppler window is centered on the trachea ("T", chin to viewer's right). The tracing shows a complex biphasic tracheal fluid flow occurring during a phase of rapid eye movements (REMs).

the level of the brainstem (8). Declining REM activity may also reflect a change in behavioral state (13). In practical terms, the presence of REMs in the fetus is reassuring; their absence should be regarded as a risk factor and prompt consideration of delivery when other features of hypoxemia are present or, alternatively, prompt percutaneous blood gas sampling for assessment of oxygenation (7) when there is diagnostic uncertainty. It may be speculated that evaluation of fetal eye movements may provide a more specific indication of fetal condition than other tests based on the demonstration of heart rate variation with activity (30). However, decreased REM activity does not appear to be limited to fetal hypoxemia and has been observed also in other conditions associated with depression of central nervous system function, e.g., the Down's syndrome (29).

Pathologic eye movements must also be considered. We have not observed nystagmus. However, we have recorded bursts of small amplitude, fluttering "pericentral" lens excursions in association with severe hydrocephalus (3), which may represent a manifestation of seizure activity. In addition, we have also observed prolonged bursts of eye movements of large amplitude that we suspect may represent analogs of infant "REM storms" (2), which have been associated with poor neurodevelopmental prognosis.

Although the pupil may be visualized by ultrasound technique (Fig. 11), it is difficult to study pupillary movements because even subtle displacements of the globe or head will shift the pupil from the field of view. In addition, the absence of functional sympathetic innervation to the iris (20) causes the pupils to remain generally small. However, dilation of the pupils may occur with fetal hypoxia when circulating catecholamine levels are elevated.

Another feature of fetal ocular dynamics that may be investigated is the relationships between lid and eye movements, e.g., lens elevation with lid closure. Forceful blinking may be observed as a component of the startle reaction elicited by administration of sudden intense sounds to the maternal lower abdomen. Repetitive auditory stimuli result generally in decremental response for most components of the startle reaction related to gestational age (4). However, the eye blink is not extinguished and persists throughout most stimulation regimes. Latencies of the order of 30 msec for auditory blink "reflexes" have been recorded in the premature infant after 36 weeks (37) and appear to correspond to the almost instantaneous response observed on fetal ultrasonic studies (sampled at 30 frames/sec). Latency appears to be longer at the beginning of the third trimester. Indeed, when a motor response can be elicited before 20 weeks gestation, the observed delay is of the order of 1 to 2 sec. The latencies for blink responses appear prolonged with hypoxia. However, further advances in instrumentation will be required to permit identification of graded patterns with diagnostic or prognostic applications. Approximately one-third of fetuses studied during the third trimester will demonstrate flurries of REMs (Fig. 12) following auditory stimulation, usually associated with yawning. Furthermore, expressive facial movements (including brow, lids, and eye movements) may be studied antenatally (Fig. 13). Post-natally, the social smile appears to develop from a combination of esophoria and knitting of the brow (25).

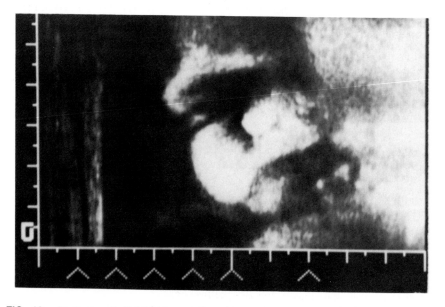

FIG. 13. An "expressive" third-trimester face (right lateral coronal view). Eye dynamics can be correlated with movements of brow, cheeks, lips, and tongue.

SUMMARY

Gross morphologic and dynamic examinations of the eye are essential elements of the newborn physical examination. Recent advances in ultrasound technique have permitted extension of the ocular examination to the human fetus. At the present time, information regarding the normal sequence of functional development of the visual system is limited. Our observations suggest that both delayed cerebral growth and functional depression of the central nervous system (with hypoxemia) may be inferred from particular ocular findings.

REFERENCES

1. Andersen, H., Ehlers, N., Matthiesen, M.E., and Claesson, M.N. (1967): Histochemistry and development of the human eyelids. II. *Acta Ophthalmol.*, 45:288–293.
2. Beckert, P.T., and Thomas, E.B. (1981): Rapid eye movement storms in infants: Rate of occurrence at 6 months predicts mental development at 1 year. *Science*, 212:1415–1416.
3. Birnholz, J.C. (1981): The development of fetal eye movement patterns. *Science*, 213:679–681.
4. Birnholz, J.C. (1984): Fetal neurology. In: *Ultrasound Annual*, edited by R.C. Saunders and M. Hill, pp. 139–160. Raven Press, New York.
5. Birnholz, J.C. (1985): Ultrasonic fetal opthtalmology. *Early Hum. Dev.*, 12:199–209.
6. Birnholz, J.C. (1988): Fetal hyaloid artery regression. *Radiology*, 166:781–783.
7. Daffos, F., Forestier, F., and Parlovsky, M.C. (1984): Fetal blood sampling during the third trimester of pregnancy. *Br. J. Obstet. Gynaecol.*, 91:118–123.
8. Dawes, G.S., Gardner, N.W., Johnston, B.M., and Walker, A. (1983): Breathing in fetal lambs: The effects of brain section. *J. Physiol. (Lond.)*, 335:535–553.
9. Demeyer, W. (1971): Classification of cerebral malformations. *Birth Defects* (Original Article Series), 7:78–93.
10. Gilles, F.H., Leviton, A., and Dooling, E.C. (1983): *The Developing Human Brain.* John Wright, Boston.
11. Goldie, L., and Hopkins, I.J. (1982): Head turning towards diffuse light in the neurological examination of newborn infants. *Brain*, 19:665–672.
12. Gottlieb, M.D., Rajaram, V., and Fugate-Weintzek, L.A. (1987): Local retinal regions control local eye growth and myopia. *Science*, 237:73–77.
13. Harding, R. (1980): State-related and developmental changes in laryngeal function. *Sleep*, 3:307–322.
14. Haynes, H., White, B.I., and Held, P. (1965): Visual accommodation in human infants. *Science*, 148:528–529.
15. Hrbek, A., Karlberg, P., and Olsson, T. (1973): Development of visual somatosensory evoked responses in preterm newborn infants. *Electroencephalogr. Clin. Neurophysiol.*, 34:225–232.
16. Isenberg, S.J., Spierer, A., and Inkelis, S.H. (1987): Ocular signs of cocaine intoxication in neonates. *Am. J. Ophthalmol.*, 103:211–214.
17. Kearsley, R.B. (1973): The newborn's response to auditory stimulation. A demonstration of orienting and defensive behavior. *Child Dev.*, 44:582–590.
18. Koos, B.J., Sameshima, M., and Power, G.C. (1987): Fetal breathing, sleep state, and cardiovascular responses to graded hypoxia in sleep. *J. Appl. Physiol.*, 62:1033–1039.
19. Lind, J., and Wegelius, C. (1953): Human fetal circulation: Changes in the cardiovascular system at birth and disturbances in the post-natal closure of the foramen ovale and ductus arteriosus. *Cold Spring Harbor Symp. Quant. Biol.*, 51:109–122.
20. Lind, N., Shinebourne, E., Turner, P., and Cotton, D. (1971): Adrenergic neurone and receptor activity in the iris of the neonate. *Pediatrics*, 47:105–112.
21. Mann, I. (1957): *Developmental Abnormalities of the Eye.* Lippincott, Philadelphia.
22. Miller, M.T., Deutsch, T.A., Cronin, C., and Keys, C.L. (1987): Amniotic bands as a cause of ocular anomalies. *Am. J. Ophthalmol.*, 104:270–279.

23. Miller, M.T., Epstein, R.J., Sugar, J., et al. (1984): Anterior segment anomalies in fetal alcohol syndrome. *J. Pediatr. Ophthalmol.,* 21:8–14.
24. Miranda, S.B., Hack, M., Fantz, R.L., Fanaroff, A.A., and Klaus, M.H. (1977): Neonatal pattern recognition: A prediction of future mental performance. *J. Pediatr.,* 91:642–647.
25. Morikawa, Y., Gato, K., Kimura, K., et al. (1983): Development of responses by facial expressions and eye movements in neonates and young infants. *Brain Dev.,* 5:278–285.
26. O'Rahilly, R., and Bossy, J. (1982): The growth of the eye: Part I—*In utero. Anal. Desarrollo,* 16:31–51.
27. Ozanics, V., and Jakobiec, F.A. (1982): Prenatal development of the eye and its adnexa. In: *Ocular Anatomy, Embryology and Teratology,* edited by F.A. Jakobiec, chap. 2. Harper and Row, Philadelphia.
28. Prechtl, H.F.R. (1974): The behavioral states of the newborn infant. (A Review). *Brain Res.,* 76:1304–1311.
29. Prechtl, H.F.R., Theorell, K., and Blair, A.W. (1973): Behavioral state cycles in abnormal infants. *Dev. Med. Child. Neurol.,* 15:606–615.
30. Rochard, F., Schifrin, B.S., Goupil, F., et al. (1976): Nonstressed fetal heart rate monitoring in the antepartum period. *Am. J. Obstet. Gynecol.,* 126:699–706.
31. Rushton, D.I. (1982): Examination of abortions. In: *Fetal and Neonatal Pathology,* edited by A.J. Barson, p. 43. Praeger, New York.
32. Scammon, R.E., and Armstrong, D. (1925): On the growth of the human eyeball and optic nerve. *J. Comp. Neurol.,* 38:165–219.
33. Sidman, R.L., and Rakic, P. (1973): Neuronal migration. *Brain Res.,* 62:1–35.
34. Stein, B.E., Clamann, H.P., and Goldberg, S.J. (1980): Superior colliculus: Control of eye movements in neonatal kittens. *Science,* 210:78–79.
35. Warburg, M. (1971): The heterogeneity of microphthalmia in the mentally retarded. *Birth Defects* (Original Article Series), 7:136–141.
36. Wiesel, T.N., and Hubel, D.H. (1965): Comparison of the effects of unilateral and bilateral eye closure on cortical unit responses in kittens. *J. Neurophysiol.,* 28:1029–1040.
37. Yamada, A. (1984): Blink reflex elicited by auditory stimulation. *Brain Dev.,* 6:45–53.

Fetal Neurology, edited by
A. Hill and J.J. Volpe.
Raven Press, New York © 1989.

Commentary on Chapter 3

*Alan Hill and **Joseph J. Volpe

*Division of Neurology, Department of Paediatrics, University of British Columbia,
British Columbia's Children's Hospital, Vancouver, British Columbia, Canada V6H 3V4;
and **Division of Pediatric Neurology, Washington University School of Medicine,
St. Louis, Missouri 63110*

The investigation of the fetal eye and eye movements represents perhaps the most striking example of the resolution and diagnostic capabilities of real-time ultrasonography. Although experience to date is limited, research has been directed toward identification and quantification of morphologic characteristics of the fetal eye at various stages of gestation and toward correlation of fetal eye movements with other parameters of behavioral states in the fetus.

Because the eye is derived embryologically from neural folds of the forebrain, it is reasonable to speculate that abnormalities of ocular size and morphology may aid in the prenatal diagnosis of cerebral malformations for which there are no genetic or enzymatic markers currently available. The eyelids and anterior portions of the eye in the fetus may be visualized consistently after 14 to 16 weeks gestational age (3). The horizontal (skull base) view provides simultaneous assessment of both eyes and permits measurement of orbital spacing. The optic nerve may be recognized on sagittal views as a central hypoechoic band within the orbital fat, which is slightly more reflective than the extraocular muscles. It is highlighted further by the pulsations of the adjacent retinal artery.

Serial studies indicate that the ocular diameter, as measured by vitreous diameter, increases progressively but not linearly during the second and third trimesters. Rapid ocular growth occurs between 16 and 20 weeks, from 28 to 32 weeks, and after 37 weeks, with relative slowing of growth from 20 to 24 weeks and 32 to 36 weeks (3). Preliminary studies suggest that eye and brain growth may be linked temporally in the fetus. Thus, assessment of the fetal eye may have potential clinical application as an indicator of cerebral growth. In this context, microphthalmia (transverse vitreous diameter <15 mm) has been associated with microcephaly, holoprosencephaly, and the fetal alcohol syndrome (3). However, it must be remembered that microphthalmia may occur as an isolated phenomenon in a significant proportion of infants who are otherwise normal neurologically. Thus, other evidence should be sought to corroborate defective cerebral growth in fetuses with diminished ocular growth, especially if termination of the pregnancy is a consideration.

Fetal eye movements have been confirmed in experimental animal studies by electrical recordings from fetal lambs (5). Investigation of eye movements in a term newborn confirmed that the movements that may be seen in the orbital region with real-time ultrasonography correspond closely to direct observation of eye movements (4).

The principal challenge in the investigation of ocular dynamics in the fetus lies in the correlation of eye movements with other parameters of fetal behavioral states. Further understanding of fetal eye movements may lead to their incorporation into composite assessments of fetal well-being, such as the "fetal biophysical profile."

The vestibular nuclei, which are considered necessary for ocular movements, are differentiated by 13 weeks of gestation in the human fetus. Slow eye movements with a single, transient linear deviation from the mid-position have been identified by 16 weeks gestation. Subsequently, between 24 and 30 weeks, rapid eye movements, involving complex sequences of deviations, including rotatory components and without apparent temporal periodicity, increase in frequency and duration. Increasing duration of eye inactivity late in the third trimester, after 36 weeks gestation, suggests the development of inhibitory mechanisms. The association of eye inactivity with sustained diaphragmatic excursions suggests that this combination may correspond to a "quiet sleep" state. This organization of behavioral states in the fetus corresponds to that observed in premature infants of comparable postconceptional age (1,6). However, it should be recognized that experience with ocular dynamics is limited and preliminary studies have revealed considerable variation in the association between eye movements and other indicators of behavioral state in the human fetus. Furthermore, fetal eye movements may not be visualized by ultrasound studies of the fetus in the prone position or may be obscured by turning of the fetal head. Further research is required before diagnostic inferences may be drawn from the apparent dissociative behavior between fetal eye movements and other parameters of behavioral state (1).

In addition to ocular dynamics, the measurement of pupillary size in the fetus may have potential value for the assessment of fetal well-being. Thus, relative miosis has been demonstrated in the third trimester, despite reduced ambient light in the intrauterine environment, and presumably results from lack of functional sympathetic control of the pupillary dilators, with consequent parasympathetic predominance. It is possible that elevated catecholamine levels in severely hypoxemic fetuses may reverse this effect to produce pupillary dilation (3).

Preliminary studies suggest a potential role for ocular dynamics in the assessment of fetal hearing. Thus, blink-startle responses to vibroacoustic stimulation may be visualized by ultrasound between 24 and 25 weeks of gestation and are consistently present after 28 weeks. Absence of a blink response under strict test conditions may indicate a serious, primary hearing impairment or significant depression of the central nervous system (2).

In summary, recent studies demonstrate that human fetal eye movements may be detected *in utero* by means of the dynamic imaging capabilities of real-time ultrasonography. Although the quantitative aspects of these observations have not been clearly defined, the objective and noninvasive recording of fetal ocular structure and dynamics adds a further variable to the techniques available for the assessment of fetal activity and well-being.

REFERENCES

1. Birnholz, J.C. (1981): The development of human fetal eye movement patterns. *Science,* 213:679–681.
2. Birnholz, J.C. (1983): The development of human fetal hearing. *Science,* 218:516–518.
3. Birnholz, J.C. (1985): Ultrasonic fetal ophthalmology. *Early Hum. Dev.,* 12:199–209.
4. Bots, R.S., Nijhuis, J.C., Martin, C.B., and Prechtl, H.F.R. (1981): Human fetal eye movements: Detection *in utero* by ultrasonography. *Early Hum. Dev.,* 5:87–94.
5. Dawes, G.S., Fox, H.E., Leduc, B.M., Liggins, G.C., and Richards, R.T. (1972): Respiratory movements and rapid eye movement sleep in the fetal lamb. *J. Physiol. (Lond.),* 220:119–143.
6. Prechtl, H.F.R., and Nijhuis, J.C. (1983): Eye movements in the human fetus and newborn. *Behav. Brain Res.,* 10:119–124.

Fetal Neurology, edited by
A. Hill and J.J. Volpe.
Raven Press, New York © 1989.

4

Antepartum Fetal Assessment: The Nonstress Test

Carl V. Smith and Jeffrey P. Phelan

Department of Obstetrics and Gynecology, University of Southern California School of Medicine, Women's Hospital, Los Angeles, California 90033

The application of the nonstress test (NST) to a high-risk obstetric population has resulted in a decrease of the fetal mortality rate to values between 2 and 3 per 1,000 live births (7,37). A discussion of this technique is relevant in a text on fetal neurology because a clear relationship exists between central nervous system function and alterations of the fetal heart rate (FHR) (32,34). This chapter traces the history of nonstress testing, reviews methods of interpretation, and describes outcome following normal and abnormal tests.

HISTORICAL PERSPECTIVES

In 1968, Hon and Quilligan (25) demonstrated the relationship between specific FHR patterns and fetal conditions. Thus, a normal FHR pattern essentially precluded an abnormal outcome. In contrast, repetitive late decelerations were associated with a significantly greater likelihood of fetal compromise. These relationships formed the basis of FHR monitoring. This new technology was applied initially only to the fetus during labor. However, investigators (43) rapidly became interested in its applications for the assessment of the antepartum fetal condition with stimulation of uterine contractions by the administration of oxytocin to the mother during pregnancy before labor. This application is the basis of the oxytocin challenge test (OCT) or contraction stress test (CST) (19), which will be discussed in the following chapter.

Other studies (29,55) reported that FHR accelerations, associated with fetal movements, were associated with a low incidence of fetal compromise. This technique was first described by Lee and colleagues, who termed the test the Fetal Activity Acceleration Determination (FAD). The FAD, which was later renamed the NST, became the primary method of fetal surveillance in many institutions.

CONTROL OF THE FETAL HEART RATE

In order to understand the clinical applications of the NST, the basic principles regarding the autonomic control of the FHR must first be discussed. As mentioned above, the basic principle underlying the NST is the relationship between the fetal central nervous system and FHR control.

Sympathetic cardioacceleratory fibers, which are under hypothalamic control, arise in the upper segments of the thoracic spinal cord. In early pregnancy, this sympathetic system is dominant, and this dominance is reflected in a slightly higher baseline heart rate. As pregnancy progresses, the parasympathetic nervous system, mediated through the vagus nerve, assumes a more important role. Consequently, many investigators (12,26,27) have documented progressive slowing of the heart rate throughout pregnancy. The interaction between the sympathetic and parasympathetic systems results in the phenomena described as long-term and short-term heart rate variability (11).

The FHR is also influenced by chemoreceptors and baroreceptors. Changes in fetal blood pressure are detected by baroreceptors located within the aortic arch and are mediated by the vagus nerve (11,26,45). Additionally, via chemoreceptors, acute arterial hypoxemia may result in increased FHR variability and/or bradycardia or late decelerations (11,26,32). Alternatively, chronic hypoxia may result in diminished FHR variability.

Thus, there is indirect evidence for a relationship between the central nervous system and FHR, i.e., a reactive NST indicates fetal well-being, as well as an intact and functional central nervous system.

SELECTION OF PATIENTS FOR NONSTRESS TESTING

All pregnancies that are at increased risk for fetal death are candidates for assessment of fetal well-being with the NST. Table 1 outlines the most common indications for nonstress testing.

The role of the NST in the low-risk population is less well defined. Schifrin and co-workers (48) studied 1,413 low-risk and 590 high-risk patients undergoing NSTs and reported no difference in the incidence of reactive tests, which were 88.3% and 86.4%, respectively. The incidence of perinatal mortality of 3 per 1,000 in the low-risk group was significantly lower than the incidence observed in the high-risk group. No difference in perinatal mortality was reported between low- and high-risk patients with nonreactive stress tests. Thus, the low-risk fetus with a nonreactive NST is as likely to die as his or her high-risk counterpart. Further data were provided by Vinacur (56), who reported the NST to be a helpful adjunct for risk assessment in 208 low-risk patients.

In summary, there is consensus concerning the benefit of antepartum fetal surveillance in high-risk pregnancies. Because of the relatively low incidence of fetal death in the low-risk population, a study population of 5,000 low-risk patients would be required to assess the effectiveness of the NST for the reduction of peri-

TABLE 1. *Current indications for fetal assessment*

Diabetics: 34 weeks, twice weekly
  Type A: 40 weeks, twice weekly
  Type A: with previous stillborn
  Type A: with additional medical problems
  Type B-R
Medical problems: 34 weeks, weekly
  Cardiac disease
  Chronic hypertension
  Preeclampsia
  Collagen-vascular disease
  Renal disease
  Thyroid disease
  Sickle cell disease
  Placenta previa-hemorrhage
Intrauterine growth retardation: at the time of diagnosis by ultrasound
Fetal arrhythmia
Decreased fetal movement
Meconium detected by amniocentesis
Previous stillborn: testing started 1 week before gestation of previous loss,
  but not earlier than 26 weeks
Rh disease: 28 weeks
Post Dates: 41 weeks, twice weekly
Spontaneous premature rupture of membranes: daily assessment

natal mortality in this group. The magnitude of perinatal resources required to address this question is enormous and, in all probability, precludes such a study. However, because the incidence of fetal death following a reactive NST is as low as 2 to 3 per 1,000, it is not inconceivable that the routine application of this test in the low-risk patient may significantly reduce perinatal mortality.

TECHNIQUES OF TESTING

The following discussion outlines the techniques and methods of interpretation of the NST at the authors' institution. Although it is recognized that institutional differences exist in testing format, the outlined approach, with some modification, has resulted in a fetal death rate of 2.6 per 1,000 over the past 8 years (51). The NST may be performed by a clinical nurse specialist with the patient in the semi-Fowler's position. Blood pressures are recorded at 10-min intervals. A test is considered reactive if there are two accelerations of at least 15 beats/min and of 15 sec in duration, within a 10-min observation period. No minimum observation period is used, but if criteria for reactivity are not met within 40 min, the test is considered nonreactive. Depending on the clinical situation, additional testing is performed, i.e., a repeat NST, a CST, or a biophysical profile (31). In general, normal tests are repeated weekly. Testing is performed twice weekly in pregnancies with increased risk, e.g., postdates and diabetes. Patients with premature rupture of the membranes are generally considered to require more frequent assessments. In this situation we advocate daily testing and assessment of amniotic fluid volume (AFV). This recommendation is based on studies by Smith et al. (50), who demonstrated rapid (within 24 hr) deterioration in a significant proportion of patients with premature rupture of membranes.

Amniotic Fluid Volume

Although the importance of AFV will be discussed primarily in the context of the fetal biophysical profile, the assessment of AFV is critical and represents such an important part of antepartum fetal surveillance that it merits additional discussion here. It has been demonstrated clearly that an inverse relationship exists between AFV and indices of perinatal morbidity and mortality. Phelan et al. (40) reported on AFV assessment of 236 postdate fetuses. AFV was classified as either adequate, adequate but decreased, or decreased (≤ 1.0 cm). There was a higher incidence of fetal distress, meconium-stained amniotic fluid, and depressed 5-min Apgar scores in the latter two groups. In addition, intrapartum decelerations and bradycardia were observed more frequently when AFV was decreased. It was concluded that even though the NST is reactive, delivery of the postmature fetus with decreased AFV should be considered.

Additional studies by Chamberlain et al. (9), utilizing AFV assessment, performed as a part of the biophysical profile, also demonstrated a higher incidence of fetal complication. Thus, there was an increased incidence of fetal mortality, intrauterine growth retardation, and congenital malformations in patients with decreased or marginal AFV. The overall incidence of abnormal AFV in this series was 3%.

A more promising, semiquantitative approach for assessment of AFV has been described by Phelan and colleagues (41), utilizing the four-quadrant amniotic fluid index (AFI) technique. This approach consists of measurement of the largest vertical diameter of a pocket of amniotic fluid in each of four quadrants of the uterus. The sum of these four numbers represents the AFI. Initially, observations were confined to pregnancies between 36 and 42 weeks gestation, in which a bell-shaped distribution was observed. A prospective comparison with the NST (46) subsequently confirmed that, irrespective of NST result, an AFI ≤ 5.0 cm was associated with an increased likelihood of complications.

In view of these observations, it appears reasonable to include AFV assessment as an integral part of antepartum fetal surveillance. The precise critical value and the optimal method of assessment of AFV remain controversial. Regardless of the method utilized, a trend of decreasing AFV should be viewed with concern. In this situation, management may include more frequent testing or delivery.

THE SIGNIFICANCE OF VARIABLE DECELERATIONS

The predictive reliability of the NST may be improved further by examination of the FHR record for other abnormalities, e.g., variable decelerations (7), which are associated with an increased likelihood of umbilical cord compression. Data are available to support the significance of variable decelerations in certain populations. Phelan and Lewis (38), reporting on 2,000 NSTs on 972 patients, observed variable decelerations in 5.5% of cases. Fetuses with variable decelerations had an increased incidence of postmaturity or growth retardation. In addition, abnormal cord position (55.3%), intrapartum persistence of variable decelerations (59.5%), cesarean delivery for fetal distress (8.5%), and intrauterine fetal death (three instances) were observed more frequently in this context. These authors concluded that the presence of variable decelerations on a NST should lead to a search for diminished AFV or abnormal cord position. Additional evaluation with a CST may also be of benefit.

A later report (39), *limited to postdate pregnancies,* observed a 20% incidence of variable decelerations. This pattern was associated with a higher incidence of cesarean delivery for fetal distress, meconium staining, and fetal death.

In addition to the association with diminished AFV, variable decelerations occur commonly in association with fetal anemia. Visser (57) correlated fetal anemia (hemoglobin <13 g/dl) with FHR patterns. The incidence of anemia was 13% in fetuses with a normal FHR pattern. Of 11 fetuses with decelerations and/or sinusoidal patterns, all were anemic.

An alternative viewpoint is presented by Meiss et al. (33), who concluded that variable decelerations were not indicative of fetal compromise. However, at least 45.8% of what was classified as variable decelerations in that study would be considered clinically insignificant by the present authors (i.e., <15 bpm in depth or lasting <15 sec). Another intriguing observation is the overall higher incidence of variable decelerations, which were reported in >50% of cases. This is in marked contrast to the previously cited work by Phelan et al. (39), who observed an incidence of 20% in postdate pregnancies, which characteristically have a high incidence of variable decelerations. Reanalysis of the data of Meiss et al. (33) with consideration of only "significant" decelerations may increase the incidence of adverse outcome to the same level reported in other studies.

Prolonged deceleration, which is perhaps more aptly termed *bradycardia,* is encountered infrequently during antepartum FHR testing. Druzin et al. (14) and Dashow and Read (10) reported incidences of 1.6% and 1.5%, respectively. These authors, as well as Phelan et al. (39), reported significant morbidity and mortality in these patients and recommended that they be considered for delivery.

More complex methods for interpretation of the NST have been proposed. Thus, Brioschi et al. (7) described tests as either reactive or nonreactive and pathologic or nonpathologic based on baseline abnormality of the FHR, alterations of variability, and the presence of variable deceleration or bradycardia. Patients with pathologic NSTs had a higher incidence of operative delivery for fetal distress, depressed 5-min Apgar scores, and fetal/neonatal acidosis. In addition to the greater morbidity, such fetuses experienced a 10-fold increase in perinatal mortality.

Whether a complex system of scoring is utilized is of little concern as long as "pathologic" features are considered in the management of high risk gravidas.

TABLE 2. *Indications for delivery*

Patient who is postdate with FHR decelerations on NST
NST demonstrating bradycardia
Biophysical profile score ≤ 4
Amniotic fluid index ≤ 5

Thus, the fetal condition should be assessed in greater detail when variable decelerations or alteration of baseline FHR occurs. With additional risk factors, e.g., postdates or intrauterine growth retardation, assessment of AFV and/or evaluation for delivery should be considered.

Table 2 outlines the current indications for delivery of a fetus with evidence of abnormal antepartum fetal surveillance.

PERINATAL MORBIDITY AND MORTALITY FOLLOWING *NORMAL* ANTEPARTUM FETAL HEART RATE TESTING

Historically, the goal of antepartum surveillance has been the prevention of intrauterine fetal death. Without question, the NST is effective in the reduction of fetal death to a reasonable minimum. Table 3 outlines the uncorrected and corrected mortality rates recently reported in several studies. Thus, on the basis of reduced fetal mortality, the NST has become an integral part of high risk prenatal care. However, mortality is only one measure of neonatal outcome, and attention must be directed also to *morbidity* following nonstress testing.

The indices of morbidity following antepartum fetal heart rate testing (AFHRT) reported most commonly include cesarean delivery rate, meconium staining, and Apgar scores. Table 4 lists perinatal morbidity following a normal (reactive) NST as reported in recent studies. It is evident that outcome is variable. In addition,

TABLE 3. *Fetal death rates following*
a reactive nonstress test

Author	Death rates/1,000	
	Uncorrected	Corrected
Phelan et al. (37)	2.6	0.6
Druzin et al. (15)	8.0	5.0
Freeman et al. (21)	7.8	—
Evertson and Paul (18)	N/A	1.6
Barrs et al. (2)	N/A	1.9
Boehm et al. (6)	N/A	1.9
Solum and Sjoberg (54)	N/A	0

TABLE 4. *Indices of perinatal morbidity following a reactive nonstress test*

	Phelan (36) (N = 1,000) (%)	Brioschi et al. (7) (N = 1,411) (%)	Freeman et al. (20) (N = 2,154) (%)	Rutherford et al. (46) (N = 250) (%)
Fetal distress	2.9	10.2	19.9	2.4
Meconium	16.0	N/A	N/A	35.6
Apgar score <7 at 5 min	N/A	3.2	3.4	2.4

not all authors provide identical information. The studies of Brioschi et al. (7) and of Rutherford et al. (46) require additional comment. These authors subdivided their data further: Brioschi, by interpreting the tests as pathologic or nonpathologic, and Rutherford, according to AFI. Brioschi reported a significant difference between pathologic and nonpathologic tests, despite the presence of a reactive NST. Similarly, Rutherford demonstrated that patients with an AFI ≤5.0 were more likely to have meconium staining and depressed 5-min Apgar scores, irrespective of NST result.

In summary, as discussed earlier, the predictive ability of the NST may be enhanced by the addition of AFV assessment and by analysis of other FHR abnormalities.

PERINATAL MORBIDITY AND MORTALITY FOLLOWING *ABNORMAL* AFHRT

There is considerable evidence to support the reliability of the NST for the prediction of fetal well-being. Thus, the reported incidence of falsely reactive NST is <5 per 1,000. The ability of an abnormal NST to predict fetal compromise is less well defined. Analysis of such data is more difficult because most studies recommend additional assessment of fetal condition in the event of a nonreactive NST. Thus, intervention based on additional investigation may improve outcome.

Table 5 summarizes the outcome data following a nonreactive NST from three recent series. In 235 patients with a nonreactive NST reported by Phelan, there was a high perinatal mortality rate as well as a significantly increased incidence of fetal distress and meconium staining. In general, the majority of patients were investigated with CST following their nonreactive NST. Similarly, Druzin and colleagues (15) reported a higher perinatal death rate in fetuses with a nonreactive NST and a subsequent negative CST. The corrected mortality rates were 5 per 1,000 and 17 per 1,000, respectively. Thus, it appears that the predictive reliability of the nonreactive NST followed by a negative CST is not identical to the purely reactive NST group. Consequently, we have adopted a policy of repeating the NST within 24 hr in patients with a nonreactive NST.

TABLE 5. *Perinatal morbidity and mortality with nonreactive nonstress test*

	Phelan (36) (N = 235) (%)	Brioschi et al. (7) (N = 141) (%)	Freeman et al. (20) (N = 245) (%)
Fetal distress	8.5	21.7	26.3
Meconium	24.3	N/A	N/A
Apgar score <7 at 5 min	N/A	21.8	13.0
Death rate/1,000	29.4	29.0	17.0

Although fetuses with a nonreactive NST appear to be at increased risk, the vast majority are normal on reevaluation. In a retrospective analysis of our population of 452 initially nonreactive tests, only 43 remained nonreactive on repeat testing on the same day (52). The incidence of a positive CST after a nonreactive NST is approximately 6.5% (36). Thus, in order to improve the ability of AFHRT to identify the compromised fetus, the incidence of persistently nonreactive tests must be reduced.

In summary, most investigators recommend additional testing when confronted with a persistently nonreactive test because it appears that the fetus may be at increased risk if left *in utero*. Management options include additional surveillance by repeat NST, biophysical profile testing, and/or CST. A final consideration is that of delivery. This becomes particularly relevant in view of the study of Brown and Patrick (8), who reported three perinatal deaths and a mean umbilical arterial pH of 6.95 in seven fetuses with nonreactive NST for >120 min.

THE PROBLEM OF THE FETUS WITH CONGENITAL ANOMALIES

Congenital malformations must be considered in the differential diagnosis of an abnormal FHR tracing. Phillips and Towell (42) reviewed the course of 3,140 patients undergoing AFHRT, 37 of whom were subsequently delivered of anomalous infants. More than 50% of these patients had abnormal FHR tracings and 48% were delivered by cesarean section because of fetal distress. Conversely, Lavery (26), in a review article, reported malformations in 23% of fetuses dying after normal antenatal fetal surveillance.

Biale and colleagues (3) performed a retrospective evaluation of FHR patterns of fetuses with "clinically" significant malformations and reported pathologic tracings in 55%. The malformations associated with the highest incidence of FHR abnormalities were those involving the central nervous system, multiple organ systems, and those associated with chromosomal abnormalities. The cesarean delivery rate (18%) and the neonatal mortality rate (38%) in these fetuses were substantially higher than in a control group.

Garite et al. (22) also reported an increased incidence of monitoring abnormalities in fetuses with malformations. The predominant FHR patterns observed in that series were decreased variability and late decelerations. Thus, an abnormal NST should increase clinical suspicion of a fetal anomaly. This relationship is further strengthened in clinical circumstances known to be associated with an increased rate of malformations, e.g., abnormal presentation, hydramnios, oligohydramnios, and intrauterine growth retardation. Real-time ultrasound evaluation is indicated in these situations.

FETAL ACOUSTIC STIMULATION TESTING

As discussed in preceding sections, the nonreactive NST not infrequently is associated with normal fetal condition on further evaluation. In an effort to improve the efficiency of AFHRT, techniques based on light, mechanical, and acoustic stimulation (16,17,35,44) have been developed. None have produced a consistent fetal response. However, we have recently reported promising experience with the application of a transabdominal vibroacoustic stimulus with an electronic artificial larynx (EAL), Model 5C (AT&T, New York, NY) (Fig. 1) (52).

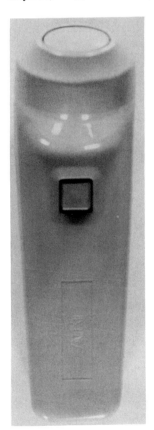

FIG. 1. An electronic artificial larynx, model 5C by AT&T, New York, New York, is pictured.

The EAL emits a fundamental frequency of 80 Hz and a sound pressure level averaging 82 dB at 1 m in air. In brief, the clinical protocol consisted of monitoring the baseline FHR for a duration of 5 min and, if the FHR remained nonreactive, a vibroacoustic stimulus was applied for ≤3 sec. If no response was observed, the stimulus was repeated on a maximum of two occasions. In a retrospective analysis, this technique reduced the incidence of nonreactive tests by approximately 50%, as compared to historical controls. Fetal death rates were comparable.

A prospective randomized clinical comparison with the more traditional NST was subsequently carried out (53). The fetal acoustic stimulation test or FAS-TEST reduced the number of nonreactive tests from 14% to 9% without changing the predictive reliability. An additional advantage of the technique was a statistically significant reduction of mean test duration.

Since the completion of this study, we have continued to use the FAS-TEST in our antenatal surveillance unit. Our experience to date includes more than 7,500 tests performed in approximately 3,500 patients with an overall fetal mortality rate of 1.9 per 1,000 within 7 days of a reactive NST (C.V. Smith, *unpublished data*). In addition, when analyzed in relation to historical controls, this rate compares favorably to those for fetuses with spontaneously reactive NSTs. Thus, because the predictive reliability of the test appears comparable to that of the NST, the FAS-TEST offers significant advantages over the more traditional NST.

One of the potential advantages of acoustic stimulation is the evaluation of the integrity of the fetal central nervous system. This dynamic method may be particularly useful in this regard in view of the consistency of certain fetal responses, e.g., movement or FHR, in response to stimulus from the EAL (Fig. 2). Divon et al. (13) reported their experience with the EAL for eliciting fetal movement. They described a startle reflex that occurred consistently despite a total of 100 successive stimuli. Other investigators, notably Birnholz and Benacerraf (4) and Gelman et al. (23), have demonstrated fetal movement in response to acoustic stimulation. Birnholz and Benacerraf (4) utilized the EAL to elicit a blink startle reflex after 28 weeks of gestation.

Although fetal movement and FHR have been extensively used for the assessment of fetal well-being, investigators have sought more sophisticated and perhaps more reproducible measurements. One such method, the auditory brainstem response (ABR), has been used in the newborn period (1,24,47). This technique is of particular interest because the auditory system appears to be exquisitely sensitive to hypoxia (24,47). Scibetta and colleagues (49) attempted to measure auditory evoked responses in the human fetus during labor but experienced difficulties with placement of electrodes and in the interpretation of many variables. Thus, transabdominal measurement of fetal brainstem electrical activity has been particularly difficult because the measured voltage is submicrovolt in amplitude.

A potential method for assessment of fetal cerebral activity before labor and rupture of membranes involves the measurement of changes in a magnetized field (5).

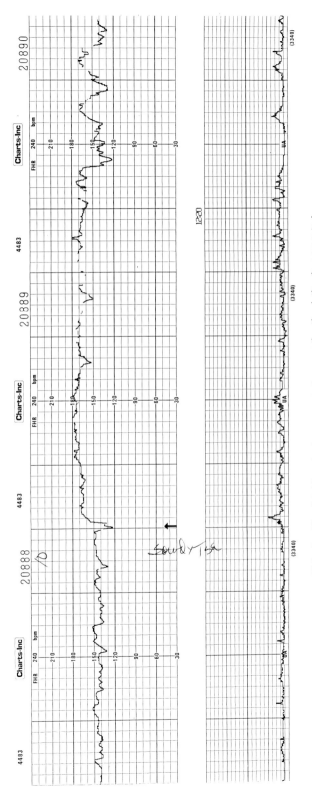

FIG. 2. The fetal heart rate response to acoustic stimulation is presented.

Furthermore, less direct methods of assessment have been proposed that involve habituation of the fetus to acoustic stimuli. Leader and co-workers (28) used a vibroacoustic stimulus (an electric toothbrush) and observed the presence or absence of response decrement (habituation) in six groups of fetuses. Habituation is considered a phenomenon mediated at the cerebral level in the newborn. Five patients with major central nervous system anomalies (four with anenecephaly, one with microcephaly) demonstrated no response. Four of five additional fetuses who showed no response decrement had normal Apgar scores. Unfortunately, additional testing was not performed during the neonatal period. In a subsequent investigation, Madison and colleagues (30) confirmed the above findings and suggested that this technique may be of value in assessing function of the fetal central nervous system.

SUMMARY

The NST is an important and reliable method for assessment of fetal well-being. Thus, the test has the capacity to predict accurately the absence of fetal death within 1 week following a reactive test. Perinatal complications are predicted less accurately. Thus, the NST or FHR monitoring alone is unreliable in the prediction of cerebral injury in the newborn infant. However, adjunctive use of ultrasound and critical evaluation of the entire FHR record as well as more dynamic assessment techniques, such as acoustic stimulation, may improve the predictive reliability of the NST.

REFERENCES

1. Artal, R., Rosen, M.G., and Sokol, R.J. (1975): Fetal response to sound. *Contemp. OB/GYN,* 5:13.
2. Barrs, V.A., Frigoletto, F.D., and Diamond, F. (1985): Stillbirth after nonstress testing. *Obstet. Gynecol.,* 65:541–544.
3. Biale, Y., Brawer-Ostrovsky, J., and Insler, V. (1985): Fetal heart rate tracings in fetuses with congenital anomalies. *J. Reprod. Med.,* 30:43–47.
4. Birnholz, J.C., and Benacerraf, B.R. (1983): The development of human fetal hearing. *Science,* 222:516–518.
5. Blum, T., Saling, E., and Bauer, R. (1985): First magnetoencephalographic recordings of the brain activity of a human fetus. *Br. J. Obstet. Gynaecol.,* 92:1224–1229.
6. Boehm, F.H., Salyer, S., Shah, D.M., et al. (1986): Improved outcome of twice weekly nonstress testing. *Obstet. Gynecol.,* 67:566–568.
7. Brioschi, P-A., Extermann, P., Terracina, D., et al. (1985): Antepartum nonstress fetal heart rate monitoring: Systematic analysis of baseline patterns and decelerations as an adjunct to reactivity in the prediction of fetal risks. *Am. J. Obstet. Gynecol.,* 153:633–637.
8. Brown, R., and Patrick, J. (1981): The nonstress test: How long is enough? *Am. J. Obstet. Gynecol.,* 141:646–651.
9. Chamberlain, P.F., Manning, F.A., Morrison, I., et al. (1984): Ultrasound evaluation of amniotic fluid volume. I. The relationship of marginal and decreased amniotic fluid volumes to perinatal outcome. *Am. J. Obstet. Gynecol.,* 150:245–249.
10. Dashow, E.E., and Read, J.A. (1984): Significant fetal bradycardia during antepartum fetal heart rate testing. *Am. J. Obstet. Gynecol.,* 148:187–190.
11. Dettaan, J., Stolte, L., Veith, A.F., et al. (1972): Die Bendentung der schnellen Osgillationen

im Kardocotachogromm des Fenen. In: *Perinatal Medizin Bnd, ill,* edited by E. Saling and J.W. Dudenhausen. p. 398, Thieme, Stuttgart.

12. DeVoe, L. (1982): Antepartum fetal heart rate testing in the preterm pregnancy. *Obstet. Gynecol.,* 60:431–436.
13. Divon, M.Y., Platt, L.D., Cantrell, C.E., et al. (1985): Evoked fetal startle response: A possible intrauterine neurologic examination. *Am. J. Obstet. Gynecol.,* 153:454–456.
14. Druzin, M.L., Gratocos, J., Keegan, K.A., et al. (1981): Antepartum fetal heart rate testing. VII. The significance of fetal bradycardia. *Am. J. Obstet. Gynecol.,* 139:194–198.
15. Druzin, M.L., Gratocos, J., and Paul, R.H. (1980): Antepartum fetal heart rate testing. VI. Predictive reliability of "normal" tests in the prevention of antepartum death. *Am. J. Obstet. Gynecol.,* 137:746–747.
16. Druzin, M.L., Gratocos, J., Paul, R.H., et al. (1985): Antepartum fetal heart rate testing. XII. The effect of manual manipulation of the fetus on the nonstress test. *Am. J. Obstet. Gynecol.,* 151:61–64.
17. Eglinton, G.S., Paul, R.H., Broussard, P.M., et al. (1984): Antepartum fetal heart rate testing. XI. Stimulation with orange juice. *Am. J. Obstet. Gynecol.,* 150:97–99.
18. Evertson, L.R., Paul, R.H. (1978): Antepartum fetal heart rate testing. The nonstress test. *Am. J. Obstet. Gynecol.,* 132:895–900.
19. Freeman, R.K. (1982): Contraction stress testing for primary fetal surveillance in patients at risk for utero placental insufficiency. *Clin. Perinatol.,* 9:265–270.
20. Freeman, R.K., Anderson, G., and Dorchester, W. (1982): A prospective multi-institutional study of antepartum fetal heart rate monitoring. I. Risk of perinatal mortality and morbidity according to antepartum fetal heart rate test results. *Am. J. Obstet. Gynecol.,* 143:771–777.
21. Freeman, R.K., Anderson, G., and Dorchester, W. (1982): A prospective multi-institutional study of antepartum fetal heart rate monitoring. II. Contraction stress test versus nonstress test for primary surveillance. *Am. J. Obstet. Gynecol.,* 143:778–781.
22. Garite, T.J., Linzey, F.M., Freeman, R.K., et al. (1979): Fetal heart rate patterns and fetal distress in fetuses with congenital anomalies. *Obstet. Gynecol.,* 53:716–720.
23. Gelman, S.R., Wood, S., Spellacy, W.N., et al. (1982): Fetal movements in response to sound stimulation. *Am. J. Obstet. Gynecol.,* 143:484–485.
24. Goldstein, P.J., Krumholz, P.J., Felix, J.K., et al. (1979): Brainstem-evoked response in neonates. *Am. J. Obstet. Gynecol.,* 135:622–628.
25. Hon, E.H., and Quilligan, E.J. (1968): Electronic evaluation of the fetal heart rate. *Clin. Obstet. Gynecol.,* 11:145–167.
26. Lavery, J.P. (1982): Nonstress fetal heart rate testing. *Clin. Obstet. Gynecol.,* 25:689–705.
27. Lavin, J.P., Miodovnick, M., and Barden, T.P. (1984): Relationship of nonstress test reactivity and gestational age. *Obstet. Gynecol.,* 63:338–344.
28. Leader, L.R., Baillie, P., Martin, B., et al. (1982): Fetal habituation in high-risk pregnancies. *Br. J. Obstet. Gynaecol.,* 89:441–446.
29. Lee, C.Y., DiLoreto, P.C., and O'Lane, J.M. (1975): A study of fetal heart rate acceleration patterns. *Obstet. Gynecol.,* 45:142–146.
30. Madison, L.S., Adubato, S.A., Madison, J.K., et al. (1986): Fetal response decrement: True habituation. *J. Dev. Behav. Pediatr.,* 7:14–20.
31. Manning, F.A., Platt, L.D., and Sipos, L. (1980): Antepartum fetal evaluation: Development of a fetal biophysical profile. *Am. J. Obstet. Gynecol.,* 136:787–795.
32. Martin, C.B., Jr. (1978): Regulation of the fetal heart rate and genesis of FHR patterns. *Semin. Perinatol.,* 2:131–146.
33. Meiss, P.J., Ureda, J.R., Swain, M., et al. (1986): Variable decelerations during nonstress tests are not a sign of fetal compromise. *Am. J. Obstet. Gynecol.,* 154:586–590.
34. Patrick, J., Fetherston, W., Vick, H., et al. (1978): Normal fetal breathing movements and gross body movements at 34–35 weeks of gestation. *Am. J. Obstet. Gynecol.,* 130:693–699.
35. Peleg, D., and Goldman, J.A. (1980): Fetal heart rate acceleration in response to light stimulation as a clinical measure of fetal well-being. A preliminary report. *J. Perinat. Med.,* 8:38–41.
36. Phelan, J.P. (1981): The nonstress test: A review of 3,000 tests. *Am. J. Obstet. Gynecol.,* 139:7–10.
37. Phelan, J.P., Cromartie, A.P., and Smith, C.V. (1982): The nonstress test: The false negative test. *Am. J. Obstet. Gynecol.,* 142:293–296.
38. Phelan, J.P., and Lewis, P.E. (1981): Fetal heart rate decelerations during a nonstress test. *Obstet. Gynecol.,* 57:228–232.

39. Phelan, J.P., Platt, L.D., Yeh, S-Y., et al. (1984): The continuing role of the nonstress test in the management of the postdates pregnancy. *Obstet. Gynecol.,* 64:624–628.

40. Phelan, J.P., Platt, L.D., Yeh, S-Z., et al. (1985): The role of ultrasound assessment of amniotic fluid volume in the management of the post dates pregnancy. *Am. J. Obstet. Gynecol.,* 151:304–308.

41. Phelan, J.P., Smith, C.V., Broussard, P.M., et al. (1987): Amniotic fluid volume assessment using the four-quadrant technique in the pregnancy between 36 and 42 weeks gestation. *J. Reprod. Med.,* 32:540.

42. Phillips, W.D.P., and Towell, M.E. (1980): Abnormal fetal heart rate associated with congenital anomalies. *Br. J. Obstet. Gynaecol.,* 87:270–274.

43. Ray, M., Freeman, R.K., Pine, S., et al. (1972): Clinical experience with the oxytocin challenge test. *Am. J. Obstet. Gynecol.,* 114:1–9.

44. Read, J.A., and Miller, F.C. (1977): Fetal heart rate acceleration in response to acoustic stimulation as a measure of fetal well-being. *Am. J. Obstet. Gynecol.,* 129:512–517.

45. Rudolph, A.M., and Heymann, M.A. (1976): Cardiac output in the fetal lamb. Effects of spontaneous and induced changes of heart rate on right and left ventricular output. *Am. J. Obstet. Gynecol.,* 124:183–192.

46. Rutherford, S.E., Phelan, J.P., Smith, C.V., et al. (1987): The four-quadrant assessment of amniotic fluid "volume"; An adjunct to antepartum fetal heart rate testing. *Obstet. Gynecol.,* 70:353–356.

47. Salamy, A., Mendelson, T., Tooley, W.H., and Chaplin, E.R. (1980): Differential development of brain-stem potentials in healthy and high risk infants. *Science,* 210:553–555.

48. Schifrin, B.S., Foye, G., Amato, J., et al. (1979): Routine fetal heart monitoring in the antepartum period. *Obstet. Gynecol.,* 54:21–25.

49. Scibetta, J.J., Rosen, M.G., Hochberg, C.J., et al. (1971): Human fetal brain response to sound during labor. *Am. J. Obstet. Gynecol.,* 109:82–85.

50. Smith, C.V., Greenspoon, J., Phelan, J.P., et al. (1987): The clinical utility of the nonstress test in the conservative management of patients with preterm rupture of the membranes. *J. Reprod. Med.,* 32:1.

51. Smith, C.V., Nguyen, H.N., Kovacs, B., McCart, D., Phelan, J.P., and Paul, R.H. (1987): Fetal death following antepartum fetal heart rate testing: A review of 65 cases. *Obstet. Gynecol.,* 70:18.

52. Smith, C.V., Phelan, J.P., Paul, R.H., et al. (1985): Fetal acoustic stimulation testing: A retrospective experience with the fetal acoustic stimulation test. *Am. J. Obstet. Gynecol.,* 153:567–569.

53. Smith, C.V., Phelan, J.P., Platt, L.D., et al. (1986): Fetal acoustic stimulation testing (The "FAS-TEST"). II. A randomized clinical comparison with the nonstress test. *Am. J. Obstet. Gynecol.,* 155:131.

54. Solum, T., and Sjoberg, N-O. (1980): Antenatal cardiotography and intrauterine death. *Acta Obstet. Gynecol. Scand.,* 59:481–487.

55. Trierweiler, M.U., Freeman, R.K., and James, J. (1976): Baseline fetal heart rate characteristics as an indicator of fetal status during the antepartum period. *Am. J. Obstet. Gynecol.,* 125:618–623.

56. Vinacur, J.C. (1980): Routine nonstress test (NST) improves the accuracy of perinatal risk scoring. In: *Proceedings of the Society for Gynecologic Investigation; 27th Annual Meeting,* p. 138.

57. Visser, G.H.A. (1982): Antepartum sinusoidal and decelerative heart rate patterns in Rh disease. *Am. J. Obstet. Gynecol.,* 143:538–544.

Fetal Neurology, edited by
A. Hill and J.J. Volpe.
Raven Press, New York © 1989.

5

Antepartum Fetal Assessment: The Contraction Stress Test

Jeffrey P. Phelan and Carl V. Smith

Department of Obstetrics and Gynecology, University of Southern California School of Medicine, Women's Hospital, Los Angeles, California 90033

The contraction stress test (CST) is of proven benefit for antepartum fetal surveillance in the management of the high risk pregnancy. The following discussion will focus on the role of the CST in the management of the high risk pregnancy and will review its advantages and disadvantages for the practicing clinician. However, it is not within the scope of this chapter to contrast the CST with other methods of antepartum fetal surveillance.

HISTORICAL PERSPECTIVE

More than two decades ago, Hon and Quilligan (21) demonstrated the relationship between intrapartum fetal heart rate (FHR) patterns and subsequent fetal outcome using continuous electronic fetal monitoring. In his atlas on FHR monitoring, Hon (20) demonstrated the association between late decelerations of the FHR and fetal hypoxia. Subsequently, these concepts led to the application of continuous electronic fetal monitoring during labor for more accurate assessment of fetal condition. In the early 1970s, Ray and associates (35) applied the principles developed by Hon (20) to a group of high risk patients before the onset of labor. The purpose was to identify those pregnancies at high risk for uteroplacental insufficiency (UPI). The theoretical basis of the CST involves the administration of oxytocin to simulate labor and thereby detect imminent fetal compromise. As soon as this relationship was demonstrated, the CST was recognized as a useful approach for clinical assessment of antepartum fetal well-being. However, because of the invasive nature of the CST, e.g., intravenous placement, use of exogenous medications, and the time-consuming nature of the test, modifications were sought. With the introduction of the nipple or breast stimulation tests

(4,9,19,22,24) (BST), the CST has become a primary method for antepartum fetal surveillance.

CONTROL OF FETAL HEART RATE (26,30)

The FHR is controlled by sympathetic and parasympathetic fibers. Cardioacceleratory fibers, which arise in the upper thoracic spinal cord, increase the FHR. In contrast, parasympathetic fibers, which are mediated by the vagus nerve, decrease the heart rate. In early pregnancy, the sympathetic system is dominant. However, with advancing gestation, the parasympathetic system assumes a greater control of the FHR. The interaction between these two opposing systems increases with advancing gestation and contributes to the recognizable changes in FHR variability.

In addition to the influence of the sympathetic and parasympathetic systems, the FHR is also controlled both by baroreceptors, located near the aortic arch, and by chemoreceptors, located within the aortic arch and carotid arteries. The baroreceptor responses, which are mediated by the vagus nerve, respond to changes in fetal blood pressure, e.g., a decrease in the FHR is observed in response to an increase in fetal systemic blood pressure. Chemoreceptors detect changes in fetal oxygenation. The response of FHR to alterations in oxygenation depends on whether the aortic or carotid chemoreceptor is stimulated. When the aortic chemoreceptors are stimulated, an increase in fetal oxygenation results in a slowing of the FHR. In contrast, stimulation of the carotid chemoreceptors produces a rise in fetal blood pressure and an increase in FHR. Thus, acute fetal hypoxemia may be manifested either by alterations in FHR variability and/or late decelerations.

The purpose of the CST is to unmask fetal hypoxia, which is caused by impaired uteroplacental perfusion. Impaired uteroplacental perfusion is manifested as late decelerations of the FHR. Late decelerations are produced by two principal mechanisms: (a) stimulation of the chemoreceptor reflex mediated by the vagus nerve, which produces cardio-inhibition (26); and (b) direct myocardial depression caused by fetal hypoxia. It is believed that during a CST, alterations in uteroplacental perfusion occur that result in cessation of intervillous blood flow and a decline in fetal oxygen transfer or uteroplacental exchange. Under normal circumstances, the fetus is able to tolerate such alterations without demonstrable changes in FHR. However, the compromised or high risk fetus is more likely to react to alterations in uteroplacental perfusion by exhibiting late decelerations or a positive CST.

Murata and associates (27) observed in a study of chronically instrumented rhesus monkeys that the appearance of late decelerations was an earlier warning sign of fetal hypoxia and acidosis than the disappearance of FHR accelerations. However, these findings may not be directly applicable to the human fetus. Thus, in the multi-institutional study of Freeman and associates (12) a significantly higher incidence of intrapartum fetal distress caused by late decelerations was reported in groups managed primarily by the CST. Furthermore, fetal acidosis generally is not observed in patients with reactive FHR patterns (5,6,38).

INDICATIONS FOR CONTRACTION STRESS TEST

Table 1 lists the current indications for CST and the gestational ages at which testing is recommended. Under certain conditions, testing may be started before 34 weeks of gestation. For example, in our institution, in patients with a prior fetal demise that occurred before 34 weeks, we begin testing 1 week before the estimated gestational age of the prior fetal demise. Testing is rarely started before 26 weeks of gestation or before a fetus has attained a fetal weight of at least 750 g based on ultrasound study. However, exceptional circumstances may dictate earlier testing. For example, evidence of intrauterine growth retardation or severe insulin-dependent diabetes mellitus may require earlier testing. If earlier testing is medically necessary before 34 weeks gestation, Gabbe and associates (15) have found the CST to be as predictive of fetal outcome as during later pregnancy. The CST is generally performed weekly unless clinical circumstances dictate more frequent testing.

The most common clinical indication for the CST is postmaturity. In this context, testing was usually started at 42 completed weeks of gestation. However, because recent data in patients beyond 40 weeks have demonstrated a significantly higher incidence of oligohydramnios (33), testing for postmaturity is now started at 41 weeks or 7 days past the patient's due date. In a series of 679 postdate pregnancies, Freeman et al. (13) found a negative CST to be highly predictive of a favorable outcome.

Contraindications to a CST relate to the presence of a prior upper segment uterine incision or to the potential for initiating premature labor. Under the circumstances listed in Table 2, a nonstress test (NST) rather than a CST is performed twice weekly to assess fetal well-being. Despite the concern that the CST may

TABLE 1. *Current indications for contraction stress testing and the gestational age when testing should be started*

Indication	Gestational age (weeks)
Diabetes mellitus	
Class A	40
Class A[a], B-R	34
Prior stillbirth	34
Medical disorders	34
Postdates	41
Rh disease	28
Decreased fetal movement	Dx
Abnormal fetal heart tones	Dx
Suspected intrauterine growth retardation	Dx

[a]Complicated.
Dx, when diagnosed.
From ref. 32.

TABLE 2. *Contraindications to the
contraction stress test*

Prior history of premature labor
Prior upper-segment uterine incision
Third-trimester bleeding
Known uterine malformation
Multiple gestation
Premature rupture of the membranes
Incompetent cervix

cipitate premature labor, persistent labor has not been reported following a CST (2,23). Nonetheless, the contraindications to the CST emphasize a major disadvantage of this testing technique, i.e., CST cannot be applied uniformly to a diverse high risk population. Thus, patients with complications listed in Table 2 cannot routinely undergo a CST for fear of potential complications, such as premature labor, persistent vaginal bleeding, or uterine rupture. As a result, alternatives, such as the NST, are used to assess fetal well-being in these circumstances.

CONTRACTION STRESS TEST TECHNIQUES

When a patient requires a CST, the customary approach is to position her in the semi-Fowler's or left lateral recumbent position. After she is comfortable, a baseline maternal blood pressure is obtained. Subsequently, the maternal blood pressure is recorded at 10-min intervals or whenever there is evidence of a FHR alteration. An external fetal monitor is then applied and a baseline FHR is recorded for 10 to 15 min. In approximately 10% of the patients (30), sufficient spontaneous uterine activity is present for an acceptable CST.

If adequate uterine activity for a CST is not present, a BST (Fig. 1) may be performed. The various techniques for conducting a CST by breast stimulation or oxytocin are illustrated in Tables 3 and 4. Breast stimulation testing offers many advantages over the oxytocin challenge test. First, there is a reduction in testing time. Moreover, there is enhanced patient acceptance because intravenous fluids, infusion pumps, and oxytocin are usually not required. This convenience makes the procedure highly acceptable to both nurses and patients. The results of the BST are similar to those obtained with the oxytocin challenge test. However, unlike other methods of fetal assessment, e.g., the NST (30), fetal biophysical profile (25), or the NST/amniotic fluid index (32), the BST should be performed in a hospital setting because of the potential risk of excessive uterine activity (Table 5) and fetal distress.

As demonstrated in Table 5, 83% of patients who underwent the BST developed sufficient uterine activity for a CST and did not require administration of oxytocin. In addition, gestational age did not seem to affect the success or failure of this approach (9). Although 17% of patients failed to produce sufficient uterine activ-

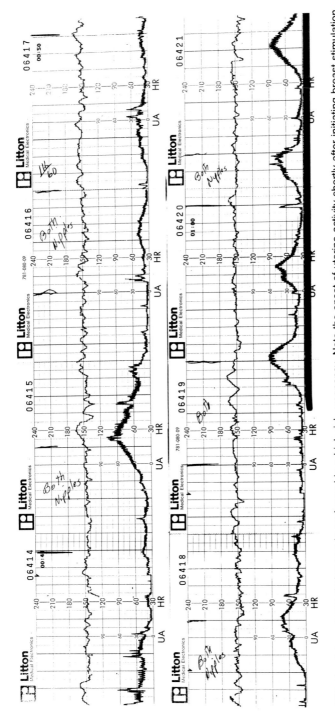

FIG. 1. A breast stimulation test is performed in a high-risk pregnancy. Note the onset of uterine activity shortly after initiating breast stimulation.

TABLE 3. *Techniques for conducting a contraction stress test by breast stimulation*

Bilateral—continuous (4,24)
   Deep palpation bilaterally for 3–5 min followed by bilateral nipple roll
   Continue breast manipulation until the first contraction
   If there is insufficient uterine activity after 10 min or less than 3 contractions after 20
     min, oxytocin infusion at 0.5 ml/min is begun
Unilateral—intermittent (22)
   Unilateral nipple stimulation for 2 min followed by a 5-min rest
   Continue nipple stimulation until the first contraction
   Repeat until an adequate contraction pattern is obtained
   If there is insufficient uterine activity for a contraction stress test within a reasonable
     number of nipple-stimulation cycles, oxytocin infusion should be started at 0.5 ml/min
Combination technique (11)
   Warm moist cloth to both breasts
   Massage and/or nipple roll one breast for 10 min until uterine activity begins
   If there is inadequate uterine activity, bilateral breast stimulation is continued until
     uterine activity is observed
   If breast stimulation fails to produce an adequate contraction pattern, oxytocin infusion
     at 0.5 ml/min is initiated

---

ity, Huddleston and associates (22) demonstrated that if breast stimulation were continued, a satisfactory CST could be obtained eventually. However, patients with inadequate uterine response to breast stimulation, who subsequently underwent oxytocin infusion, were at greater risk of excessive uterine activity (4). Thus, when a patient fails to exhibit an adequate uterine response to breast stimulation and requires oxytocin, the drug should be initiated at a low dose to reduce the risk of uterine hyperstimulation.

One of the major complications associated with nipple stimulation is excessive uterine activity, which is encountered in approximately 12% of patients (range: 0–41%). In the series of Hill and associates (19), 41% of patients had excessive uterine contractions. Of these, 10 had FHR decelerations. Nonetheless, fetuses who manifested FHR decelerations secondary to excessive uterine activity had a favorable outcome.

TABLE 4. *The performance of a contraction stress test by oxytocin infusion*

The patient is placed in the semi-Fowler's or left lateral position.
A suitable baseline fetal heart rate pattern is established for 10–30 min.
Maternal blood pressure is recorded every 10 min.
If there is sufficient spontaneous uterine activity for 3 contractions within 10 min, oxytocin
   infusion is not warranted.
If there is insufficient spontaneous uterine activity, oxytocin infusion is begun at the rate
   of 0.5 ml/min.
Oxytocin is increased at 15–20 min intervals until there are 3 contractions in a 10-min
   period.

From ref. 11.

TABLE 5. *The incidence of successful contraction stress tests and excessive uterine activity in selected reports using the breast stimulation test*

Study	No. of tests	Adequate CST (No./%)	Excessive uterine activity (No./%)
Lenke and Nemes (24)	241	189 (78)	12 (5)
Huddleston et al. (22)	345	345 (100)	7 (2)
Hill et al. (19)	185	174 (96)	76 (41)
Capeless and Mann (4)	346	239 (69)	47 (14)
Erkkola et al. (9)	76	47 (62)	0 (0)

CST, contraction stress test.

In summary, although the BST reduces overall testing time of the CST to 45 min (22), it is still twice as long as the time required to conduct a NST (39). As demonstrated by Huddleston and co-authors (22), the reduction in testing time does not cause reduction of the predictive reliability of the CST. However, as noted by the same group (24), the BST should not be performed remote from a labor and delivery suite.

INTERPRETATION

Table 6 illustrates the current criteria for interpretation of a CST. A minimum of three uterine contractions must be recorded within a 10-min period. The interpretation of a CST involves evaluation of the presence or absence of late decelerations in relation to the uterine contractions. A negative CST (Fig. 2) is the absence of late decelerations in association with three uterine contractions. A positive CST (Fig. 3) is the presence of persistent late decelerations over approximately 10 to 15 uterine contractions. If the late decelerations are not persistent, the CST is considered equivocal.

In antepartum fetal surveillance of high risk pregnancies, a *negative CST* is the most frequently encountered result, with reported incidences ranging from 60% to

TABLE 6. *Criteria for the interpretation of the contraction stress test*

Negative	Absence of late decelerations
Equivocal	Nonpersistent late decelerations
	Fetal heart rate deceleration in association with excessive uterine activity
Positive	Persistent late decelerations over 10–15 contractions
Unsatisfactory	Technically poor tracing
	Insufficient uterine contractions

From ref. 11.

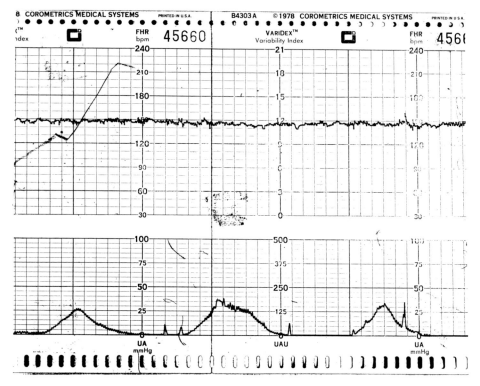

FIG. 2. A nonreactive negative contraction stress test is illustrated.

94% (2,7,22,24). A negative CST is a sign of fetal well-being and is associated with a low probability of fetal demise or distress within 7 days of the test (7,8,10,12,24). As demonstrated in Table 7, the uncorrected fetal mortality rate for a negative CST ranges from a low of 1.1 to 26 per 1,000 births (7,8,10,12,24). The higher incidence of fetal death following a negative CST reported by Druzin and associates (8) was related to the fact that these investigators limited the use of the CST to patients with a nonreactive NST. As demonstrated by these workers as well as by Phelan (30), a nonreactive NST is associated with a greater risk of fetal morbidity and mortality. The occurrence of a nonreactive negative CST, as demonstrated in Fig. 1, would necessitate either a repeat CST within 12 to 24 hr or delivery if appropriate. In addition, this FHR pattern is associated with an increased incidence of fetal anomaly (18). Thus, in addition to a repeat CST, an ultrasound evaluation should be considered to rule out the presence of fetal anomaly.

In summary, a negative CST is a sign of fetal well-being. When FHR accelerations are not observed during the CST, a repeat CST within 12 to 24 hr (8) and an ultrasound evaluation would appear to be a reasonable approach to management.

An *equivocal CST* is defined as the presence of nonpersistent late decelerations

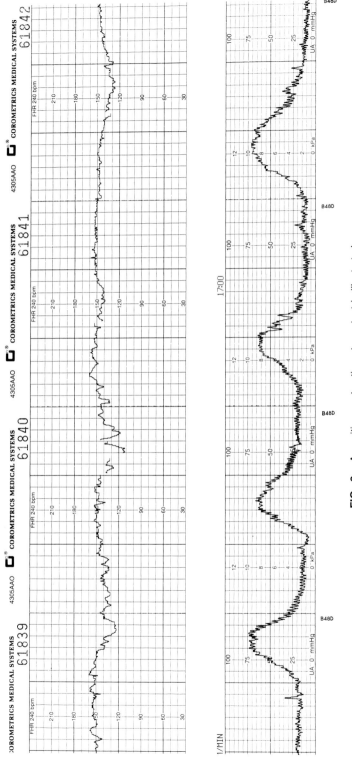

FIG. 3. A positive contraction stress test is illustrated.

TABLE 7. *Uncorrected fetal death rates following a negative contraction stress test*

Study	Patients (N)	Fetal deaths	No./1,000 births
Freeman et al. (12)	4,626	—	1.1
Collea and Holls (7)	1,739	7	4
Lenke and Nemes (24)	623	1	1.6
Everston et al. (10)	680	7	10
Druzin et al. (8)[a]	230	6	26

[a]Primary surveillance; nonstress test.

or FHR decelerations in association with excessive uterine activity (Table 6). The incidence of an equivocal CST varies from 1.7% to 28% (3,7,22,24,30). In the detailed series reported by Bruce and associates (3), 67 patients with an equivocal CST underwent a repeat CST. Of these, 54% were considered negative. However, when repeated, the incidence of a suspicious and positive CST was 39% and 7%, respectively. The overall incidence of fetal distress that required cesarean delivery was 11%. However, as emphasized by the authors, the "value of the suspicious CST is that it allows the clinician to stand back and reassess the status of the pregnancy and to consider whether delivery is indeed warranted." If delivery is not a reasonable consideration because of fetal lung immaturity, a repeat CST within 24 hr or continuous electronic fetal monitoring would appear to be reasonable alternatives. However, if there is evidence of fetal lung maturity, delivery by induction of labor with continuous electronic fetal monitoring should be considered.

A *positive CST* (Fig. 3) is a relatively uncommon occurrence. If the NST is used as the primary form of fetal surveillance, a positive CST occurs in 2.3% of patients or 1.2% of all tests performed (17,37). Of those patients with a nonreactive NST, the incidence of a positive CST approximates 6.5% (30). In contrast, if the CST is the primary form of fetal surveillance, the incidence of a positive CST varies from 1.2% (5) to 9.8% (14,29) of tests.

The conditions associated most commonly with a positive CST were postmaturity, suspected intrauterine growth retardation, hypertensive disorder of pregnancy, and diabetes mellitus (12,14,17,29,37). However, if fetal outcome in these situations is evaluated, fetuses that are small for gestational age or growth retarded are delivered most frequently. For instance, the overall incidence of intrauterine growth retardation in 229 patients with a positive CST (Table 8) was 36%. However, this incidence varied considerably from 15% to 43% in different studies. Furthermore, Slomka and Phelan (37) have demonstrated that abnormal infants have an increased incidence of abnormal FHR patterns. Thus, 17% of 41 patients with a positive CST had an abnormal fetus. Moreover, Garite and associates (16) stated that whenever "a pattern of persistent late decelerations, especially with absent reactivity and decreased fetal heart rate variability should alert the clinician to the possibility of a significant congenital anomaly." Although abnormal FHR

TABLE 8. *Outcome of pregnancy of patients with a positive contraction stress test*

	Slomka and Phelan (37)	Gauthier et al. (17)	Odendaal (29)	Freeman et al. (14)
Number	41	27	102	66
IUGR	12 (29%)	4 (15%)	41 (43%)	25 (37%)
Anomalous fetus	7 (17%)	—	—	—
Trial of labor	30	20	41	21
Late decelerations during labor	18 (60%)	21 (76%)	18 (45%)	16 (76%)
Vaginal delivery	17 (57%)	11 (55%)	24 (58%)	8 (38%)
Cesarean for fetal distress	11 (37%)	5 (19%)	18 (45%)	—
Overall cesarean delivery rate	24 (59%)	15 (56%)	78 (77%)	56 (85%)
Perinatal mortality (N/1,000)	73	74	88	132

IUGR, intrauterine growth retardation.

patterns are not associated with specific fetal anomalies, the pattern described by Garite et al. (16) is observed in approximately 50% of abnormal infants (28,34). Thus, as with a nonreactive negative CST, an ultrasound evaluation is recommended.

The high fetal morbidity associated with the specific FHR pattern just cited raises the question of vaginal delivery by induction of labor in such circumstances. Based on previous reports (14,17,29,37) (summarized in Table 8), a trial of labor would seem reasonable in a patient with a positive CST under specified conditions: (a) labor should proceed with the patient in the left lateral recumbent position; (b) oxygen should be administered via mask; (c) the cervix should be favorable for induction and permit the application of direct fetal monitoring; and (d) the hospital in which the induction is performed should have facilities for immediate cesarean section. Under these specific circumstances (Table 8), of 112 patients with positive CST who had a trial of labor, 60 (54%) delivered vaginally. During the conduct of the trial of labor, 65% manifested late decelerations. Cesarean delivery for fetal distress was necessary in approximately 35% and varied, depending on the series, from 19% to 45%.

Although these results appear favorable, not all patients with this FHR pattern should be permitted to undergo a trial of labor (1,37). As demonstrated by Braly and associates (1), the most important indicator of subsequent intrapartum fetal distress is the occurrence of a nonreactive FHR pattern during the CST. Moreover, this pattern appears to be indicative of fetuses who are less able to tolerate a trial of labor. These findings are consistent with the observations of Slomka and Phelan (37), who reported that 75% of fetuses that manifested intrapartum fetal distress were growth retarded. On the basis of this relationship, if the diagnosis of intrauterine growth retardation is established, a trial of labor should not be permitted (36). With the current availability of ultrasonography, the diagnosis of intrauterine growth retardation can be established with relative certainty. Moreover, in light of the current medical-legal climate, a more reasonable approach in the patient with a positive CST may be to limit a trial of labor to those fetuses who appear to be appropriately grown for gestational age and who do not have a nonreactive FHR pattern, as described by Braly et al. (1). Finally, as illustrated in Table 8, the clinician must be cognizant of the high perinatal mortality rate associated with these pregnancies, i.e., reported to range from 73 to 132 per 1,000 births.

In summary, a positive CST is indicative of substantial risk of fetal complications as demonstrated by the high perinatal mortality rates and cesarean delivery rates for fetal distress reported in this situation. A trial of labor is a reasonable consideration in specific situations if the infant does not have evidence of growth retardation or a nonreactive positive CST. In addition, the fetus who manifests a positive CST should have a detailed ultrasound evaluation to exclude not only intrauterine growth retardation but also major structural fetal anomalies.

MANAGEMENT

A management scheme for patients undergoing primary fetal surveillance with the CST is outlined in Fig. 4. Thus, if the patient has no contraindication to a CST, she is placed in the semi-Fowler's position and connected to an external fetal monitor. A baseline FHR is established over a 10- to 30-min period. During this time she may have sufficient uterine activity for a spontaneous CST, nipple stimulation or oxytocin will not be required, and she can be managed as outlined in Fig. 4. However, if there is inadequate spontaneous uterine activity for a CST, a BST as outlined in Table 3 is undertaken. If the patient fails to respond to breast stimulation within a reasonable period of time, oxytocin infusion, as outlined in Table 4, should be initiated. Under these circumstances, oxytocin should be started at a low dose.

When an adequate FHR pattern has been obtained, the CST should be interpreted as outlined in Table 6 and managed according to Fig. 4. If the CST is negative, it should be repeated 1 week later unless specific circumstances dictate earlier retesting. However, if the patient has a nonreactive negative CST, the CST should be repeated within 12 to 24 hr. If the patient has a persistent nonreactive negative CST 12 to 24 hr later, consideration should be given to delivery of the term infant. Similarly, if a term infant manifests a suspicious or equivocal CST, delivery should also be considered. In the preterm infant, an evaluation of the pregnancy and a repeat CST within 12 to 24 hr should be considered. The subsequent management of the preterm fetus will depend on the results of the repeat CST. If the CST is positive, delivery should be considered. Whether a trial of labor is permitted will depend on the inducibility of the cervix, the presence or absence of intrauterine growth retardation or fetal anomaly, and whether facilities for immediate cesarean section are available. If a trial of labor is deemed reasonable, the patient should be managed with direct fetal monitoring, be positioned on her left side, and receive oxygen by mask.

In summary, the CST is a valuable adjunct in the clinical management of the

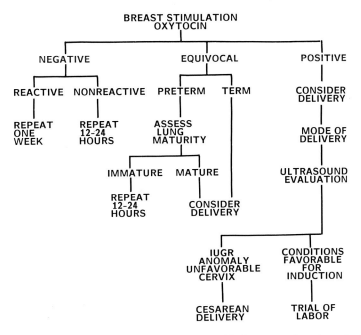

FIG. 4. Management scheme for patients managed with the contraction stress test. IUGR, intrauterine growth retardation.

high risk pregnancy. However, the CST should not serve as a replacement for good clinical judgment with careful consideration of both maternal and fetal conditions.

REFERENCES

1. Braly, P., and Freeman, R.K. (1977): The significance of fetal heart rate reactivity with a positive oxytocin challenge test. *Obstet. Gynecol.,* 50:689–693.
2. Braly, P.S., Freeman, R.K., Garite, T.J., et al. (1981): Incidence of premature delivery following the oxytocin challenge test. *Am. J. Obstet. Gynecol.,* 141:5–8.
3. Bruce, S.L., Petire, R.H., and Yeh, S.Y. (1978): The suspicious contraction stress test. *Obstet. Gynecol.,* 51:415–418.
4. Capeless, E.L., and Mann, L.I. (1984): Use of breast stimulation for antepartum stress testing. *Obstet. Gynecol.,* 64:641–645.
5. Clark, S.L., Gimovsky, M.L., and Miller, F.C. (1982): Fetal heart rate response to scalp blood sampling. *Am. J. Obstet. Gynecol.,* 144:706–708.
6. Clark, S.L., Gimovsky, M.L., and Miller, F.C. (1984): The scalp stimulation test: A clinical alternative to fetal scalp blood sampling. *Am. J. Obstet. Gynecol.,* 148:274–277.
7. Collea, J.V., and Holls, W.M. (1982): The contraction stress test. *Clin. Obstet. Gynecol.,* 25:707–717.
8. Druzin, M., Gratoacos, J., and Paul, R.H. (1980): Antepartum fetal heart rate testing: VI. The predictive reliability of "normal" tests in the prevention of antepartum death. *Am. J. Obstet. Gynecol.,* 137:746–747.

9. Erkkola, R., Rintala, H., and Gronross, M. (1984): Breast stimulation test in fetal surveillance. *Acta Obstet. Gynecol. Scand.,* 63:719–722.

10. Everston, L.R., Gauthier, R.J., and Collea, J.V. (1978): Fetal demise following negative contraction stress test. *Obstet. Gynecol.,* 51:671–673.

11. Freeman, R.K. (1982): Contraction stress testing for primary fetal surveillance in patients at high risk for uteroplacental insufficiency. *Clin. Perinatol.,* 9:265–270.

12. Freeman, R.K., Anderson, G., and Dorchester, W. (1982): A prospective multi-institutional study of antepartum fetal heart rate monitoring. I. Risk of perinatal mortality and morbidity according to antepartum fetal heart rate test results. *Am. J. Obstet. Gynecol.,* 143:771–777.

13. Freeman, R.K., Garite, T.J., Modanlou, H., and Dorchester, W. (1981): Postdate pregnancy: Utilization of contraction stress testing for primary fetal surveillance. *Am. J. Obstet. Gynecol.,* 140:128–135.

14. Freeman, R.K., Goebelsman, U., Nochimson, D., et al. (1976): An evaluation of the significance of a positive oxytocin challenge test. *Obstet. Gynecol.,* 47:8–13.

15. Gabbe, S.G., Freeman, R.K., and Goebelsman, U. (1978): Evaluation of the contraction stress test before 33 weeks gestation. *Obstet. Gynecol.,* 52:649–652.

16. Garite, T.J., Luizey, E.M., Freeman, R.K., et al. (1979): Fetal heart rate patterns and fetal distress in fetuses with congenital anomalies. *Obstet. Gynecol.,* 53:716–720.

17. Gauthier, R.J., Evertson, L.R., and Paul, R.H. (1979): Antepartum fetal heart rate testing. II. Intrapartum fetal heart observation and newborn outcome following a positive contraction stress test. *Am. J. Obstet. Gynecol.,* 133:34–39.

18. Grundy, H., Freeman, R.K., Lederman, S., et al. (1984): Nonreactive contraction stress test: Clinical significance. *Obstet. Gynecol.,* 64:337–342.

19. Hill, W.C., Moenning, R.K., Katz, M., et al. (1984): Characteristics of uterine activity during the breast stimulation stress test. *Obstet. Gynecol.,* 64:489–492.

20. Hon, E.H. (1968): *An Atlas of Fetal Heart Rate Patterns.* Harty Press, New Haven.

21. Hon, E.H., and Quilligan, E.J. (1967): The classification of fetal heart rate. II. Revised working classification. *Conn. Med.,* 31:779–784.

22. Huddleston, J.F., Sutliff, G., and Robinson, D., (1984): Contraction stress test by intermittent nipple stimulation. *Obstet. Gynecol.,* 63:669–673.

23. Knuppel, R.A., Rattan, P.K., Scerbo, J.C., et al. (1985): Intrauterine fetal death in twins after 32 weeks of gestation. *Obstet. Gynecol.,* 65:172–175.

24. Lenke, R.R., and Nemes, J.M. (1984): Use of nipple stimulation to obtain contraction stress test. *Obstet. Gynecol.,* 63:345–348.

25. Manning, F.A., Morrison, I., Lange, I.R., et al. (1985): Fetal assessment based on fetal biophysical profile scoring: Experience in 12,620 referred high-risk pregnancies. I. Perinatal mortality by frequency and etiology. *Am. J. Obstet. Gynecol.,* 151:343–350.

26. Martin, C.B., Jr. (1978): Regulation of the fetal heart rate and genesis of FHR patterns. *Semin. Perinatol.,* 2:131–146.

27. Murata, Y., Martin, C.B., Jr., Ikenoue, T., et al. (1982): Fetal heart rate accelerations and late decelerations during the course of intrauterine death in chronically catheterized rhesus monkeys. *Am. J. Obstet. Gynecol.,* 144:218–223.

28. Navot, D., Mor-Yosef, S., Granat, M., et al. (1983): Antepartum fetal heart rate pattern associated with major congenital malformations. *Obstet. Gynecol.,* 63:414–417.

29. Odendaal, H.J. (1979): The fetal and labor outcome of 102 positive contraction stress tests. *Obstet. Gynecol.,* 54:591–596.

30. Phelan, J.P. (1981): The nonstress test: A review of 3,000 tests. *Am. J. Obstet. Gynecol.,* 139:7–10.

31. Phelan, J.P. (1987): Fetal considerations in the critically ill obstetric patient. In: *Critical Care Obstetrics,* edited by S.L. Clark, J.P. Phelan, and D.B. Cotton, pp. 436–460. Medical Economics Books, Oradell, NJ.

32. Phelan, J.P. (1988): Antepartum fetal evaluation. In: *Common Problems in Ob-Gyn,* 2nd ed., edited by D.R. Mishell, Jr. and P. Brenner. Medical Economics Books, Oradell, NJ (*in press*).

33. Phelan, J.P., Smith, C.V., Broussard, P., and Small, M. (1987): Amniotic fluid volume assessment using the four quadrant technique in the pregnancy between 36 and 42 weeks gestation. *J. Reprod. Med.,* 32:540–542.

34. Phillips, W.D.P., and Towell, M.L. (1980): Abnormal fetal heart rate associated with congenital anomalies. *Br. J. Obstet. Gynaecol.,* 87:270–274.

35. Ray, M., Freeman, R.K., and Pine, S. (1971): Clinical experience with the oxytocin challenge test. *Am. J. Obstet. Gynecol.,* 114:1–9.

36. Sandenbergh, H.A., and Odendaal, H.J. (1977): Clinical experience with the contraction stress test. *S. Afr. Med. J.*, 51:660–663.

37. Slomka, C., and Phelan, J.P. (1981): Pregnancy outcome in the patient with a nonreactive nonstress test and a positive contraction stress test. *Am. J. Obstet. Gynecol.*, 139:11–15.

38. Smith, C.V., Nguyen, H.N., Phelan, J.P., et al. (1986): Intrapartum assessment of fetal wellbeing: A comparison of fetal acoustic stimulation with acid-base determinations. *Am. J. Obstet. Gynecol.*, 155:726–728.

39. Smith, C.V., Phelan, J.P., Platt, L.D., et al. (1986): Fetal acoustic stimulation testing (The FAS-TEST). II. A randomized clinical comparison with the nonstress test. *Am. J. Obstet. Gynecol.*, 155:131–134.

Fetal Neurology, edited by
A. Hill and J.J. Volpe.
Raven Press, New York © 1989.

Commentary on Chapters 4 and 5

*Alan Hill and **Joseph J. Volpe

*Division of Neurology, Department of Paediatrics, University of British Columbia,
British Columbia's Children's Hospital, Vancouver, British Columbia, Canada V6H 3V4;
and **Division of Pediatric Neurology, Washington University School of Medicine,
St. Louis, Missouri 63110*

Historically, initial attempts to identify markers of fetal disease have focused on biochemical analyses. A number of diverse compounds have been evaluated in this context, including peptide hormones (e.g., human placental lactogen), enzymes (e.g., placental alkaline phosphatase), steroids (e.g., progesterone, estriol, estrone), and specific proteins (e.g., alpha-fetoprotein). More recently, such technical advances as real-time ultrasonography have led to the replacement of these tests by more specific and direct biophysical indices of fetal integrity. Moreover, surveillance of fetal well-being by antepartum fetal heart rate monitoring has become standard obstetric practice in the management of high-risk pregnancies. Fetal heart rate responses to intrinsic stimuli such as fetal movement or spontaneous uterine contractions (nonstress test), or to extrinsic stimuli, e.g., stimulated uterine contractions (stress test), have been studied extensively as predictors of fetal outcome.

The nonstress test, which involves observation of fetal heart rate in response to spontaneous fetal movement, is most commonly used for initial evaluation (6). The principal drawback to this approach is the length of time required for the procedure. Thus, a test may be considered normal or *reactive* if two significant accelerations of the fetal heart rate are noted during 20 min of continuous observation. A test is termed abnormal or *nonreactive* only if these criteria are not fulfilled within 40 min.

The underlying principle of the nonstress test, that fetal heart rate accelerations in response to spontaneous fetal movements imply a high probability of favorable fetal outcome, has evolved principally from empiric observations. However, the neurophysiologic mechanisms that are responsible for this association of biophysical activities are poorly understood. Thus, in the human fetus it has not been clearly established whether the central nervous system controls both fetal movement and heart rate acceleration or whether fetal movements trigger a feedback mechanism that, in turn, initiates acceleration of heart rate. Because fetal movements generally precede fetal heart rate accelerations, the second explanation may be more probable.

The relationship of nonstress test results to fetal outcome has been studied extensively in high-risk pregnancies. However, application of the test in low-risk populations is controversial. Thus, although the frequency of abnormal nonstress tests is relatively high (approximately 10%) and this finding increases the presumed incidence of "fetal distress" and delivery by cesarean delivery from 2% to 30% (6), it is clear that in the majority of cases with abnormal tests there is normal fetal outcome. In an effort to improve the predictive and diagnostic accuracy of the nonstress test, modifications of the technique have been suggested, e.g., assessment of baseline variability of fetal heart rate and of heart rate response to spontaneous uterine contractions and evaluation of fetal heart rate decelerations.

Although the nonstress test has limitations, at the present time it is recommended as the initial screening procedure for assessment of fetal well-being in most clinical situations. The major advantages relate to the relatively low cost and ease of performance of the test. The predictive power of the test for fetal outcome may be improved by extending the duration of observation or by combining the technique with other testing modalities, e.g., contraction stress test or assessment of fetal breathing.

The contraction stress test is based on the evaluation of changes in fetal heart rate in response to uterine contractions, induced either by breast or nipple or oxytocin stimulation (1–3). This test is considered particularly valuable for detection of imminent fetal asphyxia related to uteroplacental insufficiency. Thus, it is most commonly used for further assessment following a nonreactive nonstress test. Experimental data suggest that late decelerations associated with uterine contractions (positive stress test) is an earlier warning sign of uteroplacental insufficiency than loss of reactive acceleration of fetal heart rate (5). The major difficulty with this method of fetal assessment relates to its large false positive rate of approximately 25% (4).

When evaluating the usefulness of both the nonstress and stress tests for antenatal fetal surveillance, it must be remembered that the tests were originally developed to detect imminent or ongoing fetal asphyxia. Thus, they were not designed to identify other serious causes of fetal compromise, e.g., congenital malformations or acquired fetal disease.

REFERENCES

1. Freeman, R.K. (1982): Contraction stress testing for primary fetal surveillance in patients at high risk for uteroplacental insufficiency. *Clin. Perinatol.,* 9:265–270.
2. Freeman, R.K., Anderson, G., and Dorchester, W. (1982): A prospective multi-institutional study of antepartum fetal heart rate monitoring. I. Risk of perinatal morbidity and mortality according to antepartum fetal heart rate test results. *Am. J. Obstet. Gynecol.,* 143:771–777.
3. Freeman, R.K., Anderson, G., and Dorchester, W. (1982): A prospective multi-institutional study of antepartum fetal heart rate monitoring. II. Contraction stress test versus non-stress test for primary surveillance. *Am. J. Obstet. Gynecol.,* 143:778–781.

4. Manning, F.A. (1985): Assessment of fetal condition and risk: Analysis of single and combined biophysical variable monitoring. *Semin. Perinatol.,* 9:168–182.
5. Murata, Y., Ikenoue, T., Hashimoto, T., et al. (1981): Fetal heart rate acceleration and late deceleration during a course of intrauterine death in chronically catheterized rhesus monkeys. *Twenty-Eighth Annual Meeting of the Society for Gynecologic Investigation,* St. Louis, MO.
6. Paul, R.H. (1982): The evaluation of antepartum fetal wellbeing using the nonstress test. *Clin. Perinatol.,* 9:253–263.

Fetal Neurology, edited by
A. Hill and J.J. Volpe.
Raven Press, New York © 1989.

6

Fetal Biophysical Score and Fetal Well-Being

Harbinder S. Brar and Lawrence D. Platt

Department of Obstetrics and Gynecology, Division of Maternal Fetal Medicine, University of Southern California School of Medicine, and Women's Hospital, Los Angeles County USC Medical Center, Los Angeles, California 90033

Improvements in the medical management of high risk pregnancies with complications such as diabetes mellitus and hypertension, as well as improvements in the understanding of the effect of maternal disease on the fetus, have resulted in a need for better assessment of fetal well-being. Similarly, significant advances in neonatal care during the past 2 decades, which have lowered the minimum gestational age for potential survival, have increased the need for early recognition and prevention of fetal morbidity. Furthermore, the expectations of modern society for a perfect outcome of a pregnancy, compounded by medico-legal concerns, have added impetus to the development of accurate and reliable diagnostic tests of fetal well-being.

BIOCHEMICAL TESTING

Initial attempts to assess the fetal condition relied heavily on the evaluation of biochemical parameters in maternal serum or urine. These tests principally focused on the integrity of the "fetoplacental unit" as an indirect measure of fetal condition, e.g., monitoring of human placental lactogen, estriol, and total estrogen. Later, "placental function tests," such as metabolic clearance rate of dehydroepiandrosterone sulfate (MCR_{DHEAS}) and the DHEAS loading tests, were described. These tests have been essentially abandoned because of difficulties with technique and interpretation as well as relatively low specificity and sensitivity in the prediction of fetal condition.

ANTEPARTUM FETAL HEART RATE TESTING

With the introduction of the nonstress test (NST) and oxytocin challenge test (OCT) for fetal monitoring, together with improvements in neonatal care, perinatal mortality has dramatically fallen to less than 12 per 1,000 live births. The ratio of stillbirth to neonatal death has reversed from 1:2 in 1970 to 2:1 in 1980 (49). Consequently, the prevention of stillbirth has become a major challenge of modern obstetrics. Although the NST and OCT are reasonably accurate in their prediction of normal outcome, they are much less accurate for prediction of poor outcome, as determined by Apgar scores, fetal distress, etc. Thus, the NST has a low false negative rate (<1%) and a high false positive rate (>75%) (21,68). The OCT has a somewhat higher false negative rate (2%–2.7%) and a false positive rate ranging from 50% to greater than 75% (13,25,62). Despite refinements to the OCT technique, e.g., use of nipple stimulation, the procedure tends to be lengthy and cumbersome and occasionally fails to identify the dying fetus (20).

DEVELOPING THE IDEAL TEST

The stillbirth rate in an unscreened population is approximately 8 per 1,000 births and accounts for at least 65% of all perinatal morbidity. Chronic intrauterine asphyxia is the single most important cause of stillbirth. Therefore, earlier detection of impending fetal asphyxia may lead to earlier intervention and should result in a reduction of perinatal mortality. Furthermore, the elimination of ongoing fetal asphyxia presumably would further reduce neonatal loss (47). The ideal method for fetal assessment would require a high specificity, sensitivity, positive and negative predictive values, and low false negative and false positive rates. True negative cases are unaffected fetuses who exhibit a normal test result, whereas true positive cases are affected fetuses with an abnormal test result. In contrast, false negatives are affected fetuses with a normal test result, and false positives are unaffected fetuses with an abnormal test (35,70). Therefore, the ideal antepartum test for fetal assessment would require high sensitivity to prevent a risk of asphyxial fetal death because of false negative results, as well as high specificity to prevent inappropriate intervention caused by false positive results.

Moreover, a useful test for fetal assessment should identify the fetus with major anomalies that are incompatible with extrauterine life and that were not detected on early ultrasound examinations. This problem is underscored by the fact that a high incidence of abnormal antepartum and intrapartum fetal heart rate patterns are reported in infants with major anomalies, and subsequent surgical intervention is more common in this group. Similarly, a high incidence of anomalies (up to 30%) has been reported in selected populations with abnormal antepartum fetal heart rate patterns (19,61).

Since detailed ultrasound examination has been combined with determination of fetal heart rate patterns, reliable fetal assessment has become a reality in the management of the high-risk pregnancy. The advantage of high resolution ultrasound imaging is the ability to visualize the fetus and monitor its activities and responses to a variety of stimuli, thus applying the time-honored principle of physical examination, albeit indirect, to the fetus (34,40). Such assessment enables the physician to intervene more appropriately in high-risk situations. Such intervention may be either early, e.g., abortion of a fetus with severe malformations, or late, e.g., delivery of a postterm infant with oligohydramnios (30,56).

FETAL BIOPHYSICAL ACTIVITIES

Numerous biophysical activities that reflect intact functioning of the central nervous system not affected by hypoxic-ischemic insult can be studied with real-time B scan ultrasound (RTBS). In addition, ultrasound permits detailed screening for anatomical abnormalities. The biophysical activities that have been described to date include the following:

1. Generalized activities, such as gross body movements, breathing movements, and fetal tone (9,52,58);
2. Specific activities, such as sucking, swallowing, micturition, and reflex activities (11);
3. Sleep states, by monitoring motion of the fetal eye movements (48);
4. Fetal heart rate (17);
5. Measurement of blood flow in umbilical vessels (4,5,8);
6. Assessment of the intrauterine environment, including quantitative determination of amniotic fluid volume (10,12,56), placental architecture, grade and pathology (27,32,54,55,73), and cord position (I.R. Lange et al., *personal communication*); and
7. Peristaltic patterns, purposeful movements, and evoked fetal reflex responses, e.g., fetal startle response evoked by the use of an artificial larynx (18).

These fetal activities vary with sleep cycles in both humans and experimental animals (16,65). The extent of assessed biophysical activities is limited most often by practicalities of time constraints placed by clinicians.

Factors Affecting Biophysical Activities

Asphyxia

Although it is well established that asphyxia may result in cerebral injury, the precise sensitivity of specific areas of the developing human brain to hypoxemia and/or acidosis is unknown (45). Under the influence of progressive asphyxia some biophysical activities cease (28). For example, the fetal tone center, which is considered to reside in the cortex-subcortical region, is the earliest to function (7.5–8.5 weeks) (28,29) but is the last function to disappear during progressively worsening asphyxia. The absence of fetal tone (FT = 0) in the biophysical profile scheme indeed was found to be associated with the highest perinatal death rate (42.8%). On the other hand, although fetal heart rate variability begins early, it matures late, i.e., at approximately 28 weeks, and thus may be predicted to be more sensitive to asphyxia. It has been suggested that the beat-beat variability is the first biophysical activity to be affected by progressively worsening asphyxia.

The spectrum of fetal asphyxia ranges from transient episodes of hypoxemia without acidosis to sustained hypoxemia with associated metabolic and/or respiratory acidosis, affecting multiple organ systems. The effect on the biophysical profile will vary depending on the extent, duration, chronicity, and frequency of the insult. For example, by stimulation of aortic body chemoreceptors, fetal hypoxemia and/or acidosis cause protective redistribution of cardiac output away from nonvital fetal organs (i.e., lung, kidney, gut) to vital fetal organs (i.e., heart, brain, adrenals, placenta). Under conditions of sustained asphyxia, the redistribution may be profound, with almost complete cessation of perfusion to lung and kidneys, resulting in decreased urine production, lung liquid flow, and subsequently oligohydramnios (14).

It must be stressed that most of the evidence supporting the effect of asphyxia on the redistribution of cardiac output and its effect on central nervous system function, as measured by biophysical parameters, is based on experimental studies. It is not clear to what extent these studies are applicable to the human fetus. For example, it is not clear whether ongoing asphyxia is associated with progressive loss of biophysical function or whether complete loss of all functions occurs at a critical level of asphyxia. Observations of the human fetus support the former notion (39,45).

Based on their association with an asphyxiating insult, the parameters of the fetal biophysical profile may be divided into two categories (39,45):

1. "Acute" effects are those that occur following a severe, acute asphyxiating insult to the fetus, e.g., fetal breathing movements, fetal tone, fetal movement, and heart rate reactivity (NST).

2. "Chronic" effects are those that occur after acute repetitive or chronic progressive hypoxic-ischemic insults and that include oligohydramnios as the only finding. Thus, oligohydramnios may be considered a "delayed" sign of asphyxia. Acute onset of asphyxia results in loss of acute variables, with normal amniotic fluid volume, whereas repetitive episodes with recovery may cause oligohydramnios, with preservation of acute variables. It must be cautioned that before attributing the absence of biophysical activities to hypoxia, other causes, such as intrinsic (biorhythms) or extrinsic factors, e.g., drugs, should be considered.

Drugs

Drugs that depress central nervous system activity, e.g., sedatives (barbiturates, diazepam), analgesics (morphine, meperidine), and anesthetics (halothane) may reduce or abolish fetal biophysical activities (2). Conversely, central nervous system stimulants, e.g., amphetamines and hyperglycemia, often result in increased fetal biophysical activities. Thus, a knowledge of maternal drug usage before fetal assessment is essential for accurate interpretation of results.

Biorhythms and Sleep-Wake Cycles

Monitoring fetal biophysical activities provides indirect information about central nervous system function. Fetal biophysical activities originate from different anatomic sites within the brain (Table 1) (76). Fetal brain electrical activity may be directly measured by electrocortical leads and may be categorized as follows (16):

1. Low frequency, high voltage pattern (quiet sleep pattern), characterized by fetal sighing and fetal breathing movements (FBM) that may be absent, isolated, or infrequent and of large amplitude. It is also associated with rapid but infrequent eye movements (REM).

2. High frequency, low voltage pattern (active REM sleep), characterized by bursts of FBM of varying frequency and amplitude and fetal REM (65).

These sleep cycles alternate during a 20- to 40-min period.

The presence of normal fetal biophysical activity indicates that at least the part of the fetal central nervous system that controls that activity is functionally intact. However, the absence of a given activity is much more difficult to interpret because it may reflect either pathological depression or normal periodicity as previously described. The periodicity has been demonstrated to be both short-term (20–80 min) and long-term, similar to circadian (diurnal) rhythms observed during extrauterine life.

TABLE 1. *Fetal central nervous system centers*

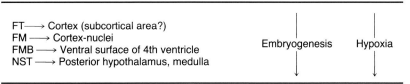

FT, fetal tone; FM, fetal movements; FBM, fetal breathing movements; NST, nonstress test.
From ref. 75.

INDIVIDUAL TESTS

Antepartum Fetal Heart Rate Testing

Nonstress Test (see also Chapter 4)

The presence of fetal heart rate accelerations in combination with fetal body movements has been associated with a high probability of favorable perinatal outcome (64). Fetal movement precedes most heart rate accelerations, thus suggesting a reflex interaction between these two variables (74). Lavery's review (33) of 11 series that employed the NST as a measure of fetal well-being in a total of 7,884 patients suggests a false negative rate (uncorrected for lethal anomalies) of 6.8 per 1,000. Among the group with abnormal tests the perinatal death rate was 12%. As previously discussed, the major advantage of the NST is its low cost and the ease of performing the testing. Major disadvantages of the NST include the following:

1. The frequency of abnormal test results is relatively high (9%–10%) (69);
2. The true positive predictive accuracy of an abnormal test is low (12%–13%) (33), although this note may be improved by extending the duration of the test (6) (to allow for sleep cycles) or combining the NST with other tests, like FBM (46) or contraction stress test (CST) (3); and
3. The false negative rate is relatively high (4–6 per 1,000) (34).

The high false positive rate caused by fetal sleep cycles may be reduced by using the fetal acoustic stimulation test to arouse the fetus (71). In a prospective randomized clinical study that compared the NST to FBM, the frequency of abnormal results with the NST were significantly higher and its positive predictive accuracy was lower (37). The negative predictive accuracy did not vary.

Contraction Stress Test (see also Chapter 5)

The CST involves the observation of periodic heart rate changes in relationship to uterine contractions. The false negative rate of this test is about 0.4 per 1,000 (24). Furthermore, fetal death during a negative test has been reported (22). False positive rates vary from 25% to 100% from study to study (13,15) but are dependent on the parameters of outcome that are used. In one study, a fetal death rate of 327 per 1,000 was reported (72). We have used other biophysical variables when a positive CST occurs in order to reduce false positive rate (42). Under these conditions, the CST appears to be a reliable and useful test.

Fetal Movement (see also Chapters 1 and 2)

Decreased fetal movement has been observed in association with increased perinatal morbidity and mortality (63,67). Fetal movements have been monitored by real-time ultrasound (44,53) and occur in 30-min cycles (with approximately 10–16 discrete movements) in each 90-min period (38). This periodicity appears to be related to sleep-wake cycles (7). Unlike breathing movements, gross body movements have little circadian periodicity and do not fluctuate with glucose levels (51). At the present time, there are two methods for evaluation of fetal movement:

1. *Subjective*. This method is based on maternal perception of fetal movement. Mothers perceiving decreased fetal movements are at higher risk for abnormal pregnancy outcomes (67). However, this technique is, of necessity, very subjective, and thereby associated with inherent error.

2. *Objective monitoring with real-time ultrasound*. In a prospective blinded study of 216 high-risk pregnancies (45), the incidence of low 5-min Apgar scores, fetal distress in labor and perinatal mortality were all significantly increased in inactive fetuses as compared to active fetuses. As with other single tests the predictive accuracy was better with a normal test result than with an abnormal result (53).

Fetal Breathing Movements (see also Chapters 1 and 2)

Rhythmic episodes of FBM *in utero* have been documented in the human fetus (26,43,50) as a function of fetal development. In the normal human fetus, FBM are episodic. The proportion of time spent breathing has a diurnal pattern. Boddy and Dawes (2) demonstrated that fetuses who spend less than 50% of the time breathing had a poor outcome. However, this study did not use real-time ultrasound. In another prospective study (59), we reported that the presence of FBM before delivery was a strong predictor of normal outcome (90%), whereas only 50% of fetuses with absent breathing activity were asphyxiated or depressed at birth. These results are similar to those reported with the NST, i.e., abnormal test results appear to be a relatively poor predictor of outcome. However, the predictive accuracy improved markedly when assessment of fetal breathing was combined with the NST (45).

Fetal Tone

Fetal tone has not been studied in detail in experimental animals. In the human fetus, normal tone may be defined as active flexion-deflexion of fetal limbs. It has been suggested that this parameter can be assessed with equal accuracy by observing the opening and closing of the fetal hand. Thus, fetal tone is considered abnormal if there is no return to a position of complete flexion after fetal movement or if the fetus remains in a deflexed position (partial or complete) in the absence of fetal movement. Loss of muscle tone in the fetus is often characterized by limb deflexion and a loss of fist formation. This phenomenon has been reported in the asphyxiated newborn (23). By this method in a blinded study of 216 high-risk pregnancies (45), fetuses with absent tone evaluated as part of the biophysical profile exhibited with a high incidence of fetal distress in labor, low 5-min Apgar score, and perinatal morbidity when compared to fetuses with normal tone on the last evaluation before delivery (45).

We believe that a more objective method for assessment of tone may be achieved by evoking a fetal startle response with an artificial larynx. This device produces a combined vibrating and auditory sensation and evokes fetal movement that lasts approximately 8.2 sec (18).

Placental Grade

Although the placenta is not a biophysical variable, it provides information about the environment of the fetus. Vintzeleos et al. (75) suggest that the placental grade be included in the composite biophysical profile scoring. These authors report an increased incidence of abnormal intrapartum fetal heart rate patterns and abruptio placenta during labor in patients with "grade 3" placentas. However, we have no personal experience with placental grade as part of the determination of fetal biophysical profile.

Amniotic Fluid Volume

The relationship between oligohydramnios and intrauterine compromise has been previously described. In a study of 120 patients, decreased amniotic fluid volume (AFV), as measured by less than a 1-cm pocket of fluid in a vertical depth on real-time ultrasound, was shown to be associated with an increased incidence of intrauterine growth retardation. Furthermore, perinatal morbidity and mortality appears to be significantly increased when oligohydramnios is present (36,41). Gross and corrected perinatal mortality in association with apparently normal AFV ranged from 4.65 per 1,000 and 1.97 per 1,000, respectively, and in association with decreased (<2 cm) AFV, from 187.5 per 1,000 and 109.4 per 1,000 (10). Other conditions associated with oligohydramnios include dysmaturity and major congenital fetal anomalies involving primarily the genito-urinary tract (i.e., renal agenesis) (41).

Recently, four-quadrant assessment of AFV by ultrasound has been used to assess oligohydramnios. The sum of the total depth of amniotic fluid in four quadrants has been called the amniotic fluid index. An index of 5 or less is associated with a higher incidence of meconium, fetal distress in labor, and low 5-min Apgar score (66).

THE COMBINED BIOPHYSICAL SCORE

We have assessed the predictive value of individual biophysical variables for fetal outcome. The common denominator is that a normal test is a much better predictor of normal fetal condition than is the abnormal test a predictor of fetal compromise. Individual variables are consistently associated with false negative results, e.g., a rate of 4 to 6 per 1,000 for NST (33), as well as unacceptably high false positive rates (30%–70%).

Because an abnormal variable may be explained on the basis of either fetal compromise caused by asphyxia or a normal fetal sleep-wake cycle, it is necessary to develop a method of fetal assessment that can differentiate between these two conditions. This diagnostic dilemma may be resolved by using several biophysical variables in concert as well as by extending the period of observation beyond a sleep-wake cycle. This has led to the development of a combined biophysical profile of the fetus (46). Currently, there are two scoring systems reported in the literature:

1. The first system was initially described by Manning et al. (46). In this score, each variable is recorded as either normal (score = 2) or abnormal (score = 0), as described in Table 2; and
2. In the second system, developed by Vintzileos et al. (76), each variable receives a score of 0, 1, or 2, as shown in Table 3.

TABLE 2. *Biophysical profile scoring: techniques and interpretation*

Biophysical variable	Normal (score = 2)	Abnormal (score = 0)
FBM	At least 1 episode of FBM of at least 30-sec duration in 30-min observation	Absent FBM or no episode of ≥30 sec in 30 min
Gross body movement	At least 3 discrete body/limb movements in 30 min (episodes of active continuous movement considered as single movement)	2 or fewer episodes of body/limb movements in 30 min
Fetal tone	At least 1 episode of active extension with return to flexion of fetal limb(s) or trunk. Opening and closing of hand considered normal tone	Either slow extension with return to partial flexion or movement of limb in full extension or absent fetal movement
Reactive FHR	At least 2 episodes of FHR acceleration of ≥15 beats/min and of at least 15-sec duration associated with fetal movement in 30 min	Less than 2 episodes of acceleration of FHR or acceleration of <15 beats/min in 30 min
Qualitative AFV	At least 1 pocket of AF that measures at least 1 cm in two perpendicular planes	Either no AF pockets or a pocket <1 cm in two perpendicular planes

FBM, fetal breathing movement; FHR, fetal heart rate; AFV, amniotic fluid volume; AF, amniotic fluid.
From ref. 45.

TABLE 3. *Criteria for scoring biophysical variables*

Nonstress test (NST)
    Score 2 (NST 2): 5 or more fetal heart rate (FHR) accelerations of at least 15 bpm in
        amplitude and at least 15-sec duration associated with FM in a 20-min period
    Score 1 (NST 1): 2–4 accelerations of at least 15 bpm in amplitude and at least 15-
        sec duration associated with fetal movements in a 20-min period
    Score 0 (NST 0): 1 or fewer accelerations in a 20-min period
Fetal movements (FM)
    Score 2 (FM 2): At least 3 gross (trunk and limbs) episodes of fetal movements within
        30 min—Simultaneous limb and trunk movements counted as a single movement
    Score 1 (FM 1): 1 or 2 fetal movements within 30 min
    Score 0 (FM 0): Absence of fetal movements within 30 min
Fetal breathing movements (FBM)
    Score 2 (FBM 2): At least 1 episode of fetal breathing of at least 60-sec duration within
        a 30-min observation period
    Score 1 (FBM 1): At least 1 episode of fetal breathing lasting 30–60 sec within 30 min
    Score 0 (FBM 0): Absence of fetal breathing or breathing lasting <30 sec within 30 min
Fetal tone (FT)
    Score 2 (FT 2): At least 1 episode of extension of extremities with return to position of
        flexion, also 1 episode of extension of spine with return to position of flexion
    Score 1 (FT 1): At least 1 episode of extension of extremities with return to position of
        flexion or 1 episode of extension of spine with return to position of flexion
    Score 0 (FT 0): Extremities in extension—Fetal movements not followed by return to
        flexion—Open hand
Amniotic fluid (AF) volume
    Score 2 (AF 2): Fluid evident throughout the uterine cavity—A pocket that measures
        ≥2 cm in vertical diameter
    Score 1 (AF 1): A pocket that measures <2 cm but >1 cm in vertical diameter
    Score 0 (AF 0): Crowding of fetal small parts—Largest pocket <1 cm in vertical
        diameter
Placental grading (PL)
    Score 2 (PL 2): Placental grading 0, 1, or 2
    Score 1 (PL 1): Placenta posterior difficult to evaluate
    Score 0 (PL 0): Placental grading 3

NST, nonstress test; FHR, fetal heart rate; bpm, beats per minute; FM, fetal movements;
FBM, fetal breathing movements; FT, fetal tone; AF, amniotic fluid; PL, placental grading. Maxi-
mal score, 12; minimal score, 0.
From ref. 75.

FETAL BIOPHYSICAL PROFILE AND FETAL SURVEILLANCE
(CLINICAL STUDIES)

Table 4 summarizes the published studies on the fetal biophysical profile. In an
initial study involving 216 patients (58) in which only the NST was used for management of the pregnancy, there was a direct correlation between an abnormal biophysical score and low 5-min Apgar scores, fetal distress in labor, and antepartum
and perinatal death rates. A combination of individual parameters in the profile
always resulted in improved positive predictive accuracy for both normal and abnormal test results. The maximal positive predictive accuracy for a normal test oc-

TABLE 4. Cumulative results of fetal biophysical profile for antepartum fetal assessment

Study population	No. of patients	High risk (%)	No. of tests				Crude PNM[a]		Corrected PNM[b]		False negative rate	
			Total	Normal (%)	Equivocal (%)	Abnormal (%)	No.	Rate	No.	Rate	No.	Rate
Manitoba general population 1979–1982 (34)	65,979	20	—	—	—	—	943	14.1	586	8.81	—	—
Manitoba prospective study (40)	12,620	100	26,257	97.52	1.72	0.76	93	7.37	24	1.90	8	0.643
Baskett et al. (1)	2,400	100	5,618	97.1	1.70	1.2	23	9.20	11	4.40	1	0.500
Platt et al. (57)	286	100	1,112	94	3.5	2.4	4	14.00	2	7.00	2	7.400
Schifrin et al. (70)	158	Most	240	—	—	—	7	44.00	2	12.60	1	6.300
Vintzileos et al. (75)	150	100	342	94.9	2	3.1	5	33.30	4[c]	26.60	0	0
Total	15,614	>90	33,569	>95	2	1	132	8.40	43	2.70	12	0.770

[a]PNM, perinatal mortality.
[b]Corrected to exclude death from lethal anomaly or Rh disease.
[c]All neonatal deaths.

curred when all variables were normal and the maximal predictive accuracy for abnormal tests occurred when all tests were abnormal. The perinatal death rate when all variables were normal (combined score = 10) was zero, as compared with 400 per 1,000 when all variables were abnormal (score = 0).

In a follow-up study, Manning et al. (35) reported 5,182 fetal biophysical profile scores in 1,184 consecutive high-risk pregnancies (38). Unlike earlier studies, the scores were used in clinical management according to the protocol outlined in Table 5. Only one fetus suffered unpredictable and unpreventable death, producing a true false negative rate of 0.8 per 1,000. Six perinatal deaths occurred, producing a corrected perinatal mortality rate of 5.06 per 1,000, which is a lower rate than would be predicted even in a low-risk population. In addition, 13 fetuses with major congenital anomalies were detected, eight of which were lethal.

Baskett et al. (1) reported a similar prospective study of 2,400 high-risk pregnancies. The perinatal death rates ranged from 0.3 per 1,000 when the biophysical score was 10 (false negative rate) to 292 per 1,000 when the score was 0. The corrected perinatal mortality rate was 2.8 per 1,000.

The largest reported antenatal experience has been that recently recorded by Manning et al. (39) and included a total of 26,257 tests performed in 12,620 referred high-risk pregnancies. Ninety-three perinatal deaths occurred (gross perinatal mortality rate of 7.37 per 1,000). Only 24 deaths occurred among structurally normal, nonisoimmunized fetuses who were presumed to be asphyxiated, i.e., corrected perinatal mortality rate 1.9 per 1,000. Eight structurally normal fetuses died within 1 week of a normal test result (corrected false negative rate of 0.634 per 1,000); 97.52% of tests were normal and only 0.75% received a score of 4 or less. The same authors managed 307 consecutive postterm pregnancies with biophysical profile scores performed twice weekly. Decreased AFV was considered one abnormal test. These scores accurately differentiated normal fetuses from those at risk

TABLE 5. *Biophysical profile scoring: management protocol*

Score	Interpretation	Management
10	Normal infant, low risk for chronic asphyxia	Repeat testing at weekly intervals. Repeat twice weekly in diabetics and patients ≥42 week gestation.
8	Normal infant, low risk for chronic asphyxia	Repeat testing at weekly intervals. Repeat testing twice weekly in diabetics and patients ≥42 week. Oligohydramnios an indication for delivery.
6	Suspect chronic asphyxia	Repeat testing in 4–6 hr. Deliver if oligohydramnios present.
4	Suspect chronic asphyxia	If ≥36 week and favorable, then deliver. If <36 week and L/S[a] 2.0, repeat test in 24 hr. If repeat score ≤4, deliver.
0–2	Strong suspicion of chronic asphyxia	Extend testing time to 120 min. If persistent score ≤4, deliver regardless of gestational age.

[a]L/S, amniotic fluid lecithin: spingomyelin.
From ref. 38.

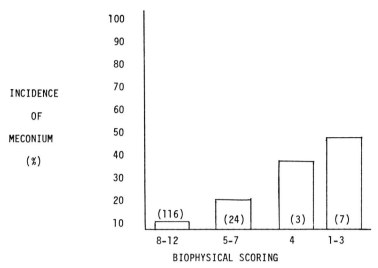

FIG. 1. The relationship of fetal biophysical scoring to incidence of fetal distress. Number of patients is shown in parentheses.

for intrauterine hypoxia. Thus, when the profile score is normal, waiting for spontaneous labor results in healthy neonates and much lower rates of cesarean section (15% versus 42% with "prophylactic" induction) (31).

Vintzileos et al. (75) reported their experience with 150 high-risk pregnancies and a total of 342 examinations. There was a strong correlation between abnormal scores and abnormal intrapartum fetal heart rate patterns, the presence of meconium and fetal distress during labor, and perinatal mortality. As previously reported, predictive values improved when individual variables were combined (Figs. 1–4). The predictive value of biophysical scoring with a nonreactive NST in 33 patients is shown in Table 6. Seven patients had a score of 1–3 and, as a group, accounted for 57.1% of neonatal deaths. Thus, a protocol for antepartum fetal evaluation was recommended by the authors as outlined in Fig. 5.

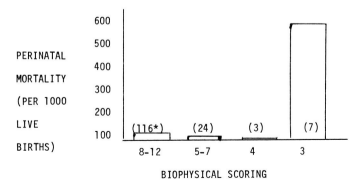

FIG. 2. The relationship of fetal biophysical scoring to perinatal mortality. Number of patients is shown in parentheses. *, one case of Potter's syndrome.

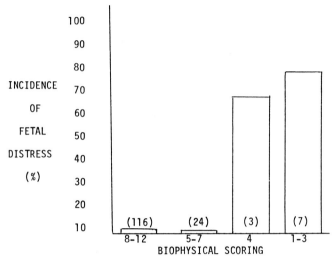

FIG. 3. The relationship of fetal biophysical scoring to incidence of meconium in labor. Number of patients is shown in parentheses.

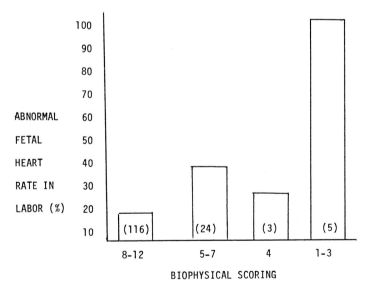

FIG. 4. The relationship of fetal biophysical scoring to incidence of abnormal fetal heart rate patterns in labor. Number of patients is shown in parentheses.

TABLE 6. *Predictive value of biophysical scoring with nonreactive nonstress test*[a]

No. of biophysical scores	Percentage	Score	Outcome
13/33	39.3	8–12	Good 100%
10/33	30.3	6–7	Good 80%; fetal distress 20%
3/33	9.0	4	Fetal distress 100%; no neonatal deaths
7/33	21.2	1–3	Good 14%; fetal distress 28.5%; neonatal deaths 57.1%

[a]Zero to one accelerations every 20 min. As the biophysical score decreases, the incidence of good outcome decreases while fetal distress increases (P < 0.00005).
From ref. 75.

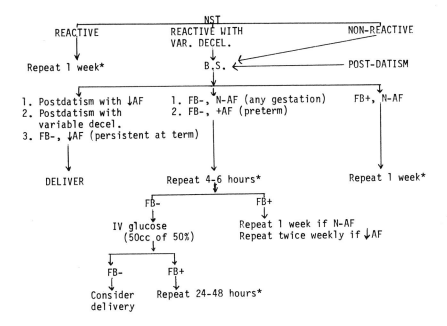

FIG. 5. Protocol of antepartum fetal evaluation. *, repeat fetal evaluation starting with nonstress test; ↓ AF, decreased amniotic fluid volume; N-AF, normal amniotic fluid volume; FB−, fetal breathing absent; FB+, fetal breathing present; BS, biophysical scoring.

These studies indicate the strong predictive value of the normal biophysical score for good neonatal outcome. In contrast, each abnormal variable was associated with a high false positive rate. The absence of fetal movements was the best predictor of abnormal heart rate patterns in labor (80%); the nonreactive NST was the best predictor of fetal distress (37.5%); and poor fetal tone was the best predictor of perinatal death rate.

Platt and co-workers (57), in a study of biophysical scores of 286 fetuses, reported a corrected perinatal mortality rate of 7.0 per 1,000 compared to 22.6 per 1,000 for all patients in their institution. Although they confirmed the predicted values of an abnormal score, they challenged the concept that the predictive value of a normal score exceeds that of the NST. In this regard, it is interesting to note that the combined studies of fetal biophysical profile scoring from other institutions have consistently yielded a false negative rate of less than 1 per 1,000, whereas cumulative studies of the NST alone yield a false negative rate of 4 to 6 per 1,000 (33). In a subsequent study, Platt et al. (60) randomized patients into two groups, one of which was managed by the NST alone and the other by biophysical profile. There was no significant difference in the negative predictive value, the sensitivity or the specificity of the two tests in the prediction of overall abnormal outcome as measured by perinatal mortality, the presence of fetal distress in labor, low 5-min Apgar score, or low birth weight. The corrected perinatal mortality in the group evaluated by biophysical profile was 5 per 1,000 as compared to 7 per 1,000 in the group managed by NST. A statistically significant difference was found only between the biophysical profile and NST for positive predictive value in the determination of whether a patient will have any abnormal outcome parameter.

FETAL BIOPHYSICAL PROFILE AND AMNIOTIC INFECTION

Vintzileos et al. (76) described a most intriguing use of the fetal biophysical profile. They assessed serially a modified fetal biophysical profile in 73 patients with ruptured membranes who were not in labor. They assumed that rupture of membranes alone should not alter the biophysical activity of the healthy fetus. A score of ≥8 was associated with an infection rate of 2.7%, whereas a score of ≤7 was associated with an infection rate of 93.7%. Thus, a low score of ≤7 was a good predictor of impending fetal infection, and the biophysical activities in this group were altered in a manner similar to that observed with uteroplacental insufficiency. The first manifestations of impending fetal infection were nonreactive NST and absent fetal breathing. It has been hypothesized that fetal breathing ceases secondary to release of prostaglandins by the bacteria responsible for the intra-amniotic infection. Loss of fetal motion and poor fetal tone were late manifestations. The presence of fetal breathing had the highest specificity for predicting the *absence* of fetal infection, i.e., no cases of fetal infection were identified when fetal breathing was present during the 24 hr before delivery. The hypothesized mechanism by which fetal infection diminishes fetal biophysical activities appears

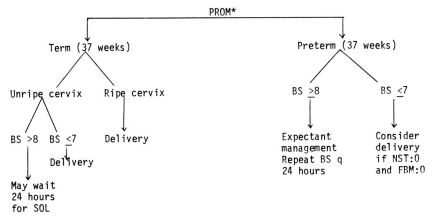

FIG. 6. Proposed protocol for management of premature rupture of the membranes. *, premature rupture of the membranes; BS, biophysical scoring; NST 0, nonreactive nonstress test; FMB 0, fetal breathing absent; SOL, spontaneous onset of labor.

to involve an increase of fetal oxygen demands, which lead to local tissue hypoxia and which in turn alter the central nervous system centers that control reflex biophysical activities (75). In view of these results, the authors recommended a protocol for management of patients with premature rupture of membranes as outlined in Fig. 6.

In a later prospective study of 58 patients with premature rupture of membranes (A.M. Vintzileos et al., *personal communication*), amniocentesis was compared with daily fetal biophysical profile for prediction of infection. The fetal biophysical profile had a sensitivity, specificity, positive predictive value, and negative predictive value of 80%, 97.6%, 92.3%, and 93.2%, respectively, in predicting infection as compared to 60%, 81.3%, 52.9%, and 85.3%, respectively, for results of Gram stain obtained at the time of amniocentesis.

ADVANTAGES OF FETAL BIOPHYSICAL PROFILE

Fetal assessment by means of the fetal biophysical profile offers several potential advantages in clinical practice:

1. The average time required to complete the test when performed by specially trained personnel is approximatley 20 min;
2. The test can be widely applied in a high-risk population;
3. Use of the score appears to result in a substantial reduction of false positive results. The rate of false negative results appears comparable to that observed with the use of the OCT;
4. The score may provide additional useful information with regard to the fetus, e.g., fetal number, placental location, and structure. The potential impact of this information is difficult to determine clearly but is likely to be beneficial.

However, it must be emphasized that at the present time, early ultrasound examination is the investigation of choice in the high-risk fetus;

5. Assurance of fetal well-being in high-risk pregnancies permits conservative management in many instances, thus minimizing the risk of failed induction and iatrogenic prematurity; and

6. The test is of potential benefit in the monitoring of patients with premature rupture of membranes for impending infection, thereby preventing neonatal and maternal sepsis as well as reducing the need for diagnostic amniocentesis.

LIMITATIONS OF THE FETAL BIOPHYSICAL PROFILE

1. The long-term developmental sequelae of fetuses with low biophysical scores is unknown;

2. The effect of duration and frequency of hypoxemia on the various CNS centers responsible for individual biophysical activities of the fetus is unknown; and

3. Further studies are required to determine whether there is any value in "disease-specific testing" with regard to timing, duration, and specific parameters to be tested.

SUMMARY

Antepartum detection, classification, determination of injury, and, ultimately, treatment of the high risk fetus forms the basis of modern fetal medicine. Recent experience indicates that the determination of fetal biophysical profile score appears to be an acceptable means for surveillance of fetal well-being. The assessment of multiple biophysical variables, combined with the observation of responses of the fetus to intrinsic and extrinsic stimuli, enables the differentiation of a normal sleeping fetus from an asphyxiated fetus. However, further studies of different variables or reclassification of existing variables will undoubtedly lead to refinement of the existing fetal biophysical score.

REFERENCES

1. Baskett, T.G., Gray, J.H., Prewett, S.J., et al. (1984): Antepartum fetal assessment using a fetal biophysical profile. *Am. J. Obstet. Gynecol.,* 148:630–633.
2. Boddy, K., and Dawes, G.S. (1975): Fetal breathing. *Br. Med. Bull.,* 31:3–7.
3. Braly, P., and Freeman, R.K. (1977): The significance of fetal heart rate reactivity with a positive oxytocin challenge test. *Obstet. Gynecol.,* 50:689–693.
4. Brar, H.S., Platt, L.D., DeVore, G.R., and Horenstein, J.H. (1986): Surveillance of pregnancies complicated with placenta previa using fetal umbilical velocimetry and placental resistance (Abstract). Presented at the 31st Annual Meeting of the American Institute of Ultrasound in Medicine, Las Vegas, NV, Sept. 16–19.
5. Brar, H.S., Platt, L.D., DeVore, G.R., and Horenstein, J.H. (1986): Analysis of placental vascular resistance using umbilical artery velocimetry in patients with late decelerations, *ACOG.* (Abstract).

6. Brown, R., and Patrick, J.E. (1981): The non-stress test: How long is enough? *Am. J. Obstet. Gynecol.*, 141:646–651.

7. Campbell, K. (1980): Ultradian rhythms in the human fetus during the last 10 weeks of gestation: A review. *Semin. Perinatol.*, 4:301–309.

8. Campbell, S., Griffin, D.R., Pearce, J.M., et al. (1983): New doppler technique for assessing utero placental blood flow. *Lancet*, 1:675–677.

9. Chamberlain, P.F., and Manning, F.A. (1984): Ultrasound: Fetal movements and fetal condition. In: *Principles and Practice in Obstetrics and Gynecology* (3d ed.). pp. 175–188. Appleton/Century Crofts, New York.

10. Chamberlain, P.F., Manning, F.A., Morrison, I., et al. (1984): Ultrasound evaluation of amniotic fluid volume. I. The relationship of marginal and decreased amniotic fluid volume to perinatal outcome. *Am. J. Obstet. Gynecol.*, 150:245–249.

11. Chamberlain, P.F., Manning, F.A., Morrison, I., et al. (1984): Circadian rhythm in bladder volume in the term human fetus. *Obstet. Gynecol.*, 674:657–660.

12. Chamberlain, P.F., Manning, F.A., Morrison, I., et al. (1984): Ultrasound evaluation of amniotic fluid: II. The relationship of increased amniotic fluid to perinatal outcome. *Am. J. Obstet. Gynecol.*, 150:250–254.

13. Christie, G.B., and Cudmore, D.W. (1974): The oxytocin challenge tests. *Am. J. Obstet. Gynecol.*, 118:327–330.

14. Cohn, H.E., Sachs, E.T., Heyman, M.A., et al. (1974): Cardiovascular responses to hypoxemia and acidemia in fetal lambs. *Am. J. Obstet. Gynecol.*, 120:817–824.

15. Collea, J.V., and Holls, W.M. (1982): The contraction stress test. *Obstet. Gynecol.*, 25:707–717.

16. Dawes, G.S., Fox, H.E., Leduc, B.M., et al. (1972): Respiratory movements and rapid eye movement sleep in the fetal lamb. *J. Physiol. (Lond.)*, 220:119–143.

17. DeVore, G.R., Donnelstein, R.L., Kleinman, C.S., Platt, L.D., and Hobbins, J.C. (1982): Fetal echocardiography. I. Normal anatomy using realtime directed M-mode ultrasound. *Am. J. Obstet. Gynecol.*, 144:249–260.

18. Divon, M.Y., Platt, L.D., Cantrell, C.J., et al. (1985): Evoked fetal startle response. A possible intrauterine neurological examination. *Am. J. Obstet. Gynecol.*, 153:454–456.

19. Druzin, M., Gratacos, J., Keegan, K., et al. (1981): Antepartum fetal heart rate testing. VII. Significance of fetal bradycardia. *Am. J. Obstet. Gynecol.*, 139:194–198.

20. Evertson, L.R., Gauthier, R.J., and Collea, J.V. (1978): Fetal demise following negative contraction stress tests. *Obstet. Gynecol.*, 51:671–673.

21. Evertson, L.R., Gauthier, R.J., Schifrin, B.S., et al. (1979): Antepartum fetal heart rate testing. I. Evaluation of the nonstress test. *Am. J. Obstet. Gynecol.*, 133:29–33.

22. Flood, B., and Lee, J. (1978): Fetal death during a negative contraction stress test. *Obstet. Gynecol. (Suppl.)*, 52:41–52.

23. Freeman, J.M., and Brann, A.W., Jr. (1977): Central nervous system disturbances. In: *Neonatal-Perinatal Medicine. Disease of the Fetus and Infant*, edited by R.E. Behrman, p. 799. Mosby, St. Louis.

24. Freeman, R.K., Anderson, G., Dorchester, W., et al. (1982): A prospective multi-institutional study of antepartum fetal heart rate monitoring. Risk of perinatal mortality and morbidity according to AFHR test results. *Am. J. Obstet. Gynecol.*, 143:771–777.

25. Gauthier, R.J., Evertson, L.R., and Paul, R.H. (1979): Antepartum fetal heart rate testing. II. Intrapartum fetal heart rate testing and neonatal outcome following a positive contraction stress test. *Am. J. Obstet. Gynecol.*, 133:34–39.

26. Golde, S.H., Petrucha, R., Meade, K.W., and Platt, L.D. (1982): Fetal lung maturity: The adjunctive use of ultrasound. *Am. J. Obstet. Gynecol.*, 142:445–447.

27. Grannum, P.A.T., Berkowitz, R.L., and Hobbins, J.C. (1979): The ultrasonic changes in the maturity placenta and their relationship to fetal pulmonic maturity. *Am. J. Obstet. Gynecol.*, 133:915–922.

28. Humphrey, T. (1978): Function of the nervous system during prenatal life. In: *Perinatal Physiology*, edited by S. Uwe, p. 651. Plenum, New York.

29. Ianniruberto, A., and Tejani, E. (1981): Ultrasonographic study of fetal movements. *Semin. Perinatol.*, 5:175–181.

30. Johnson, J., Harman, C.R., Lange, I.R., et al. (1988): Fetal biophysical profile scoring in the management of post date pregnancy. A prospective study. *Am. J. Obstet. Gynecol. (in press)*.

31. Johnson, J.M., Harman, C.R., Lange, I.R., and Manning, F.A. (1986): Biophysical profile scoring in the management of the post term pregnancy. An analysis of 307 patients. *Am. J. Obstet. Gynecol.*, 154:269–273.

32. Kaufman, A.J., Fleisher, A.C., Thieme, G., et al. (1985): Separated choric amnion and elevated chorion. Sonographic features and clinical significance. *J. Ultrasound Med.*, 4:119–125.

33. Lavery, J.P. (1982): Non-stress fetal heart rate testing. *Clin. Obstet. Gynecol.*, 25:689–705.

34. Manning, F.A., (1985): Assessment of fetal condition and risk: Analysis of single and combined biophysical variable monitoring. *Semin. Perinatol.*, 9:168–183.

35. Manning, F.A., Baskett, T.F., Morrison, I., et al. (1981): Fetal biophysical profile scoring. A prospective study in 1,184 high risk patients. *Am. J. Obstet. Gynecol.*, 140:289–294.

36. Manning, F.A., Hill, L.M., and Platt, L.D. (1981): Qualitative amniotic fluid volume determination by ultrasonic antepartum detection of intra uterine growth retardation. *Am. J. Obstet. Gynecol.*, 139(3):254–258.

37. Manning, F.A., Lange, I.R., Morrison, I., et al. (1984): Fetal biophysical profile score and the NST: A comparative trial. *Obstet. Gynecol.*, 64:326–331.

38. Manning, F.A., Morrison, I., and Lange, I.R. (1981): Fetal biophysical profile and scoring: A prospective study of 1,184 high risk patients. *Am. J. Obstet. Gynecol.*, 140:289.

39. Manning, F.A., Morrison, I., Lange, I.R., et al. (1985): Fetal assessment based on fetal biophysical profile scoring: Experience in 12,620 referred high risk pregnancies. I. Perinatal morbidity by frequency and etiology. *Am. J. Obstet. Gynecol.*, 151:343–350.

40. Manning, F.A., Morrison, I., Lange, I.R., and Harman, C. (1982): Antepartum determination of fetal health composite biophysical profile scoring (Symposium on fetal monitoring). *Clin. Perinatol.*, 9(2).

41. Manning, F.A., and Platt, L.D. (1979): Qualitative assessment of amniotic fluid volume—A rapid screen for detecting the small for gestational age fetus (abstract). In: *Proceedings of the Twenty-sixth Annual Meeting of the Society for Gynecological Investigation*, p. 128. Society for Gynecological Investigation, San Diego.

42. Manning, F.A., and Platt, L.D. (1979): Fetal breathing movements and the abnormal contraction stress test. *Am. J. Obstet. Gynecol.*, 133:590–593.

43. Manning, F.A., and Platt, L.D. (1980): Human fetal breathing monitoring—Clinical considerations. *Semin. Perinatol.*, 4:311–318.

44. Manning, F.A., Platt, L.D., and Sipos, L. (1979): Fetal movements in human pregnancies in the third trimester. *Am. J. Obstet. Gynecol.*, 54:699–702.

45. Manning, F.A., Platt, L.D., and Sipos, L. (1980): Antepartum fetal evaluation. Development of a fetal biophysical profile score. *Am. J. Obstet. Gynecol.*, 136:787–795.

46. Manning, F.A., Platt, L.D., Sipos, L., et al. (1979): Fetal breathing movements and the non-stress test in high risk pregnancies. *Am. J. Obstet. Gynecol.*, 135:511–515.

47. Martin, C.B., and Schifrin, B.S. (1976): In: *Perinatal Fetal Monitoring*, edited by S. Aladjem and A. Brown. C.V. Mosby Co, St. Louis.

48. Martin, C.B., Jr. (1981): On behavioral states in human fetus. *J. Reprod. Med.*, 26:425–432.

49. Morrison, I. (1985): Perinatal morbidity. *Semin. Perinatol.*, 9(4).

50. Patrick, J.E., Campbell, K., Carmichael, L., et al. (1980): A definition of human fetal apnea and the distribution of fetal apneic intervals during the last 10 weeks of pregnancy. *Am. J. Obstet. Gynecol.*, 136:471–477.

51. Patrick, J.E., Campbell, K., Carmichael, I., et al. (1982): Patterns of gross fetal body movements over 24 hour observation intervals during the last 10 weeks of pregnancy measured with a real time scanner. *Am. J. Obstet. Gynecol.*, 142:363–371.

52. Patrick, J.E., and Challis, J.R.G. (1980): Measurement of human fetal breathing in healthy pregnancies using real time ultrasound. *Semin. Perinatol.*, 4:275–286.

53. Patrick, J., Fetherston, W., Vick, H., et al. (1978): Human fetal breathing movements and gross body movements at weeks 34–35 of gestation. *Am. J. Obstet. Gynecol.*, 130:693–699.

54. Petrucha, R., Golde, S.H., and Platt, L.D. (1982): Real-time ultrasound of the placenta in assessment of fetal pulmonic maturity. *Am. J. Obstet. Gynecol.*, 142:463–467.

55. Petrucha, R.A., Golde, S.H., and Platt, L.D. (1983): The use of ultrasound in the prediction of fetal lung maturity. *Am. J. Obstet. Gynecol.*, 144:931–934.

56. Phelan, J.P., Platt, L.D., and Yeh, S. (1985): The role of ultrasound assessment of amniotic fluid volume in the management of the post date pregnancy. *Am. J. Obstet. Gynecol.*, 151:304–308.

57. Platt, L.D., Eglington, G.S., Sipos, L., et al. (1983): Further experience with the fetal biophysical profile score. *Obstet. Gynecol.*, 61:480–485.

58. Platt, L.D., and Manning, F.A. (1980): Fetal breathing movements. An update. *Clin. Perinatol.*, 7:423–433.

59. Platt, L.D., Manning, F.A., and LeMay, M. (1978): Fetal breathing movements: The relationship to fetal condition. *Am. J. Obstet. Gynecol.*, 132:514–518.

60. Platt, L.D., Walla, C.A., Paul, R.H., et al. (1985): A prospective trial of fetal biophysical profile versus the non stress test in the management of high risk pregnancies. *Am. J. Obstet. Gynecol.*, 153:624–633.

61. Powell-Phillips, W.D., and Towell, M.E. (1980): Abnormal fetal heart rate associated with congenital anomalies. *Br. J. Obstet. Gynaecol.*, 87:270–274.

62. Ray, M., Freeman, R., Pine, S., et al. (1972): Clinical experiences with the oxytocin challenge test. *Am. J. Obstet. Gynecol.*, 114:1–9.

63. Rayburn, W.F. (1982): Antepartum fetal assessment: Monitoring fetal activity. *Clin. Perinatol.*, 9:231.

64. Rochard, F., Schifrin, B.S., Goupil, F., et al. (1976): Nonstressed fetal heart rate monitoring in the antepartum period. *Am. J. Obstet. Gynecol.*, 126:699–706.

65. Ruckebusch, Y., Gaujoux, M., and Eghbali, B. (1977): Sleep cycles and kinesis in the fetal lamb. *Electroencephalogr. Clin. Neurophysiol.*, 42:226–237.

66. Rutherford, S.E., Smith, C.V., Broussard, P., et al. (1986): The four quadrant assessment of amniotic fluid "volume": An adjourn to antepartum fetal heart rate testing (Abstract). In: *Proceedings of the 6th Meeting for the Society of Perinatal Obstetricians*, vol. 53. San Antonio, Texas.

67. Sadovsky, E., and Polishuk, W.Z. (1977): Fetal movements *in utero:* Nature, assessment, prognostic value, timing of delivery. *Obstet. Gynecol.*, 50:49–55.

68. Schifrin, B.S. (1979): The rationale of antepartum fetal heart rate monitoring. *J. Reprod. Med.*, 23:213–221.

69. Schifrin, B.S., Foye, G., Amatao, J., et al. (1981): Routine fetal heart rate monitoring in the antepartum period. *Obstet. Gynecol.*, 57:320.

70. Schifrin, B.S., Guntes, V., Gergely, R.C., et al. (1981): The role of real time scanning in antenatal fetal surveillance. *Am. J. Obstet. Gynecol.*, 140:525–530.

71. Smith, C.V., Phelan, J.P., and Paul, R.H. (1986): Fetal acoustic stimulation testing. III. The predictive value of a reactive test (Abstract). In: *Proceedings of the 6th Annual Meeting for the Society of Perinatal Obstetricians*, vol. 54. San Antonio, Texas.

72. Staisch, K.J., Westlake, J.R., and Bashore, R.A. (1980): Blind oxytocin challenge test and perinatal outcome. *Am. J. Obstet. Gynecol.*, 138:399–403.

73. Tahilramaney, M.P., Golde, S.H., and Platt, L.D. (1988): The use of femur length by ultrasound in the prediction of fetal lung maturity. *Am. J. Obstet. Gynecol. (in press)*.

74. Timor-Tritsch, T.E., Dierker, L.J., Sador, I., et al. (1978): Fetal movement associated with fetal heart rate accelerations and decelerations. *Am. J. Obstet. Gynecol.*, 131:276–280.

75. Vintzileos, A.M., Campbell, W.A., Ingardia, C.J., and Nochimson, D.J. (1983): The fetal biophysical profile and its predictive value. *Obstet. Gynecol.*, 62:271–278.

76. Vintzileos, A.M., Campbell, W.A., Nochimson, D.J., et al. (1985): The fetal biophysical profile in patients with premature rupture of membranes—An early predictor of fetal infection. *Am. J. Obstet. Gynecol.*, 152:510–516.

Fetal Neurology, edited by
A. Hill and J.J. Volpe.
Raven Press, New York © 1989.

Commentary on Chapter 6

*Alan Hill and **Joseph J. Volpe

*Division of Neurology, Department of Paediatrics, University of British Columbia,
British Columbia's Children's Hospital, Vancouver, British Columbia, Canada V6H 3V4;
and **Division of Pediatric Neurology, Washington University School of Medicine,
St. Louis, Missouri 63110

Recent experience has demonstrated that irrespective of the method used for assessment of fetal well-being, e.g., nonstress test, contraction stress test, or determination of fetal movement, a single abnormal test predicts abnormal outcome accurately in generally less than 30% of cases (6). Variability in results most commonly reflects alterations in sleep-wake cycles of the fetus and presumed variations in patterns of hypoxic-ischemic cerebral insult.

At the present time, the optimal method for antepartum identification of the fetus at risk for cerebral injury is unknown. Such a method should have the capacity to detect the diverse causes of fetal compromise, including major developmental anomalies as well as fetal asphyxia. A recent approach to reduction of this diagnostic uncertainty involves measurement of several fetal biophysical parameters in concert, i.e., a composite fetal biophysical profile. In the preceding chapter, Brar and Platt discussed the fetal biophysical score, which is based on real-time ultrasound assessment and the scoring of five fetal variables. The latter includes four variables that reflect the acute fetal condition: fetal movement, fetal breathing, fetal heart rate reactivity, and fetal tone, in addition to a fifth variable, i.e., amniotic fluid volume, that is an indicator of long-term fetal condition.

Several studies support the notion that monitoring of fetal biophysical activities may play a major role in the early identification and prevention of fetal asphyxia. Thus, in a study of 12,620 high-risk pregnancies monitored by fetal biophysical profile, the overall fetal mortality rate fell significantly along with the asphyxial fetal death rate, whereas the relative proportion of fetal death caused by congenital anomalies more than doubled (5). The rationale for use of the biophysical profile in the assessment of fetal asphyxia is strengthened by the fact that the various measures reflect activity of several levels of the central nervous system, including cerebrum, diencephalon, and brainstem. It is known from experimental animal studies that the manifestations of fetal asphyxia vary depending on the severity, duration, and chronicity of the asphyxial insult and on the gestational age of the fetus. Although the variations in sensitivity of specific regions of the fetal brain exposed to acute, total asphyxia or prolonged, partial asphyxia have been documented extensively in experimental animal studies (2,7–9), these variables remain to be defined in the human fetus. Careful assessment of abnormalities of the parameters in the biophysical profile may provide valuable insight into patterns of cerebral injury associated with hypoxic-ischemic insults in the human fetus.

Similarly, it is not clear whether increasing severity of hypoxic-ischemic insult results in progressive loss of individual biophysical functions or whether all functions are lost simultaneously after a critical level of insult is reached. Preliminary observations of alterations in the biophysical profile support a graded and individualized response, i.e., fetal breathing movements disappear earlier in the course of hypoxemia than does fetal movement (5,6).

With respect to chronic asphyxial insult, the unique protective reflex of the fetus whereby there is redistribution of cardiac output from nonvital organs (lung, kidney, gut) toward vital organs (brain, heart, adrenals, placenta) causes decreased urine production and lung liquid flow with eventual diminished amniotic fluid production and oligohydramnios. This physiological phenomenon provides the basis for the value of measurement of amniotic fluid volume as an indicator of chronic fetal condition. However, at the present time, the usefulness of this measurement is limited because, although amniotic fluid volume is known to vary throughout gestation, longitudinal studies are not available and the time scale of normal variation is unknown. Furthermore, the variation of amniotic fluid volume with multiple pregnancies has not been established (3).

The fetal biophysical profile may find further application in the study of fetal recovery following hypoxic-ischemic insult. At present, the temporal aspects of the recovery of fetal central nervous system function following asphyxia have not been clearly defined. However, it appears that recovery of biophysical function may be delayed relative to the recovery of blood gases (1).

The precise advantages of the biophysical profile over individual fetal biophysical parameters for prediction of outcome have not been established. Several studies suggest that the biophysical profile has a higher positive predictive accuracy than the nonstress test, for example (4,10). However, although the fetal biophysical profile is a reasonably accurate method for detection of fetal anomalies as well as of fetal asphyxial states, its false positive predictive accuracy of 43.5% is still far from ideal (4). It remains to be determined whether the use of additional variables or refinement of existing variables will improve the predictive accuracy of the technique. With further experience, perhaps alterations in fetal sleep-wake states, determined by peristalsis and evoked reflex responses, may be included in the assessment. Nevertheless, the principle that the greatest accuracy in prediction of fetal compromise is achieved when multiple fetal and environmental parameters are considered in combination will likely remain valid.

REFERENCES

1. Boddy, K., Dawes, J.S., Fisher, R., et al. (1974): Fetal respiratory movements, electrocortical and cardiovascular responses to hypoxemia and hypercapnia in sheep. *J. Physiol. (Lond.)*, 243:599–618.
2. Brann, A.W., and Myers, R.E. (1975): Central nervous system findings in the newborn monkey following severe *in utero* partial asphyxia. *Neurology*, 25:327–338.
3. Chamberlain, P. (1985): Amniotic fluid volume: Ultrasound assessment and clinical significance. *Semin. Perinatol.*, 9:163–167.
4. Manning, F.A., Lange, I.R., Morrison, I., and Harman, C.R. (1984): Fetal biophysical profile score and the nonstress test: A comparative trial. *Obstet. Gynecol.*, 64:326–331.
5. Manning, F.A., Morrison, I., Lange, I.R., et al. (1985): Fetal assessment based on fetal biophysical profile scoring: Experience in 12,620 referred high risk pregnancies. I. Perinatal mortality by frequency and etiology. *Am. J. Obstet. Gynecol.*, 151:343–350.
6. Manning, F.A., Platt, L.D., and Sipos, L. (1980): Antepartum fetal evaluation: Development of a fetal biophysical profile score. *Am. J. Obstet. Gynecol.*, 136:787–795.
7. Myers, R.E., (1972): Two patterns of perinatal brain damage and their conditions of occurrence. *Am. J. Obstet. Gynecol.*, 112:246–276.
8. Myers, R.E. (1975): Four patterns of perinatal brain damage and their conditions of occurrence in primates. *Adv. Neurol.*, 10:223–234.
9. Myers, R.E. (1975): Fetal asphyxia due to umbilical cord compression. *Biol. Neonate*, 26:21–43.
10. Platt, L.D., Walla, C.A., Paul, R.H., et al. (1985): A prospective trial of the fetal biophysical profile versus the nonstress test in the management of high-risk pregnancies. *Am. J. Obstet. Gynecol.*, 153:624–633.

Fetal Neurology, edited by
A. Hill and J.J. Volpe.
Raven Press, New York © 1989.

7

Fetoplacental and Uteroplacental Blood Flow in Pregnancy

*Dermot E. FitzGerald and **Bernard T. Stuart

*Angiology Research Group, Vascular Medicine Laboratory, St. Mary's Hospital, Dublin 20, Ireland; and **Coombe Lying-in Hospital, Dublin 8, Ireland*

In common with all embryos that employ hemochorial placentation, the human fetus depends for its survival on the early establishment and maintenance of adequate vascular communications with the maternal circulation. Toward this end, by the third week after implantation, angiogenesis within the placental villi is sufficiently developed to establish a fetoplacental circulation in intimate contact with the maternal uteroplacental vessels. Because of their inaccessibility, little was known until recently about the vascular physiology of these circulations, and most of the knowledge that was available was inferred from animal studies that used invasive techniques unsuitable for use in the human (4,8,14). The first attempt to measure umbilical blood flow used Ludwig's stromuhr on the exteriorized fetal lamb. Barcroft et al. (2) measured the cardiac output of seven exteriorized fetal goats by means of a "cardiometer," a tambour that recorded stroke output, and calculated that cardiac output per unit fetal weight remains constant throughout pregnancy at 180 ml/kg/min. The first systematic observations on fetoplacental blood flow at various gestational ages were those of Cooper et al. (12), who calculated that flow increased with advancing gestational age to reach a value of 104 to 279 ml/kg/min in the fetal lamb in good condition near term. Dawes and Mott (14) obtained a flow rate of 104 ml/kg/min with a velodyne flowmeter inserted into the umbilical vein of fetal lambs at term and a rate of 170 ml/kg/min with a cannulated electromagnetic flowmeter.

The first method of measuring umbilical blood flow *in utero* was developed by Barron et al. (3), who used a constant infusion technique based on the Fick principle of steady-state diffusion. More recently, radioisotopes have been used by several investigators to study both umbilical blood flow and the regional distribution of fetal cardiac output (10,35,38).

The first successful measurement of umbilical blood flow in humans was made on early aborted fetuses by Assali et al. (1), who used an electromagnetic flow-meter to obtain mean flow rates of 110 ml/kg/min on 10 fetuses of between 10 and 28 weeks gestation. Other studies on fetoplacental blood flow in the mature human fetus were performed immediately after delivery because no method was available at that time to assess fetal blood flow *in utero* (31,41).

Although Doppler ultrasound was developed some 30 years ago (40) and has been extensively used in the investigation of the peripheral circulation in the adult, it was not until 1977 that continuous wave Doppler ultrasound was employed to study fetoplacental blood flow *in utero* by a noninvasive technique (19). The fol-lowing year McCallum et al. (31) used range-gated, pulsed Doppler ultrasound to obtain sonograms of umbilical blood flow. In 1980 Stuart et al. (43), using contin-uous wave Doppler ultrasound, published the first systematic study of fetoplacental blood flow throughout normal pregnancy. There are now numerous centers using the same or similar techniques to study fetal blood flow, although its place in prac-tical clinical obstetrics remains to be established.

Pulsed Doppler ultrasound, which can be depth gated, has been combined with ultrasonic imaging to permit blood flow signals to be obtained from any vessel that can be visualized. This technique has been employed to study the volume of blood flow in the fetal aorta (18) and umbilical vein (24) and qualitative blood flow in the arcuate arteries of the uteroplacental circulation (7). Initial studies on the feto-placental circulation with continuous wave Doppler ultrasound (21) and on the uteroplacental circulation with pulsed Doppler ultrasound (25) have suggested that these techniques may be of value in assessing intrauterine growth retardation (IUGR), although further study is needed before they can be applied to clinical practice.

THE DOPPLER EFFECT

In 1842 Christian Doppler, an Austrian physicist, described the effect of motion on the frequency of wave emissions. This effect, the Doppler effect, also pertains to ultrasound waves and means that when an ultrasound beam strikes a moving reflector the frequency of the reflected beam is slightly altered in accordance with the Doppler formula.

$$f = 2 \cdot F \cdot V \cdot \cos \theta / C$$

where f is the frequency of the Doppler shift, F the emitted frequency, V the ve-locity of the reflector, C the velocity of ultrasound in tissue, and θ the angle of the intersection of the emitted ultrasonic beam with the reflector. If the target is moving toward the source of the ultrasound, the Doppler shift will have a positive value; if the movement is away from the source of ultrasound, the Doppler shift will be negative. Red blood cells act as ultrasonic reflectors, and therefore ultra-sound reflected from moving blood will exhibit a Doppler shift.

With a large reflector, such as the fetal heart, the ultrasound beam has to be at right angles to the direction of movement in order to detect the reflected Doppler shifted signals. However, because the size of a red blood cell is small (7 μm) in relation to the wavelength of ultrasound commonly used in blood flow detection (300 μm at 5 MHz), the ultrasound energy is scattered omnidirectionally so that the emitting and receiving transducers of continuous wave (CW) Doppler blood flow detectors can be sited adjacent to each other (Fig. 1). Ultrasonic blood flow detectors can use either CW or pulsed wave (PW) Doppler ultrasound.

Continuous Wave Doppler Ultrasound

The simplest form of Doppler ultrasound is CW, where two transducers, an emitting transducer and a receiving transducer, are located side by side, usually inclined slightly toward each other. In this device, ultrasound is emitted continuously from one transducer, and the resultant Doppler shifted signals are constantly received by the other (Fig. 2). Instruments of this type work in a fashion analogous to shining a torch in the dark in that reflections will be received from all moving objects in the path of the beam and no ranging is possible. In addition, it is generally impossible to measure the beam/vessel angle (θ of the Doppler equation) so that it is not possible with CW Doppler ultrasound to make any quantitative measurements of absolute Doppler shift values, blood velocity, or volume flow. In spite of these limitations, CW Doppler ultrasound has been used extensively for nearly 30 years and has yielded much useful information on qualitative blood flow in peripheral vessels. In most applications, these disadvantages are more than offset by the relative inexpensiveness and simplicity of the instrument and the ease with which it can be used. CW Doppler ultrasound is perfectly satisfactory for the qualitative study of fetoplacental and uteroplacental blood flow.

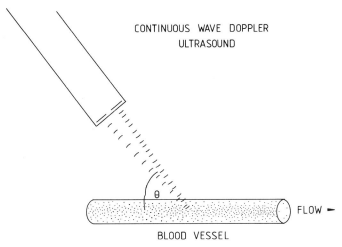

FIG. 1. Doppler blood flow detection. The angle θ is the angle between the Doppler beam and the axis of flow.

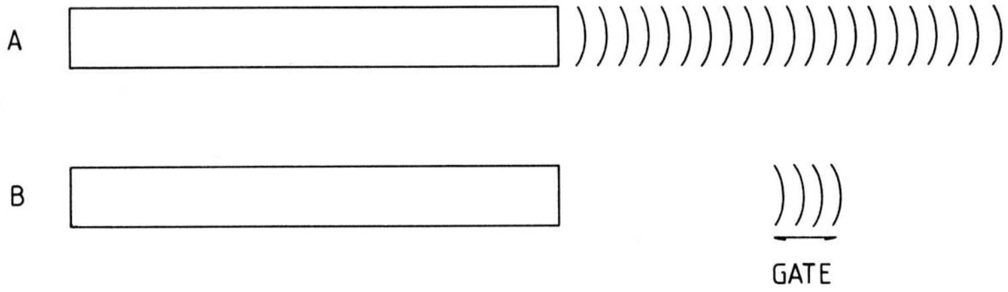

FIG. 2. A continuous wave Doppler beam **(A)** receives signals from everything in the path of the beam, whereas in a pulsed Doppler system **(B)** both the range and sample volume (gate) can be varied.

Pulsed Wave Doppler Ultrasound

PW Doppler ultrasound resembles PW imaging ultrasound in that a single transducer is used to both emit and receive the ultrasonic waves. In the Doppler instrument ultrasound is emitted in short pulses and a time delay is applied before the transducer is switched to the receive mode to obtain the back-scattered Doppler shifted signals (Fig. 2).

Because the velocity of ultrasound in biological tissue is fairly constant at approximately 1,540 m/sec, for each 10-μsec time delay applied, the ultrasonic beam will have traveled 15 mm, representing 7.5 mm to the target and 7.5 mm back to the receiving transducer. Thus, if a 100-μsec time delay was applied, Doppler shifted signals would be obtained only from structures lying at a depth of 7.5 cm. PW Doppler ultrasound can therefore be range or depth gated to obtain signals only from a selected distance from the transducer. A further advantage of PW Doppler ultrasound is that by varying the duration for which the transducer is in the receive mode (the gate), the sample size from which Doppler signals can be obtained is readily adjustable. By adjusting the size of the gate, it is therefore possible to obtain Doppler signals from across the entire lumen of a vessel or from selected points within the vessel.

Combining a PW Doppler ultrasound transducer with a linear array real-time imaging ultrasound device (18) produced a duplex scanner capable of imaging the blood vessel from which Doppler signals were being obtained and of measuring the beam/vessel angle. This combination made it possible to obtain quantitative measurements of Doppler shift (blood velocity). By gradually stepping the gate across the lumen of the vessel, the velocity of flow at many points within the vessel could be measured (velocity profile) and mean blood flow velocity calculated. By measuring the diameter of the vessel with imaging ultrasound (using either M- or B-mode), it was then possible to calculate volume flow from the equation

$$Q = vr^2$$

where Q represents volume flow in ml/min, v mean velocity, and r the radius of the blood vessel.

PW Doppler instruments do, however, have several inherent disadvantages when compared with the simpler CW devices. They are far more costly and complex to operate. The depth from which signals can be obtained is limited by the pulse repetition frequency (PRF) of the instrument, which is itself optimized, depending on the expected maximum Doppler shift (blood velocity). At a typical PRF of 5 to 7.5 MHz, the range of these instruments is limited to 10 to 15 cm. A more serious problem, however, is the limited accuracy of these instruments in the measurement of either velocity or flow caused by the inherent difficulty of accurately measuring the beam/vessel angle and, more particularly, the diameter of the blood vessel. Most duplex systems operate with an angle of insonation of 50° to 55°, and in practice, the error in measuring velocity does not exceed 10% (11). Because the radius of the vessel is squared in calculating volume flow, small errors in the measurement of vessel diameter result in large inaccuracies in volume flow estimation, such that an error of 0.5 mm in the diameter of a 4-mm vessel results in a 23% inaccuracy in estimation of volume of flow. For these reasons, although velocity measurements may be acceptably accurate, volume flow estimations are probably too inaccurate to be clinically useful.

Processing Doppler Signals

The output from a Doppler instrument can be represented by the equation

$$f = F_1 - F_0$$

where f is the Doppler shift frequency, F_1 the emitted frequency, and F_0 the reflected frequency. Where the reflector is a single structure, F will have a single constant value corresponding to the velocity of the reflector. Blood flowing in a vessel, however, consists of many cells, with each cell acting as an omnidirectional scatterer of ultrasonic energy and traveling at many different velocities. As each velocity will yield a different Doppler shift value, a Doppler blood flow signal is a complex signal of many frequencies representing different blood flow velocities. Conveniently, using Doppler ultrasound with a frequency of 2 to 10 MHz, physiological blood flow velocities yield Doppler shift frequencies that are within the audible spectrum to the human ear. Much information can be obtained by a trained observer listening to such blood velocity signals, although serious study of Doppler signals requires more complex analysis, which is usually performed on either a zero-cross detector or frequency spectrum analyzer.

Zero-cross Detector

The zero-cross detector or "velocimeter" is a simple instrument that displays the instantaneous mean of all received Doppler frequencies. Although such instruments are relatively inexpensive, they have several inherent disadvantages that limit their practical usefulness. In particular where blood flow signals are of poor quality (high signal-to-noise ratio) or where there is a large variation in observed blood velocities (broad Doppler spectrum), the zero-cross detector will tend to overestimate the average velocity. In addition, the zero-cross detector yields no information concerning the velocity distribution of cells within the blood vessel. For these reasons, formal spectral analysis is the preferred method of processing Doppler signals.

The velocity profile across a small artery (e.g., the umbilical artery) is such that the cells at the center of the stream have a greater velocity than those at the vessel wall that are slowed because of viscous drag (Fig. 3). The velocities may vary between zero and V_{max}; the corresponding Doppler shifted frequencies will vary between zero and F_{max} and may in addition have both positive and negative components. Doppler ultrasound signals are therefore complex signals containing many different frequency components.

Frequency Spectrum Analysis

A spectrum analyzer yields information on all the frequencies contained in the Doppler signal. The output is in the form of a sonogram, a display of frequency (velocity) plotted against time (Fig. 4). Early frequency analyzers (Kay Sonograph 6061B) printed hard copies, off line, on heat-sensitive paper, whereas more recent examples (Doptek 9012) have a variety of output options including audio, TV monitor, computer interface, and direct printer output. These instruments can also display both positive and negative Doppler shifts and can therefore display both forward and receding blood flow when used with directionally sensitive Doppler devices.

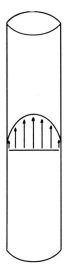

FIG. 3. Blood cells at the center of the stream have a greater velocity than those at the vessel wall, giving a roughly parabolic velocity profile.

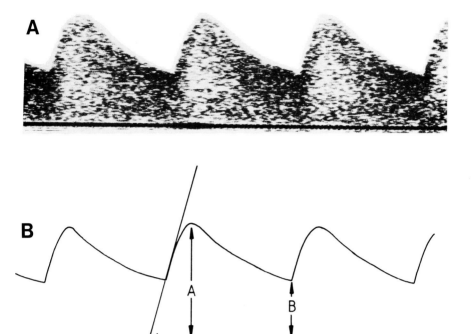

FIG. 4. The sonogram **(A)** plots all the frequencies in the Doppler spectrum against time. The maximum frequency envelope **(B)** yields a blood velocity waveform.

The Sonogram

The sonogram is a display of frequency (velocity) on the ordinate plotted against time on the abscissa (Fig. 4A). The intensity (amplitude) of the signal corresponds to the number of red blood cells traveling at the corresponding velocity and is usually displayed as either shades of gray or in different colors. The maximum frequency envelope of the sonogram (Fig. 4B) yields a blood velocity waveform (BVW) containing information on vascular hemodynamics.

The shape of the waveform reflects the characteristics of the circulation from which it was obtained, and whereas arterial flow is pulsatile, venous flow is continuous and nonpulsatile (Fig. 5), although frequently modulated by breathing.

Cardiac contraction causes a force in the form of pressure to be applied to the blood cells in the arterial tree. A high forward pressure gradient is generated, and the cells accelerate rapidly and produce the rising slope of the waveform. The rate of acceleration depends on the density of the blood, elasticity of the vessel wall, and the pressure gradient generated (32). As the pressure wave moves distally, the gradient is reversed, acceleration ceases, and the blood reaches its greatest systolic velocity. The shape of the diastolic component of the waveform depends on peripheral vascular impedance that determines the magnitude of pressure waves reflected from the peripheral circulation. Where peripheral resistance is high, large

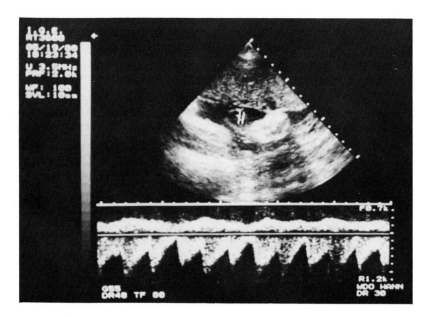

FIG. 5. Blood velocity signals obtained from the umbilical vessels with a pulsed Doppler system. The on-line spectrum analyzer is displaying both umbilical venous *(upper)* and arterial *(lower)* signals.

reflected pressure waves cause rapid deceleration with the waveform returning to the baseline (zero flow line). In high resistance peripheral vessels (such as the femoral artery), the reflected pressure waves may be of such magnitude as to cause a temporary reversal of flow so that blood flows back toward the heart (Fig. 6). Where peripheral resistance is low, however, forward flow continues throughout diastole with the waveform remaining elevated above the baseline, so that there is a significant end diastolic flow. Whereas systolic flow is independent of peripheral resistance and depends on the capacitance of blood vessels, diastolic flow is an accurate reflection of peripheral (downstream) vascular impedance (34).

In most studies with CW Doppler ultrasound, the angle between the Doppler beam and the blood vessel is not known (θ of the Doppler equation) and therefore neither frequencies nor velocities can be measured quantitatively. Qualitative information can, however, be extracted from the waveform by a variety of techniques that compare various factors within the waveform and are therefore angle independent. A comprehensive review of the techniques used in BVW analysis is beyond the scope of this chapter but, with particular reference to the fetal umbilical artery, is to be found in a number of recent publications (30,44). In relation to the fetoplacental and uteroplacental circulations, most interest has been focused on those parameters that describe the shape of the waveform in terms of peripheral resistance. The simplest of these are the A/B ratio [the ratio of maximum systolic flow (A) to end diastolic flow (B)] (43,45) and the resistance index [(A-B)/A] (36), whereas the most accurate in describing the waveform is the pulsatility index

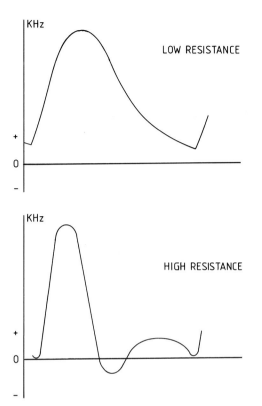

FIG. 6. Schematic representation of blood velocity waveforms obtained from arteries of high resistance (femoral artery) and low resistance (umbilical artery).

(PI), which, however, necessitates the computation of the mean Doppler shift throughout the cardiac cycle, a capability not available on all spectrum analyzers (Fig. 7).

BLOOD FLOW IN NORMAL PREGNANCY

Umbilical Blood Flow

The umbilical circulation is unique in that a readily accessible arterial system supplies a single organ (the placenta). Furthermore, the umbilical cord lies in the amniotic fluid, and there are no other vessels in the vicinity to contaminate the signal. Because of this relative ease of access to the umbilical arteries, they were the first fetal vessels studied *in utero* in the pilot study of ref. 19. This study demonstrated that using a combination of pulsed echo imaging to locate the umbilical cord and CW Doppler ultrasound, satisfactory blood flow velocity signals could be obtained from the umbilical artery *in utero* from the 12th week of pregnancy onward. McCallum et al. (31), using a range-gated, pulsed Doppler system, obtained both umbilical arterial and venous flow signals and demonstrated that abnormalities in pregnancy may be associated with changes in the umbilical arterial BVW.

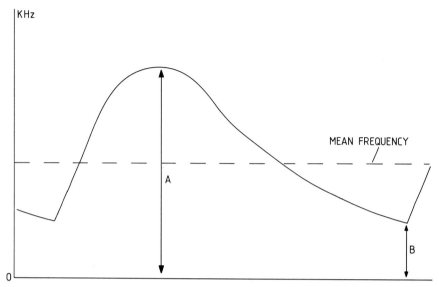

FIG. 7. Three main methods are used to describe the waveform: A:B ratio (A/B) (ref. 43); resistance index ([A-B]/A) (ref. 36); and pulsatility index ([A-B]/Mean) (ref. 20).

The first longitudinal study of umbilical artery BVWs in normal pregnancy was published by our group (43), and the results of this study have been both confirmed and amplified by several other groups (11,25,37,45). In our initial studies, a real-time imaging system was used to locate the umbilical cord within the amniotic fluid, but further experience has shown that although such a system is useful and probably saves time, satisfactory umbilical artery BVWs can be obtained in the majority of patients without using an imaging system.

The primary feature of the umbilical artery BVW after the 16th week of gestation is that there is continuous diastolic flow, indicating low placental vascular resistance. Furthermore, pulsatility decreases significantly with advancing gestational age whether it is measured by the A/B ratio (43) or the PI (37). The results of our own investigations are shown in Figs. 8 and 9, and both of these studies indicate that the major reduction in placental vascular impedance occurs in the period 16 to 28 weeks, with no significant change occurring after the 36th week. A similar pattern of decreasing placental resistance to fetoplacental blood flow, most pronounced in the earlier stages of gestation, had been observed previously during experiments on fetal sheep (13). The advantage of this hemodynamic change to the fetus is that it can thus increase placental blood flow without increasing mean arterial driving pressure or cardiac workload.

Cardiac contractility is reflected in the rising slope of the waveform (32), and in a study in which the acceleration slope of the waveform was measured throughout pregnancy, Stuart (42) found that no significant difference occurred with advancing gestational age. McCallum et al. (31) had noted previously that there was no significant difference in the percentage of the cardiac cycle the waveform spent in systole between normal and complicated pregnancies. Because placental vascular

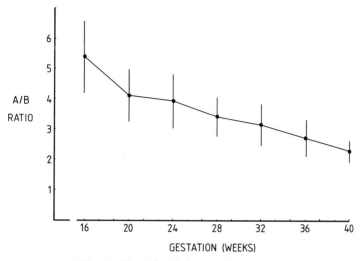

FIG. 8. The A:B ratio in normal pregnancy.

resistance does not appear to be significantly influenced by either neurohormonal (16,17,28) or biochemical (29) changes in the fetal circulation, it has been suggested that the fall in umbilical vascular resistance with advancing gestational age may be caused by physical growth of the placenta and the associated expansion of the circulation in the fetal villi (9). The early studies in human pregnancy showed that umbilical blood flow per unit weight remained constant throughout pregnancy (1,39), and this constancy has recently been confirmed noninvasively with a combination of PW Doppler ultrasound and B-mode imaging (18,24). New fetal villi

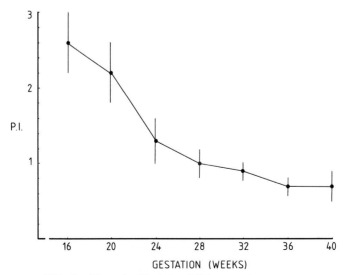

FIG. 9. The pulsatility index (PI) in normal pregnancy.

are known to grow throughout pregnancy, and in all species in which it has been studied there is a positive correlation between fetal and placental weights (13). Many of the new blood vessels that grow with the villi are short and of wide caliber and can therefore be considered as an arteriovenous anastomosis, which offers little resistance to flow (20,27).

Analysis of the umbilical BVW has also yielded information concerning the flow velocity profile across the umbilical artery. Thompson et al. (44), by averaging the velocity across the vessel lumen and assuming axisymmetric flow and a round arterial cross section, mathematically computed that the velocity profile was more blunt than parabolic, although not flat. Reuwer et al. (37) measured the profile ratio, the value of the maximum envelope divided by the spectral value, and reached the same conclusion.

Thompson et al. (44) also evaluated the relative flow rates in the umbilical artery before and after peak systolic velocity and found that the ratio of the average rate of flow before the peak to the average after the peak remained constant at about 1.33 throughout the third trimester, so that fetal cardiac systole increases flow rate by one-third.

Uteroplacental Blood Flow

Normal human placentation is associated with structural changes in the walls of the maternal uterine spinal arteries in which, following trophoblast invasion, the musculoelastic elements are replaced by a nonresponsive fibrinoid material (6). This results in vasodilation and increased uterine blood flow caused by, as in the case of fetoplacental blood flow, reduced peripheral (in this case, uteroplacental) vascular resistance, which is characteristic of hemochorial placentation (33). Campbell et al. (7) were the first to apply Doppler ultrasound to the study of uteroplacental blood flow in the maternal spiral arteries by using a duplex scanner originally developed by Eik-Nes et al. (18). This system allows the imaging of the spiral arteries by B-mode ultrasound and on-screen range gating of the PW Doppler system across the imaged vessel, thus permitting sonograms to be obtained. Arcuate artery sonograms in normal pregnancy are of the low resistance type with considerable diastolic flow and can be obtained as early as 18 weeks gestation (25).

Fetal Aortic Flow

The fetal aorta is easily visualized, relatively lengthy and of large caliber. It can therefore be studied readily by the duplex scanning technique (18,25) and also with CW Doppler. Different workers have obtained diverse results because of the use of high pass filters of differing values. Eik-Nes' group used a high pass filter of 600 Hz, and because all Doppler shifted values below this level were excluded, the fetal aortic BVW appeared to have no diastolic flow. Reducing the high pass filter to 150 Mz, however, reveals low frequency aortic diastolic flow throughout diastole in normal pregnancy (25) with the PI in the third trimester having a value of 1.83 ± 0.29 (SD). This low resistance pattern most likely arises because the low resistance placental circulation is supplied from this vessel.

COMPLICATED PREGNANCY

Umbilical Blood Flow

The earliest reports on the use of Doppler ultrasound as a tool to investigate fetal blood flow commented on the potential value of this method of investigation in pregnancies complicated by various problems (19). It was noted by McCallum et al. (31) that where pregnancy was complicated by premature rupture of the membranes, the fetal umbilical BVW changed to a highly pulsatile form with the waveform returning to the zero flow line midway through the cardiac cycle. They obtained similar BVWs from pregnancies complicated by hypertension and diabetes and noted that in these pregnancies the PI was elevated from a normal value of 0.6 to 1.5 to a value of >1.6 and that PI values of >2.4 were often associated with adverse outcome of pregnancy. Because signals were obtained with a range-gated, pulsed Doppler system, their origin from the umbilical artery cannot be doubted.

Other studies have shown that pregnancies complicated by IUGR are frequently associated with abnormal fetal umbilical BVW. Trudinger et al. (45), in a large study of 168 patients at high risk of IUGR, showed that 75% of patients yielded BVWs in which the A/B ratio was above the normal range, whereas our group (21) found that the A/B ratio was increased in excess of two standard deviations above the mean in 77% of cases of IUGR. More importantly we found that in all cases where intrauterine death occurred as a result of "placental insufficiency," the fetal BVW was altered to the high pulsatility, zero diastolic flow pattern (Fig. 10). These changes in the fetal umbilical BVW indicate raised placental vascular impedance. Several abnormalities of the vessels of the fetal villi have been found in association with IUGR. Of these, the most important are avascularity of the villi (26) and obliterative endarteritis of the fetal stem arteries (22). A reduction in the number of vessels in the tertiary villi has been noted in infants found to have abnormal BVWs (23).

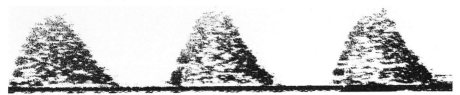

FIG. 10. A typical umbilical artery sonogram in a case of severe intrauterine growth retardation. There is complete absence of flow in diastole, indicating increased placental vascular resistance.

Although it has now been shown that IUGR is frequently associated with umbilical BVW, indicating raised placental vascular impedance, the value of this technique in fetal assessment in clinical practice has yet to be established.

Aortic Blood Flow

IUGR results in changes in the aortic BVW similar to those noted in the umbilical artery and probably of similar etiology. These changes are characterized by absent diastolic flow and elevated PI values, reflecting the increased placental vascular impedance.

Uteroplacental Flow

Uteroplacental blood flow in complicated pregnancies has been studied with both CW Doppler ultrasound (45) and PW Doppler ultrasound (11,15), and the results indicate a pattern similar to that found in the fetoplacental circulation. In the Trudinger et al. study (45), 15 of 25 (60%) growth-retarded fetuses demonstrated a pattern of low diastolic flow consistent with increased uteroplacental vascular resistance and reduced uterine artery perfusion, whereas the remaining 10 (40%) had normal uterine artery BVWs. It was suggested that these two groups corresponded to what has been called asymmetrical and symmetrical IUGR, in that the former is owing to "placental insufficiency" and the latter to an inherently reduced-growth potential in the fetus. Similar results were obtained from the study of Cohen-Overbeek et al. (11), who divided patients with complicated pregnancies into two groups; Group 1 had normal arcuate artery BVW, and Group II abnormal arcuate BVW. The patients with abnormal arcuate BVW had a higher incidence of pregnancy-induced hypertension, were delivered at an earlier mean gestational age, and had a higher incidence of IUGR.

It has been noted (5) that in approximately 50% of pregnancies associated with IUGR, the normal physiological adaptative changes that occur in the maternal spiral arteries either fail to develop or only partially develop, with the vasodilatation not progressing beyond the level of the decidual-myometrial junction so that there is narrowing of the vessels at this junction with consequent placental hypoperfusion. Experimental work in animals has yielded further information on the role of uteroplacental ischemia in the etiology of IUGR. Microsphere embolization of the uteroplacental circulation of the fetal lamb, sufficient to cause a reduction in placental blood flow, results in growth retardation. Furthermore, the same investigators demonstrated a significant correlation between uteroplacental and fetoplacental blood flow in that chronic placental ischemia ultimately results in reduced fetoplacental blood flow because of an increase in placental vascular resistance. In human pregnancy complicated by IUGR, the increase in placental resistance has been shown to be associated with a reduction in the number of small arteries in the tertiary placental villi, presumably because of a placental hypoxia (23).

CONCLUSIONS

The study of the fetoplacental and uteroplacental circulations with Doppler ultrasound is now well established and has yielded valuable information concerning fetal and placental vascular physiology *in utero*. Being noninvasive, the technique allows these circulations to be studied under physiological conditions. Its current status as a clinically useful tool is uncertain, and it may be considered as complementary to more established techniques of monitoring fetal well-being. It has been established that IUGR is frequently associated with demonstrable changes in both the uteroplacental and fetoplacental circulations and that these changes precede clinical signs of reduced fetal growth. It remains to be demonstrated whether this technique will prove useful as a screening test for IUGR.

ACKNOWLEDGMENTS

The authors wish to acknowledge the generous support of a Florence and William Blair-Bell Memorial Research Fellowship from the Royal College of Obstetricians and Gynecologists (to B.S.), of the Coombe Lying-in Hospital Development Trust, and of the Irish Foundation for Human Development.

REFERENCES

1. Assali, N.S., Morris, J.A., and Beck, R. (1960): Measurement of uterine blood flow and uterine metabolism. *Am. J. Obstet. Gynecol.,* 79:86–98.
2. Barcroft, J., Kennedy, J.A., and Mason, M.F. (1939): The direct determination of the oxygen consumption of the fetal sheep. *J. Physiol.,* 95:269–275.
3. Barron, D.H., Meschia, G., Cotter, J.R., and Breathnach, C.S. (1965): The hemoglobin, oxygen, carbon dioxide and hydrogen ion concentrations in the umbilical blood of sheep and goats as sampled via indwelling plastic catheters. *Q. J. Exp. Physiol.,* 50:185–195.
4. Brennan, S.C., McLaughlin, M.K., and Chez, R.A. (1977): Effects of prolonged infusion of B-adrenergic agonists on uterine and umbilical blood flow in pregnant sheep. In: *Hypertension in Pregnancy,* edited by M.D. Linheimer, p. 363. Wiley, New York.
5. Brosens, I., Dixon, H.G., and Robertson, W.B. (1977): Fetal growth retardation and the arteries of the placental bed. *Br. J. Obstet. Gynaecol.,* 84:656–663.
6. Brosens, I., Robertson., W.B., and Dixon, H.G. (1967): The physiological response of the vessels of the placental bed to normal pregnancy. *J. Pathol.,* 93:569–579.
7. Campbell, S., Diaz-Recasens, J., Griffin, D.R., et al. (1983): New Doppler technique for assessing utero-placental blood flow. *Lancet,* 1:675–677.
8. Clapp, J.F. (1978): The relationship between blood flow and oxygen uptake in the uterine and umbilical circulations. *Am. J. Obstet. Gynecol.,* 132:410–413.
9. Clapp, J.F., Szeto, H.H., Larrow, R., Hewitt, J., and Mann, L. (1980): Umbilical blood flow response to embolisation of the uterine circulation. *Am. J. Obstet. Gynecol.,* 138:60–67.
10. Clavero, J.A., Negueruela, J., Ortiz, I., and De Los Heros, J.A. (1973): Blood flow in the interville space and fetal blood flow. *Am. J. Obstet. Gynecol.,* 116:340–346.
11. Cohen-Overbeek, T., Pearce, M.J., and Campbell, S. (1985): The antenatal assessment of utero-placental and feto-placental blood flow using Doppler ultrasound. *Ultrasound Med. Biol.,* 11:329–339.
12. Cooper, K.E., Greenfield, A.D.M., and Huggett, A. St. G. (1949): The umbilical blood flow in the fetal sheep. *J. Physiol.,* 108:160–166.
13. Dawes, G.S. (1968): *Fetal and Neonatal Physiology.* Year Book Publishers Inc., Chicago.

14. Dawes, G.S., and Mott, J.C. (1959): The increase in the oxygen consumption of the lamb after birth. *J. Physiol.,* 170:524–540.
15. Drumm, J. (1977): The prediction of delivery date by ultrasonic measurement of crown-rump length. *Br. J. Obstet. Gynaecol.,* 84:1–5.
16. Ehrenkranz, R.A., Hamilton, L.A., Brennan, S.C., Oakes, G.K., Walker, A.M., and Chez, R.A. (1977): Effects of salbutamol and isoxuprine on uterine and umbilical blood flow in pregnant sheep. *Am. J. Obstet. Gynecol.,* 128:287–293.
17. Ehrenkranz, R.A., Walker, A.M., Oakes, G.K., Hamilton, L.A., and Chez, R.A. (1977): Effect of Fenoterol infusion on uterine and umbilical blood flow in pregnant sheep. *Am. J. Obstet. Gynecol.,* 128:177–182.
18. Eik-Nes, S., Brubakk, A., and Ulstein, M. (1980): Measurement of human blood flow. *Br. Med. J.,* 1:283.
19. FitzGerald, D.E., and Drumm, J.E. (1977): Non-invasive measurement of the fetal circulation using ultrasound; a new method. *Br. Med. J.,* 2:1450–1451.
20. FitzGerald, D.E., Gosling, R.G., and Woodcock, J.P. (1971): Grading dynamic capability of arterial collateral circulation. *Lancet,* 1:66–67.
21. FitzGerald, D.E., Stuart, B., Drumm, J.E., and Duignan, N.M. (1984): The assessment of the feto-placental circulation with continuous wave Doppler ultrasound. *Ultrasound Med. Biol.,* 10:371–376.
22. Fox, H. (1978): *Pathology of the Placenta.* W.B. Saunders Co., London.
23. Giles, W.B., Trudinger, B., and Baird, P.J. (1985): Fetal umbilical artery flow velocity waveforms and placental resistance: Pathological correlation. *Br. J. Obstet. Gynaecol.,* 92:31–38.
24. Gill, R.W., Trudinger, B.J., Garrett, W.J., Kossoff, G., and Warren, P.S. (1981): Fetal umbilical venous flow measured *in utero* by pulsed Doppler and B mode ultrasound. *Am. J. Obstet. Gynecol.,* 139:720–725.
25. Griffin, D., Cohen-Overbeek, T., and Campbell, S. (1983): Fetal and utero-placental blood flow. *Clin. Obstet. Gynaecol.,* 10:565–602.
26. Gruenwald, P. (1961): Abnormalities of placental vascularity in relation to intrauterine deprivation and retarded fetal growth; significance of avascular chorionic villi. *NY State J. Med.,* 61:1508–1513.
27. Hamilton, W.J., and Boyd, J.D. (1970): Development of the human placenta. In: *Scientific Foundations of Obstetrics and Gynecology,* edited by E.E. Philipp, J. Barnes, and M. Newton, pp. 185–254. William Heinemann Medical Books Ltd., London.
28. Hollingworth, M. (1974): Electrical stimulation and drug responses of isolated human umbilical blood vessels. *Eur. J. Pharmacol.,* 27:140–141.
29. Johnson, G.H., Brinkman, C.R., and Assali, N.S. (1972): Effects of acid and base infusin on umbilical hemodynamics. *Am. J. Obstet. Gynecol.,* 112:1122–1128.
30. Maulik, D., Saini, V.D., Nanda, N.C., and Rosenzweig, M.S. (1982): Doppler evaluation of fetal hemodynamics. *Ultrasound Med. Biol.,* 8:705–710.
31. McCallum, W.D., Williams, C.S., Napel, S., and Daigle, R.E. (1978): Fetal blood velocity waveforms. *Am. J. Obstet. Gynecol.,* 132:425–429.
32. McDonald, D.A. (1974): *Blood Flow in Arteries,* 2nd ed. Edward Arnold Publishers Ltd., London.
33. Moll, W., Kunzel, W. (1973): Blood pressure in arteries entering the placentae of guinea pigs, rats, rabbits and sheep. *Pflugers Arch.,* 338:125–131.
34. Olson, R.M., and Cooke, J.P. (1975): Human carotid artery diameter and flow by a non-invasive technique. *Med. Instrum.,* 9:99–102.
35. Paton, J.B., Fischer, D.E., De Lannoy, C.W., and Behrman, R.E. (1973): Umbilical blood flow, cardiac output and organ blood flow in the immature baboon fetus. *Am. J. Obstet. Gynecol.,* 117:560–566.
36. Planiol, T., and Pourcelot, L. (1975): Doppler effect study of the carotid circulation. In: *Proceedings of the 2nd World Congress of Ultrasonics in Medicine,* edited by M. De Vlieger, D.N. White, and P. McCreedy. American Elsevier, New York.
37. Reuwer, P.J.H.M., Nuyen, W.C., Beijer, H.J., et al. (1984): Characteristics of flow velocities in the umbilical arteries, assessed by Doppler ultrasound. *Eur. J. Obstet. Gynecol. Reprod. Biol.,* 17:397–408.
38. Rudolf, A.M., and Heymann, M.A. (1967): The circulation of the fetus *in utero;* methods for studying distribution of blood flow, cardiac output, and organ blood flow. *Circ. Res.,* 21:163–184.

39. Rudolf, A.M., Heymann, M.A., Teramo, K.A.W., Barnett, C.T., and Raiha, N.C.R. (1971): Studies on the circulation of the pre-viable human fetus. *Pediatr. Res.,* 5:452–465.
40. Satomura, S., Matsubara, S., and Yoshioka, M. (1956): A new method of mechanical vibration measurement and its application. *Memoirs of the Institute of Industrial Research, Osaka University,* 13:125–133.
41. Stembera, Z.K., Hodra, J., and Jandra, J. (1965): Umbilical blood flow in healthy newborn infants during the first few minutes after birth. *Am. J. Obstet. Gynecol.,* 91:568–574.
42. Stuart, B. (1982): A study of the feto-placental circulation using Doppler ultrasound. M.A.O. Thesis, National University of Ireland.
43. Stuart, B., Drumm, J.E., FitzGerald, D.E., and Duignan, N.M. (1980): Fetal blood velocity waveforms in normal pregnancy. *Br. J. Obstet. Gynaecol.,* 87:780–785.
44. Thompson, R.S., Trudinger, B.J., and Cook, C.M. (1985): Doppler ultrasound waveforms in the fetal umbilical artery: Quantitative analysis technique. *Ultrasound Med. Biol.,* 11:707–718.
45. Trudinger, B.J., Giles, W.B., Cook, C.M., Bombardieri, J., and Collins, L. (1985): Fetal umbilical artery flow velocity waveforms and placental resistance: Clinical significance. *Br. J. Obstet. Gynaecol.,* 92:23–30.

Fetal Neurology, edited by
A. Hill and J.J. Volpe.
Raven Press, New York © 1989.

Commentary on Chapter 7

*Alan Hill and **Joseph H. Volpe

*Division of Neurology, Department of Paediatrics, University of British Columbia,
British Columbia's Children's Hospital, Vancouver, British Columbia, Canada V6H 3V4;
and **Division of Pediatric Neurology, Washington University School of Medicine,
St. Louis, Missouri 63110*

This chapter provided a valuable overview of an exciting new area of study of the fetus and the fetoplacental units.

Because an important portion of the neuropathology that occurs *in utero* appears to be caused by derangements of blood flow, a means for assessing fetal and placental blood flow would be a major advance indeed. In this chapter, the reader was provided with the perspective of a research group that includes experts in vascular physiology and obstetrics. The initial work is most promising.

Recent advances in ultrasound technology have created new possibilities for noninvasive evaluation of the hemodynamic status of the fetus. The initial studies of FitzGerald and Drumm in 1977 (3) recorded blood flow velocity waveforms from the arteries of the intrauterine umbilical cord by continuous wave Doppler ultrasound with velocity frequency spectrum analysis. Later studies have applied pulsed wave Doppler ultrasound to obtain volume blood flow estimations from the fetal umbilical vein (1,2,6,8) and fetal aorta (1,2). Although early studies were involved principally with volume flow estimations, the relatively large errors associated with estimation of vessel size appear to have altered the direction of studies toward the analysis of blood flow velocity waveforms. Other sources of error associated with estimation of volume of blood flow include localization of the vessel, measurement of the beam-vessel angle, measurement of mean blood velocity over the vessel's cross-sectional area, and the estimation of fetal weight from biparietal diameter and abdominal diameter measurements (4).

Analysis of the flow velocity waveform of the umbilical artery provides information concerning the vascular resistance of the fetoplacental circulation. The index commonly used to define the blood flow velocity waveform is the pulsatility index (PI). This reflects the resistance of the vascular bed downstream to the umbilical artery, i.e., the placental bed. In normal pregnancies, the values for the PI decrease with increasing gestational age, indicating a gradual decrease in the vascular resistance of the placental bed (16,18).

It has been recently recognized that umbilical artery blood flow is influenced not only by the resistance of the placental bed but also by fetal physiological variables.

Thus, the PI has been studied in relation to fetal breathing movements, fetal heart rate, and fetal behavioral states in the normal term fetus. The blood flow velocity waveform is altered by fetal breathing movements, and an inverse relationship has been established between fetal heart rate and PI, independent of fetal behavioral state. Thus, umbilical artery blood flow measurements should be performed in the absence of fetal breathing (which causes irregularity of the blood flow velocity waveform) and body movements (because of the accompanying accelerations in fetal heart rate). Furthermore, the fetal heart rate should be taken into account when evaluating fetal blood flow, and the PI should be expressed as a function of fetal heart rate or corrected to a fixed rate (140 bpm) (14,19).

The value of fetal blood flow measurements has been demonstrated in the clinical management of pregnancies complicated by fetal cardiac arrhythmias (11) and in pharmacological studies for the evaluation of the effect of drugs on fetal circulation (10,17).

Major attention has been directed toward the application of fetal blood flow measurements in the early detection of fetal compromise or intrauterine growth retardation. A decrease in volume of placental flow has been reported in association with fetal growth failure (7). Velocity waveforms in the umbilical artery have demonstrated a decrease in the diastolic blood flow velocity relative to the systolic velocity in pregnancies with fetal growth failure, presumably because of increased resistance of the placental bed (4). Histological studies of the placentae from such pregnancies reveal obliteration of the small arterial vessels of the tertiary stem villi (5).

Measurement of fetal cerebral blood flow has been attempted. Examination of blood flow in the common carotid (13) and internal carotid (20) arteries has been accomplished. In the internal carotid artery, there is elevation of blood flow velocity profile above the baseline throughout the cardiac cycle in the normal population, confirming the existence of low peripheral cerebrovascular resistance in the fetus, especially during the third trimester. In the growth-retarded fetus, the PI was decreased in the internal carotid artery and increased in the descending aorta and umbilical artery, suggesting an increase in peripheral vascular resistance in the fetal body and placenta and a compensatory reduction in vascular resistance in the fetal brain, i.e., a brain-sparing effect in the presence of fetal hypoxia. Perhaps of greatest interest, Huch and collaborators (9) have studied blood flow velocity in the middle cerebral artery of the fetus. Employing the resistance index of Pourcelot, they have shown a progressive decrease in the index with advance of normal pregnancy (as shown also in the studies of the carotid arteries). Still more interesting, they have demonstrated a greater decrease in the index in severe fetal distress and in the postterm pregnancy and suggest that this phenomenon reflects an exaggeration of the normal decrease in fetal cerebrovascular resistance late in gestation.

This further decrease in cerebrovascular resistance may reflect an adaptive response to lowered oxygen delivery to brain, caused either by impaired cerebral blood flow (e.g., severe fetal distress) or by impaired arterial oxygen content (e.g., postterm pregnancy with placental insufficiency). (Recall that oxygen delivery relates to cerebral blood flow × arterial oxygen content.) If reproducible study of blood flow velocity in the middle cerebral artery of the fetus can be accomplished, an enormous advance in fetal surveillance will be effected.

In addition to study of umbilical vessels in growth-retarded fetuses with chronic hypoxia, fetal blood flow studies of these vessels may be of value in instances in which the episode of hypoxia is more acute (12). In addition to the absence of aortic blood flow velocity during diastole previously described, abnormalities in blood flow in the umbilical vein have been recorded. Blood flow in the umbilical vein is typically nonpulsatile and continuous. Pulsation in the intraabdominal umbilical vein has been observed in fetuses who are exposed to an asphyxiating intrauterine insult (15). Changes in the aortic blood flow velocity waveform of fetuses with imminent intrauterine asphyxia have been detected before the recording of pathological fetal heart rate patterns. This finding suggests that blood flow changes may provide an early warning signal of impending asphyxia, which, in turn, may lead to intensification of fetal surveillance by other methods, e.g., nonstress and stress tests. Evaluation of vessel diameter displayed in the real-time image may also reflect disturbed fetal circulation, e.g., the aorta normally has a smaller diameter than the umbilical vein, but this relationship may be reversed in asphyxiated fetuses (12). Clearly, there is a need for further studies to elucidate the time relationships between the onset of fetal blood flow changes and the occurrence of other signs of fetal asphyxia.

REFERENCES

1. Eik-Nes, S.H., Brubakk, A.O., and Ulstein, M.K. (1980): Measurement of human fetal blood flow. *Br. Med. J.*, 280:283–284.
2. Eik-Nes, S.H., Marsal, K., Brubakk, A.O., Kristoffersen, K., and Ulstein, M. (1982): Ultrasonic measurement of human fetal blood flow. *J. Biomed. Eng.*, 4:28–36.
3. FitzGerald, D.E., and Drumm, J.E. (1977): Non-invasive measurement of human fetal circulation using ultrasound: A new method. *Br. Med. J.*, 2:1450–1451.
4. Giles, W.B., Lingman, G., Marsal, K., and Trudinger, B.J. (1986): Fetal volume blood flow and umbilical artery flow velocity waveform analysis: A comparison. *Br. J. Obstet. Gynaecol.*, 93:461–465.
5. Giles, W.B., Trudinger, B.J., and Baird, P.J. (1985): Fetal umbilical artery flow velocity-time waveforms and placental resistance: Pathological correlation. *Br. J. Obstet. Gynaecol.*, 92:31–38.
6. Gill, R.W., Trudinger, B.J., Garrett, W.J., and Kossoff, G. (1981): Fetal umbilical venous flow measured *in utero* by pulsed Doppler and B-mode ultrasound. I. Normal pregnancies. *Am. J. Obstet. Gynecol.*, 139:720–725.
7. Jouppila, P., and Kirkinen, P. (1984): Increased vascular resistance in the descending aorta of the human fetus in hypoxia. *Br. J. Obstet. Gynaecol.*, 91:853–856.
8. Kirkinen, P., and Jouppila, P. (1983): Ultrasonic measurement of human umbilical circulation in various pregnancy complications. In: *Ultrasound Annual*, edited by R.C. Saunders and M. Hill, pp. 153–162. Raven Press, New York.
9. Kirkinen, P., Muller, R., Baumann, H., et al. (1987): Fetal cerebral vascular resistance. *Lancet*, 11:392.
10. Lindblad, A., Marsal, K., Venersson, E., and Renck, H. (1984): Fetal circulation during epidural analgesia for caesarean section. *Br. Med. J.*, 288:1329–1330.
11. Lingman, G., Dahlstroem, J.A., Eik-Nes, S.H., Marsal, K., Ohlin, P., and Ohrlander, S. (1984): Hemodynamic evaluation of fetal heart arrhythmia. *Br. J. Obstet. Gynaecol.*, 91:647–652.

12. Lingman, G., Laurin, J., and Marsal, K. (1986): Circulatory changes in fetuses with imminent asphyxia. *Biol. Neonate,* 49:66–73.
13. Marsal, K., Lingman, G., and Giles, W. (1984): Evaluation of the carotid, aortic and umbilical blood velocity. *Proceedings from the Society for the Study of Fetal Physiology, XI Annual Conference,* Oxford.
14. Mulders, L.G.M., Muijsers, G.J.J.M., Jongsma, H.W., Nijhuis, J.G., and Hein, P.R. (1986): The umbilical artery blood flow velocity waveform in relation to fetal breathing movements, fetal heart rate and fetal behavioural states in normal pregnancy at 37 to 39 weeks. *Early Hum. Dev.,* 14:283–293.
15. Reuss, M.L., Rudolpe, A.M., and Dae, M.W. (1983): Phasic blood flow patterns in the superior and inferior venae cavae and umbilical vein of fetal sheep. *Am. J. Obstet. Gynecol.,* 145:70–78.
16. Reuwer, P.J.H.M., Bruinse, H.W., Stoutenbeck, P., and Haspels, A.A. (1984): Doppler assessment of the fetoplacental circulation in normal and growth-retarded fetuses. *Eur. J. Obstet. Gynecol. Reprod. Biol.,* 18:199–205.
17. Sindberg Erickson, P., and Marsal, K. (1984): Acute effects of maternal smoking on fetal blood flow. *Acta Obstet. Gynecol. Scand.,* 63:391–397.
18. Trudinger, B.J., Giles, W.B., Cook, C.M., Bombardieri, J., and Collins, L. (1985): Fetal umbilical artery flow velocity waveforms and placental resistance: Clinical significance. *Br. J. Obstet. Gynaecol.,* 92:23–30.
19. Van Eyck, J., Wladimiroff, J.W., Noordam, M.J., Tonge, H.M., and Prechtl, H.F.R. (1986): The blood flow velocity waveform in the fetal descending aorta; its relationship to behavioral states in the growth-retarded fetus at 37–38 weeks of gestation. *Early Hum. Dev.,* 14:99–107.
20. Wladimiroff, J.W., Tonge, H.M., and Stewart, P.A. (1986): Doppler ultrasound assessment of cerebral blood flow in the human fetus. *Br. J. Obstet. Gynaecol.,* 93:471–475.

Fetal Neurology, edited by
A. Hill and J.J. Volpe.
Raven Press, New York © 1989.

8

The Diagnosis and Treatment
of Fetal Distress

Barry S. Schifrin

AMI–Tarzana Regional Medical Center, Tarzana, California 91356

''Fetal distress'' during labor constitutes a major reason for surgical intervention in pregnancy. Thus, many techniques have been developed to enable early recognition of this condition and hopefully to prevent subsequent disability or fetal death. These techniques include observation (of the number of fetal movements and meconium), palpation (of fundal height), auscultation of fetal heart tones, electronic fetal monitoring (EFM), and fetal blood sampling (FBS).

The term *fetal distress* is used generally to connote fetal asphyxia. Unfortunately, there is no clinical technique available, at the present time, that accurately predicts fetal asphyxia. Thus, the principal value of EFM and FBS lies in the confirmation of fetal well-being rather than in the prediction of fetal asphyxia.

CLASSIC SIGNS OF FETAL DISTRESS

Before discussing the benefits of new techniques, it is necessary to understand the limitations of the older methods. Auscultation of fetal heart rate (FHR) is used most frequently in the evaluation of fetal well-being. The technique was first promulgated in the early 1800s, shortly after the discovery of the stethoscope by Laennec (126). The clinical criteria of fetal distress that prevailed for almost a century, i.e., a FHR greater than 160 bpm or less than 120 bpm, were described in the 1890s. Since that time there has been little improvement in the technique of auscultation or in the auscultatory criteria used to diagnose fetal distress.

The technique of auscultation has several distinct disadvantages. Thus, assessment is limited to the time between contractions, and inaccuracies may arise because of listener bias and the short period of time during which the rate is counted and averaged (35). Profound FHR changes often do not correlate with genuine fetal disturbance, whereas important but subtle abnormalities, e.g., poor variability, late decelerations, that indicate fetal distress may be overlooked. Because of these problems, auscultation must be considered of limited practical value for the prediction of early fetal distress (11,151).

MECONIUM STAINING OF AMNIOTIC FLUID

It is well recognized that perinatal mortality and morbidity are increased in fetuses who pass meconium before delivery (9,58). This sign occurs commonly with placental insufficiency (growth retardation, postdates) and almost invariably accompanies death in the term fetus. Recent studies have reported fetal acid-base disturbances during labor in approximately 20% of the fetuses who have passed meconium (133). Theoretically, hypoxia causes the fetus to pass meconium by increasing peristalsis of the gastrointestinal tract and perhaps by simultaneously relaxing the anal sphincter (57).

However, current data do not support a close relationship between the passage of meconium and fetal hypoxia (69,107). Indeed, many neonates who are apparently normal are meconium stained at delivery. Furthermore, meconium is considered a normal finding with breech presentation, and the significance of this finding during early gestation is not known. Although resorption may eventually occur, meconium tends to remain in the amniotic fluid for a considerable period of time. Thus, because its presence may relate to transient fetal compromise, the isolated finding of meconium during labor is seldom, if ever, considered an indication for immediate delivery (41).

The passage of meconium may result from increased vagal tone associated with fetal maturation, rather than from fetal hypoxia (69). Meconium is observed only rarely before 36 weeks gestation but occurs frequently thereafter. Meconium-stained amniotic fluid is found in about 10% to 15% of pregnancies at term and in approximately 25% to 50% of postdate pregnancies (9,56).

In an extensive study, Miller and colleagues (107) concluded that in the absence of abnormal FHR patterns or acidosis determined in fetal scalp blood, the presence of meconium does not appear to prejudice outcome. Moreover, they did not find a higher incidence of abnormal FHR patterns in patients with meconium. On the other hand, when abnormal FHR patterns were observed in the presence of meconium, acidosis and neonatal depression were more severe than in the absence of meconium. Thus, it appears that meconium acts as a foreign body in the tracheobronchial tree that interferes with neonatal respiratory adaption. When the normal, reflex mechanisms for cleansing the tracheobronchial tree (coughing, etc.) are depressed as a result of hypoxia, the adverse effects of meconium are enhanced.

In practical terms, the presence of meconium without other signs of fetal distress should not influence the conduct of labor. Of course, every attempt should be made to minimize asphyxia and to avoid difficult or traumatic delivery. In addition, the presence of meconium requires that trained personnel be available at delivery for aggressive neonatal resuscitation. Although aspiration of the upper airway of the infant as the head emerges and the shoulders are delivered greatly reduces the risk of meconium aspiration (21,58,69), this approach probably does not entirely eliminate complications.

Reliance on the color of amniotic fluid and intermittent auscultation of the FHR for evaluation of the fetus during labor has resulted in arbitrary criteria for the clinical diagnosis of intrapartum fetal distress. Obstetric management based on these criteria alone did not result in significant improvement of fetal outcome. More recently, the assessment of fetal well-being has been refined by the availability of EFM and FBS (Table 1). The application of these techniques during labor will be discussed separately and then followed by discussion of their complementary role in the clinical management of fetal distress.

ELECTRONIC FETAL MONITORING

Several unique features of EFM account for its considerable value in fetal assessment: (a) the continuous recording of FHR, (b) the correlation of FHR with uterine contractions (UC), and (c) the permanent printed record. The FHR may be obtained electronically with a variety of transducers, including ultrasound, microphone, and electrodes that record from the surface of the maternal abdomen or directly from the fetus. There are practical and technical benefits and limitations to each method (4) (Tables 2–6). Because the fetal scalp electrode provides definition of the fetal QRS complex, it is most accurate technique for recording FHR.

TABLE 1. *Specificity of FHR and FBS indicators of distress*

Factor contributing to low Apgar	Specific FHR pattern	Specific pH pattern
Hypoxia	Late decelerations	Acidosis
Congenital anomaly	Occasionally	None
Infection	Nonspecific	Nonspecific
Trauma	Nonspecific	Nonspecific
Drugs	Nonspecific	Nonspecific

TABLE 2. *Monitoring techniques*

FHR	UC
Auscultation	Palpation
Direct ECG	Intrauterine catheter
Ultrasound	Extraovular catheter
Microphone	Tocodynamometer (EMG)
Abdominal ECG	

TABLE 3. *Practicality of external FHR transducers*

Transducer	Potential trace quality	Satisfactory tracing
Ultrasound	3	1 (95%)
Microphone	2	2 (85%)
Abdominal ECG	1	3 (75%)

TABLE 4. *Errors in determining FHR*

Technique	Cause
Direct ECG	Rate >250 bpm—half count
	Complex fetal ECG
	Maternal ECG
Ultrasound	Rate <70 bpm—double count
	Rate >180 bpm—half count
	Fetal movement
	Maternal signal
Microphone	Rate <70 bpm—double count
	Rate >180 bpm—half count
	Fetal movement
	Maternal signal
Abdominal ECG	Prominent maternal ECG
	Low-amplitude fetal ECG
	Multiple gestation

TABLE 5. *Errors in determining FHR variability*

Source	Increase variability	Decrease variability
Patient	Complex signal	Not applicable
	Low-amplitude ECG	
	Arrhythmia	
Transducer	Noisy electrode	Not applicable
	Ultrasound	
	Microphone	
Detector/tachometer	"Jitter"	Missed beats
	Polarity switch	Averaged rate
Recorder	"Jitter"	Slow response
		"Overshoot"

TABLE 6. *FHR monitoring pitfalls and recommendations*

Source of error	Solution
Electrical or signal errors	
Faulty electrode, legplate, or monitor	Replace defective parts
Fetal ECG voltage too low	Use Doppler method
60-cycle interference	Ground the machine
Interference from maternal signal (maternal ECG, movement, or UCs)	Recognize
Limitations of machinery	
Penlift (switch on back of certain machines that omits FHR >30 bpm different from preceding beat, so it may omit arrhythmias)	Leave penlift out Record strip of fetal ECG from back of machine
Averaging (may smooth variability)	Recognize that some ultrasound monitors take a running average of 2 or 3 beats
Halving or doubling [very slow rates may be doubled and very fast rates (>240 bpm) may be halved by machine]	Auscultation
Short-term variability in Doppler signal caused by indistinct FHR signal	Realize that one cannot determine short-term variability with a Doppler method
Interpretative errors	
Maternal signal being picked up because fetus is dead	Compare FHR pattern with maternal rate
Maternal signal being picked up because electrode is on cervix	Compare FHR pattern with maternal rate
Scaling error (using both speeds on some machines, which are capable of 1 and 3 cm/min)	Recognize that FHR pattern changes with recording rate, and use one rate all the time, preferably 3 cm/min
Nonrecognition of artifact (good variability may really be a noisy signal, especially with Doppler method)	Recognize
Arrhythmias (tend to be regular)	Record fetal ECG from back
Artifact (tends to be irregular)	of machine

Techniques

The fetal monitor "counts" and displays the FHR differently from conventional techniques. In fact, the monitor determines the interval between consecutive heart beats and plots a "rate" on the graph, which projects the number of beats that would occur in 1 min if all intervals were the same as the calculated interval (Fig. 1). Thus, if the interval is 500 msec (0.5 sec), the machine plots the rate at 120 bpm. If the next interval is 400 msec, the machine plots a rate of 160 bpm, and so on. With the direct scalp electrode, the monitor has no memory for the last interval, and therefore there is no smoothing of the sequential rate plots. By responding to each new interval between heart beats, the monitor produces a detailed

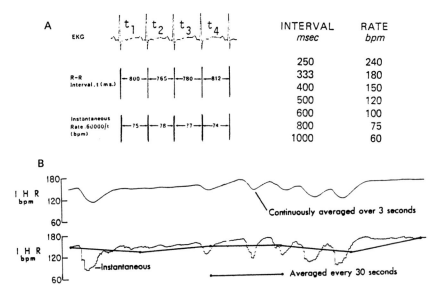

FIG. 1. A: Technique of counting. Machine detects fetal cardiac complex (ECG) and determines the interval (R-R) between consecutive beats, then plots the instantaneous rate according to the formula rate = 60,000/t (msec). Note that each interval is calculated and plotted anew without influence from the previous rate. **B:** Cardiotachometry: comparison of techniques for obtaining fetal heart rate. *Top panel:* Heart rate averaged over 3 sec. Note smooth tracing and loss of detail compared to instantaneous rate *(bottom panel)*. Averaging every 30 sec eliminates all detail about both decelerations and variability.

record of the subtle changes in the FHR, i.e., the beat-to-beat interval. By plotting the information in this format, this technique provides information not only about baseline FHR but also about the rhythm (or variability) of the changes.

EFFECTS OF UTERINE CONTRACTIONS

Maximum information about fetal condition may be obtained by correlating changes of the FHR pattern with UCs. Contractions may be recorded by means of external devices or by an internal catheter attached to a suitable strain gauge. Uterine contractions represent both a repetitive stimulus and stress to the fetus. In the responsive fetus, UCs are frequently accompanied by fetal cardiac accelerations, which are most pronounced before labor or with nonvertex presentation. In addition, UCs may exert pressure on the fetal presenting part, which may contribute to increased intracranial pressure and trauma. UCs may also trap the umbilical cord between the fetal body and extremities or between the fetus and uterine wall and thereby reduce umbilical blood flow. However, the most consistent effect of UCs is the impairment of uterine blood flow in direct proportion to their duration and amplitude (60,101). Thus, the longer and stronger the UC, the greater the impairment of uterine blood flow. For example, with UCs above 50 mm Hg, the fetus essentially is functionally isolated from the mother. This decrease in oxygen availability during UCs is usually well tolerated, and there is little evidence that the effect is cumulative. However, excessive UCs may compromise even an otherwise healthy fetus. For example, when uterine blood flow to the intervillous space is chronically impaired, e.g., in preeclampsia, or if there is maternal or fetal anemia, UCs may cause a decrease in blood oxygen content sufficient to result in fetal distress.

CONTROL OF FETAL HEART RATE

The FHR is regulated by intrinsic and extrinsic factors (20,32,61,76, 77,103,104,119,129,134,140,144,149). Although any region of the heart may serve as pacemaker, the sinoatrial (SA) node predominates because its spontaneous discharge frequency is faster than any other focus. If this pacemaker is depressed, other pacemaker cells including the atrioventricular (AV) node or the ventricular myocardium may incite a cardiac contraction.

Similar to the adult, the fetal heart responds predictably to numerous neural, humoral, physical, and pharmacological influences. Thus, automonic drugs, temperature, electrolytes, oxygenation, acid-base balance, hormonal milieu, fetal activity and stimulation, and maternal smoking all influence cardiac rate or rhythmicity (81,101,153,154). These responses, in turn, depend on the gestational age and the maturation of the fetal central nervous system.

The FHR correlates closely with *gestational age*. Thus, as the fetus matures, the baseline FHR decreases, variability increases, and epochs of activity become better defined (19,54,74,104,148,149). In the very immature fetus, the average FHR is approximately 160 bpm. At term, the range has decreased to between 110 and 150 bpm or lower in the normal postterm fetus. Before term, fetal sleep/wake cycles are poorly defined, and fetal movement may precipitate minor accelerations or decelerations of FHR. By term, movements are well organized and are associated with discrete accelerations and increased variability.

The *central control* for the modulation of the FHR and circulation originates primarily in the medulla, although some integration also occurs at spinal cord level (29,101). The medulla is influenced in turn by the hypothalamus and the cerebral cortex. Experimental and clinical experience in both the fetus and neonate shows that decerebration from hypoxia, anencephaly, or intracranial hemorrhage eliminates reflex decelerations, rest/activity cycles, and variability (1,34,36,85,144, 147,163).

The heart rate is controlled principally by the *autonomic nervous system* (26,32,52,103,129,134,153,154). Both sympathetic and parasympathetic influences are well developed in the term fetus. Acetylcholine, the cholinergic transmitter of the *parasympathetic system* slows the FHR and regulates short-term variability as well as most of the decelerations recorded during labor. These reflex decelerations are an immediate response to stress that may be either abrupt or gradual in onset. Acetylcholine, with its extremely rapid onset and brief duration of action, is ideal for rapid regulation of the FHR responses.

The *sympathetic nervous system* with its transmitter norepinephrine increases the FHR in a more sustained fashion. Unlike acetylcholine, norepinephrine is not metabolized locally, and therefore produces a more graded response with slower onset and longer duration of action (153,154). The balance between the two opposing influences of the automonic system results in the baseline FHR and its variability.

Variability may be divided into two components. *Beat-to-beat variability* represents the differences in time intervals between consecutive cardiac contractions and reflects parasympathetic control. *Long-term variability* refers to the gentler oscillations in the FHR pattern that occur with frequency of about two to six cycles per minute and an amplitude of 5 to 15 bpm. This long-term variability is controlled partially by sympathetic tone. This FHR periodicity is related to rest/activity (state) and fetal breathing pattern. In addition, there is a circadian periodicity of FHR that parallels a similar periodicity in the maternal heart rate (61,104,120,121,149).

Several factors influence the output of the autonomic nervous system. Thus, the baroreceptors, which are active in the fetus after 20 weeks of gestation, play an important role in the regulation of both FHR and its variability. The baroreceptors respond to changes in blood pressure with alteration of heart rate and peripheral vascular tone (76,77,102,103,140). When the blood pressure decreases, the baroreceptors induce vasoconstriction with increased vascular resistance and heart rate. When the blood pressure rises, the heart rate decreases with a tendency toward vasodilatation. Although the role of central and peripheral chemoreceptors in the fetus are less well defined, they appear to affect the FHR and blood pressure in response to changes in hydrogen ion concentration, CO_2 tension, or oxygen content.

As mentioned previously, the fetus has *sleep/wake (rest/activity) cycles* similar to those observed in the normal newborn, which influence both the heart rate and the variability, as well as the responsiveness to stimulation and, perhaps, hypoxia (104,149,150). While the fetus is awake and active, long-term variability, including accelerations and decelerations, dominate the FHR tracing. Fetal breathing increases the beat-to-beat variability by alteration of intrathoracic pressure and carotid blood pressure. With increased intrathoracic pressure, pulse pressure decreases and the heart rate increases. With decreased intrathoracic pressure, the opposite occurs (32,104). With transition from wakefulness to non-rapid eye movement (REM) sleep with regular breathing movements and absent body movement, heart rate variability diminishes. These effects become increasingly obvious as the fetus matures. Thus, electrocortical activity modulates the activity of the fetal autonomic nervous system. Although the fetus rarely breathes during UCs, fetal breathing movements may precipitate reflex, late decelerations that cease when breathing activity ceases.

In addition to intrinsic factors, the FHR is also subject to *external influences*.

Thus, the active fetus responds to sound and tactile stimulation of the head or body with FHR acceleration. There is distinctly diminished response in the sleeping state. Stimulation of the face or injection of cold saline into the uterus around the face or the cord produces prompt deceleration of FHR. Maternal ingestion of glucose also increases the reactivity of the fetus (104).

Uterine contractions increase both sympathetic and parasympathetic tone in the fetus (20,128,129,132). Contractions stimulate cortical centers in the fetal brain and provoke accelerations of FHR via the cardiac nerves and perhaps the adrenal medulla. In addition, when the fetal head is engaged in the maternal pelvis, UCs may increase intracranial pressure and cause a reflex slowing of the FHR. In general, during labor, these opposing influences on the FHR are balanced, and there is either no observable change in the FHR pattern during UCs or, at most, some increased variability (40). These opposing influences may be uncovered by pharmacologic blockage of the fetal automonic nervous system. Administration of atropine increases the FHR (rarely more than 155–160 bpm) and diminishes variability, as well as causing accelerations during UCs. For practical purposes, fetuses with nonvertex presentations or those at high station display FHR accelerations during contractions.

Hypoxemia alters peripheral resistance both by direct effect on the vascular beds and indirectly via the baro- and chemoreceptors (26–28,76,103,119,140). By these mechanisms, hypoxemia influences the FHR and its variability as well as the blood pressure and distribution of blood flow in the fetus. The precise effect varies, depending on the nature of the insult, its rapidity of onset, and the presence or absence of UCs.

The response of a fetus who becomes *mildly hypoxemic* during a UC involves an increase in blood pressure and variability and a decrease of the FHR to produce a late deceleration. The delayed onset of the deceleration is related in part to the transit time through the umbilical circulation. There is more rapid onset when the acidosis becomes more severe (111). As the fetal pH decreases, the FHR rises and the frequency followed by the amplitude of the oscillations decreases. These decelerations in the mildly hypoxemic fetus are of reflex (vagal) origin and may be blocked experimentally by atropine (65,103,140). *Chronic hypoxia* depresses these reflexes and thus results in diminished variability and late decelerations; the latter cannot be blocked by atropine because they are due to a direct hypoxic effect on the myocardium.

Variable decelerations are the most frequent decelerations encountered during labor. This FHR pattern is precipitated commonly by umbilical cord compression and is rarely associated with fetal hypoxia (18,23,76,96,101). With *frequent and prolonged decelerations,* the fetus will most probably become hypoxic (43).

The placenta receives about half of the fetal cardiac output via the umbilical circulation. When umbilical cord occlusion occurs, there is an increase in peripheral resistance and in blood pressure, an activation of the baroreceptors, and a precipitous decrease in FHR. Activation of the chemoreceptors and the sympathetic system maintains the FHR and blood pressure. When the cord occlusion is released, fetal hypertension diminishes as the FHR returns to its baseline level. The duration of a variable deceleration is not related exclusively to the duration of cord compression. Delayed recovery following a variable deceleration suggests that the stimulus activated the sympathetic system, which resulted in vasoconstriction that disappears only slowly. An immediate return of the FHR to baseline with normal variability suggests that the stimulus was not severe enough to produce the significant vasoconstriction. Alternatively, when there is return of the FHR to baseline with absent variability and rebound accelerations, it is probable that sympathetic reserve has been depleted. As fetal acidosis worsens, the decelerations become broader and smoother in contour, provoking less elevation of blood pressure, and are less amenable to pharmacological manipulation. Decelerations of the FHR are generally considered to be ''protective'' for the fetus. However, FHR changes are of little practical benefit as long as the pressor response is maintained. Thus, atropine may block or delay the decelerations caused by brief cord occlusion, but this effect of atropine does not generally affect outcome (8). In contrast, with adrenergic blockade, e.g., by propranolol, the fetus is unable to withstand even transient hypoxia, and there is an immediate, profound slowing of the FHR, which results in cardiac arrest (104). These observations are analogous to the manipulation of the dive reflex in mammals. Immersion of the seal or the trained diver results in peripheral vasoconstriction, hypertension, and bradycardia. These responses redistribute cardiac output away from nonvital organs (skin, intestines, lungs) and to vital organs (heart, brain, placenta) (28). This response may be impaired significantly by blockade of the pressor response.

Decelerations and bradycardia occur commonly during the second stage of labor (13,67). The observed decelerations are of variable shape and are related to the frequency of contractions, the position of the head and cord in the pelvis, and the amount of expulsive effort. In general, these decelerations appear to be reflex FHR patterns that are rarely accompanied by significant metabolic acidosis. *As long as FHR variability is maintained, fetal well-being is assured* (14).

In summary, these diverse responses demonstrate that many factors not necessarily related to hypoxia may influence FHR and variability. Thus, auscultation of FHR is of limited value for the assessment of fetal well-being. In terms of current knowledge, it is oversimplistic to assume that all bradycardia or tachycardia imply fetal distress.

TERMINOLOGY OF FHR MONITORING

The interpretation of FHR monitoring requires more rigorous terminology than that used in the context of auscultation. *Baseline* features refer to changes in FHR that occur between contractions, whereas *periodic* changes are related directly to contractions. Thus, *bradycardia, tachycardia,* and *variability* refer to baseline changes, whereas *accelerations* and *decelerations* describe changes during the UC cycle.

The fetal monitor readily displays the long- and short-term variability of the FHR pattern (Fig. 2). Short-term variability represents *nonpredictable,* abrupt

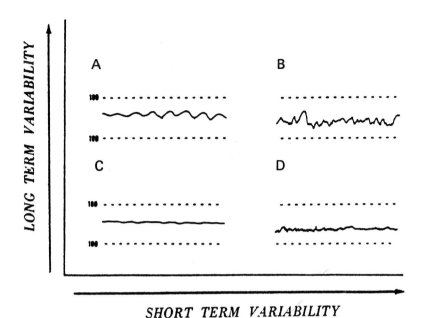

SHORT TERM VARIABILITY

FIG. 2. Illustration of long- and short-term variability. Under normal conditions both long- and short-term variability change concomitantly. Long-term variability describes predictable unduions in the range of two to six cycles per minute and amplitude 5–15 bpm. Short-term variability describes unpredictable changes in interval from beat to beat. "Normal Variability" represents adequate short-term variability *(B,D)*. Diminished short-term variability *(A,C)* prevails irrespective of presence of long-term variability.

changes in rate from beat to beat. Long-term variability reflects undulating, *predictable* oscillations with a period of two to six cycles per minute and an amplitude of 5 to 15 bpm. Although these indices of variability generally change together and in the same direction, they may vary independently. As discussed previously, short-term variability is almost exclusively a parasympathetic function and may be considered the single most important indicator of fetal well-being (14,24).

As mentioned previously, the FHR responses to hypoxia depend not only on the rapidity of onset and the intensity of the asphyxial episode but also on the frequency and intensity of concomitant contractions (Table 7). In the absence of significant uterine activity, the fetus responds to *asphyxia of gradual onset* with (relative) tachycardia (rarely more than 160 bpm) and decreased variability, both of which responses are presumably mediated through release of sympathomimetic amines from the adrenal medulla. In this situation, tachycardia represents early, compensatory response to hypoxia. When this compensation fails, the FHR becomes unstable, slows, and death ensues. On the other hand, the earliest signs of *distress during labor* are late or variable decelerations that, in turn, are followed by elevation of the baseline FHR and loss of variability. If the insult is *very acute and/or profound,* the fetus will respond with bradycardia irrespective of uterine activity.

TABLE 7. *FHR responses to hypoxia*

	Uterine contractions	
Onset of hypoxia	Present	Absent
Acute	Bradycardia	Bradycardia
Chronic	Late decelerations	Tachycardia

DIAGNOSIS AND TREATMENT OF FETAL DISTRESS USING FHR PATTERNS

The clinical features of FHR evaluation during labor may be classified into five categories, as outlined in Table 8. Note that this classification requires evaluation of both baseline and periodic features (24) in each instance.

Reassuring Patterns

As discussed previously, the presence of adequate short-term variability usually presages a good outcome even in the presence of other FHR abnormalities that may be consistent with hypoxia, e.g., tachycardia, bradycardia, or decelerations. Early decelerations imply uniform, symmetrical decelerations that mirror the UC in both amplitude and timing. They are not accompanied by change in baseline rate or variability. They are caused by compression of the fetal head (Fig. 3) (71)

TABLE 8. *Classifications of FHR patterns*

	Clinical features	
Patterns	Baseline	Periodic
Reassuring	Average variability	Absent
	Stable FHR	Early decelerations
		Mild variable decelerations
		Uniform accelerations
Suspicious	Tachycardia (>150 bpm)	Decelerations absent
	Bradycardia (<110 bpm)	
	Decreased variability	
Threatening	Stable rate	Late decelerations
	Variability average	Variable decelerations
		Prolonged decelerations
Ominous	Absent variability	Late decelerations
	Unstable rate	Variable decelerations
	Bradycardia	Rebound accelerations
	Tachycardia	
Chronic	Absent variability	Variable decelerations
	Tachycardia (>150 bpm)	Rebound accelerations

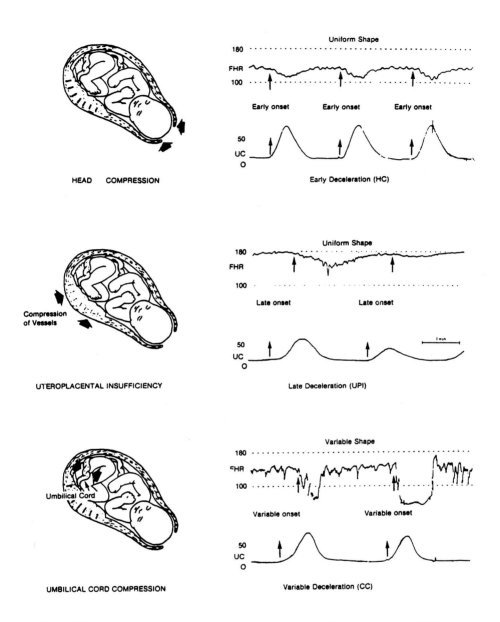

FIG. 3. Diagrammatic representation of proposed pathogenetic mechanism of fetal heart rate (FHR) deceleration patterns. In early decelerations caused by head compression, onset of deceleration *(arrows)* coincides with rise in intrauterine pressure *(arrows)*. Uniform shape of deceleration reflects shape of associated uterine pressure curve. Late decelerations caused by uteroplacental insufficiency are characterized by uniform shape and onset late in contraction. Variable decelerations caused by umbilical cord compression are of variable shape and do not reflect shape of associate intrauterine pressure curve; onset is variable in relationship to onset of contraction. (From ref. 71.)

and are not associated with hypoxia or adverse fetal outcome. Similarly, small variable decelerations, which are often indistinguishable from early decelerations, are totally innocuous, especially if associated with mild variable accelerations ("shoulders") before and after the deceleration (106). Uniform accelerations (Fig. 4) invariably signify a healthy, reactive fetus (5,53,63,64,90,94). These accelerations may occur either with contractions or as a result of fetal movement or stimulation of the fetus during vaginal or abdominal examination. Accelerations with UCs are seen more frequently in early labor before descent or with nonvertex presentation. Irrespective of the timing or association of acceleration with stimulation, movement, or UCs, the FHR between accelerations has normal variability. Neurologically abnormal, but well-oxygenated fetuses may exhibit FHR accelerations with fetal movements or UCs but will not exhibit variability between accelerations. Isolated compression of the umbilical vein may also produce uniform accelerations and may precede the onset of variable decelerations (79). However, as long as accelerations are present, the condition of the fetus is uniformly good. The presence of this reassuring pattern suggests strongly that there is no fetal indication for intervention (87,89).

Suspicious Patterns

Although the above baseline changes may be associated with fetal hypoxia during labor, in the absence of decelerations, they suggest a mechanism other than hypoxia (24,125). Clinically, maternal fever, secondary to amnionitis, is the most common recognizable cause of fetal tachycardia (Table 9). In this instance, the fetal and maternal heart rates rise in direct proportion to the degree of fever. However, fetal tachycardia, caused by fetal infection, may precede maternal fever. Elevated FHR >150 bpm in the postdate fetus suggests nutritional deficiency (130). An elevated FHR generally responds to treatment of the underlying cause or by cooling of the mother if the fever is very high. Drugs, especially atropine and beta-sympathomimetics, as well as fetal tachyarrhythmias may also be causes of fetal tachycardia.

Baseline bradycardia, as opposed to prolonged decelerations, is a late sign of fetal asphyxia (Table 9). Although fetuses who are near death will invariably have bradycardia (along with absent variability), the majority of fetuses with persistent heart rates between 90 and 120 bpm are postdates, demonstrate average baseline variability, are not asphyxiated, and demonstrate no objective signs of compromise (Fig. 5) (160). Baseline bradycardia in the range of 50 to 80 bpm with absent variability may represent profound asphyxia (unstable rate-sinus rhythm) or may signal the presence of complete heart block with idioventricular rhythm-stable rate. The diagnosis of heart block is facilitated by ultrasound scanning or examination of the fetal electrocardiogram (ECG). Fetal heart block, in turn, requires search for congenital heart disease, which has an incidence of approximately 20% in the fetus/newborn, as well as examination of the mother for collagen-vascular disease, especially lupus, or for significant infection, e.g., cytomegalovirus (139).

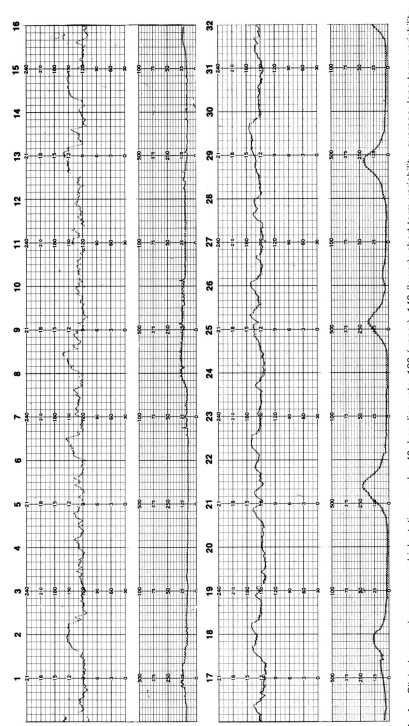

FIG. 4. Clinical: normal pregnancy, high station; weeks: 40; baseline rate: 120 (upper), 140 (lower); short-term variability: average; long-term variability: average; decelerations: none; accelerations: periodic, variable; uterine contraction: sporadic (upper), oxytocin (lower); outcome: normal, cesarean section, failure of descent. Comment: This tracing reveals effective medication that smoothes out the accelerations and decreases variability. Note effect of contraction on maternal breathing pattern (lower panel).

TABLE 9. *Etiologies of tachycardia,*
bradycardia, and decreased variability

Tachycardia
  Asphyxia
  Idiopathic
  Maternal fever
  Fetal infection
  Prematurity
  Drugs, e.g., atropine, isoxsuprine
  Arrhythmia
  Maternal anxiety
  Maternal throtoxicosis
Bradycardia
  Asphyxia (late)
  Arrhythmia
  Drug effect
  Hypothermia
Decreased variability
  Asphyxia
  Drugs
    Atropine—Scopolamine
    Tranquilizers—Diazepam
    Narcotics
    Barbiturates
    Local anesthetics
  Prematurity
  Tachycardia
  Physiologic? "sleep"
  Anesthesia
  Cardiac and CNS anomalies
  Arrhythmias—especially nodal

Decreased variability, signifying loss of autonomic control of the heart rate, may be a result of several causes (Table 9). Although acute hypoxia may increase baseline variability transiently, significant chronic hypoxia is associated invariably with diminished, short-term variability. Decreased variability during labor may be observed despite adequate oxygenation in premature fetuses or when drugs are administered to the mother during labor. All barbiturates, tranquilizers, and local or general anesthetics may reduce variability (Fig. 6). This is a predictable pharmacological response, the duration and extent of which varies in direct proportion to the amount of drug administered. During physiologic periods of rest or sleep, there is diminished variability. Stimulation of such fetuses, either by vaginal examination and abdominal palpation, or by scalp sampling, will often provoke a transient increase in variability or an acceleration, responses that suggest that the decreased variability is not the result of hypoxia or neurologic compromise. When asphyxia is present, decreased variability is associated with late or variable decelerations

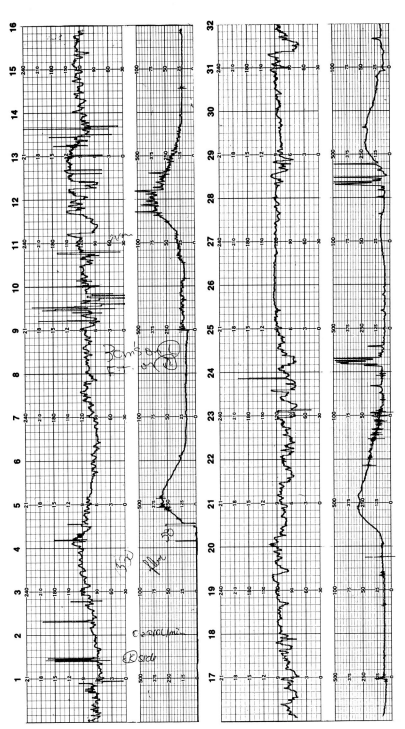

FIG. 5. Clinical: postdate pregnancy, early labor, oligohydramnios; weeks: 43; baseline rate: 110 to 120; short-term variability: average/increased; long-term variability: average; decelerations: prolonged, variable; accelerations: variable; uterine contraction: irregular; outcome: Meconium stained, normal outcome, postmaturity syndrome. Comment: Typical postdate pattern including low baseline rate, normal to increased variability, and broad shallow decelerations and variable decelerations. Anticipate more decelerations later in labor. This pattern is not an indication for intervention.

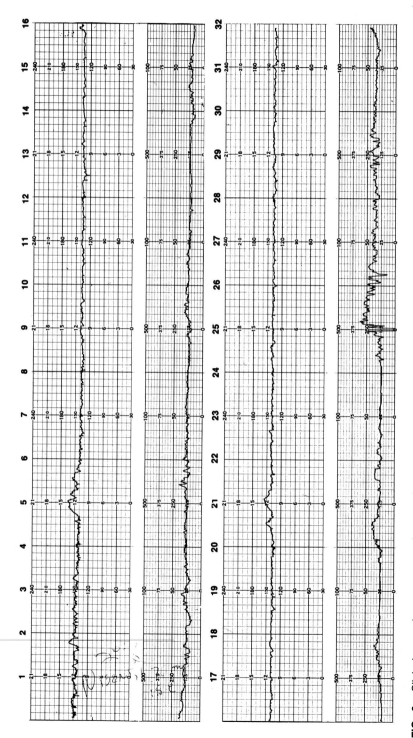

FIG. 6. Clinical: normal pregnancy; weeks: term; baseline rate: 140; short-term variability: average to decreased; long-term variability: decreased; decelerations: none; accelerations: none; uterine contraction: none; uterine contraction: sporadic, occasional; outcome: normal. Comment: This represents effect of medication that decreases both variability and frequency and angularity of accelerations of fetal movement.

(see ominous patterns section). In the moribund fetus, absent variability may represent an agonal pattern. Under these circumstances, decelerations may be absent (Fig. 7). Alternatively, absent variability without decelerations may provide a clue to neurologic compromise or congenital anomaly unrelated to asphyxia (48).

To minimize uncertainty regarding the significance of decreased variability, we recommend that monitoring be initiated before the administration to the mother of any medication that has the potential for altering FHR patterns. We emphasize that decreased variability in the absence of decelerations is almost invariably related to an etiology other than asphyxia—usually medication. If an asphyxial insult is superimposed in a baby whose variability is diminished by medication, decelerations will appear.

Suspicious patterns usually require no intervention, but a search for the underlying cause should be undertaken. If hypoxia cannot reasonably be excluded, a fetal blood sample may be obtained and will be normal in more than 95% of cases. If a suspicious FHR pattern is recognized, potentially compromising drugs or anesthetics should be avoided until a clear explanation other than hypoxia has been identified.

Threatening Patterns

Threatening patterns imply unequivocal fetal insult related to impaired uterine blood flow (late decelerations) or impaired umbilical blood flow (variable decelerations). Although other mechanisms have been proposed for these decelerations, their relationship to compromised blood flow is well established by clinical observations (2,71,140).

Late decelerations are considered to be related to impaired uteroplacental exchange. Late decelerations have a uniform appearance and are repetitive, beginning after the onset of the contraction and returning to the baseline after the contraction subsides. The amplitude and duration of the late deceleration is generally proportional to the amplitude and duration of the underlying contraction (Fig. 8). In the normal fetus, late decelerations may be precipitated acutely by anesthesia (epidural or spinal), excessive uterine activity, or supine hypotension. They occur more frequently in the fetus with chronic placental insufficiency, e.g., intrauterine growth retardation. Frequently, late decelerations may be ameliorated by cessation of the oxytocin infusion and turning the mother to her side. Although late decelerations associated with good variability may be associated with episodes of compromise in a fetus with a previously normal FHR pattern, they usually respond to conservative measures. During recovery there may be a transient rise in FHR and decreased variability as the decelerations diminish in amplitude. The duration of these changes is proportional to the duration of the hypoxemic episode. If the hypoxemic stimulus is not removed, late decelerations exhibit progressive increase in amplitude with decreasing variability and a rising baseline rate. In this instance, surgical intervention for nonremediable fetal distress should be considered.

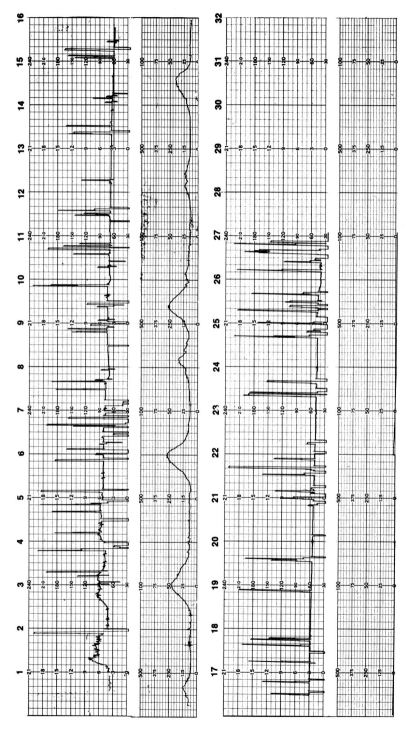

FIG. 7. Clinical: no fetal movements; weeks: 36; baseline rate: 70 and falling slowly; short-term variability: absent; long-term variability: absent; decelerations: mild unclassified (M2–3); accelerations: absent; outcome: fetal death. Note deterioration of baseline heart rate but generally absent variability and absent decelerations as fetus dies *in utero*. Vertical spikes in record represent artifact, not arrhythmia. Electrocardiogram (ECG) reveals sinus rhythm until death.

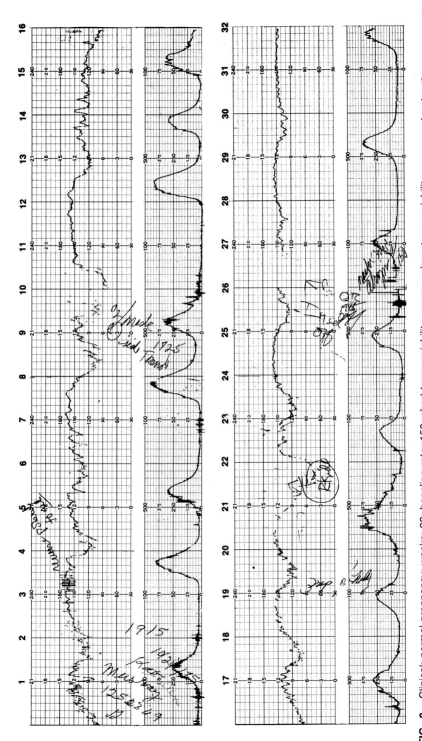

FIG. 8. Clinical: normal pregnancy; weeks: 38; baseline rate: 150; short-term variability: average; long-term variability: average; decelerations: recurrent variable; accelerations: sporadic; uterine contraction: late labor, coupling of contractions, oxytocin effect; outcome: emergency cesarean section, Apgars 7–9. Comment: Despite frequent contractions and variable decelerations, note the stability of the baseline rate and the maintenance of baseline variability.

Variable decelerations are observed commonly (Fig. 9) (49). They frequently develop without warning late in the first stage of labor and are often related to cord compression. They can be produced in experimental animals or humans by occlusion of the umbilical cord. They may be precipitated or relieved by maneuvers that enhance amniotic fluid buffering of the cord or by alteration of the relationship of the cord, the fetus, and the uterine wall (46). In the absence of cord prolapse, variable decelerations are not associated with fetal distress, i.e., sudden death during an episode of variable decelerations is virtually unknown (18,82).

Variable decelerations may be associated with cord compression, vasa previa, nuchal, short or prolapsed cord and decreased amniotic fluid volume (ruptured membranes, oligohydramnios), descent of the fetus, and head compression, especially with occiput-posterior pattern (75). However, any significant alteration in uteroplacental perfusion may precipitate variable or prolonged decelerations (12).

During the second stage of labor, variable decelerations are common and predominantly related to head compression. These occur generally during pushing and occur more commonly when the head is in an occiput-posterior position rather than in an occiput-anterior position (75). Figure 10 illustrates the decelerations in the FHR pattern associated with bearing down efforts of the mother during the second stage of labor (Fig. 10). Cessation of expulsive efforts will diminish both the severity and amplitude of the decelerations. This maneuver plays an important role in both the prevention and treatment of fetal distress.

Variable decelerations are generally inconsistent in onset and duration in relation to the underlying UCs. Consecutive decelerations tend to differ in appearance but they may mimic early or late decelerations. They are best classified according to the ''company they keep.'' In the majority of instances, no obvious explanation for variable decelerations is found. However, as the frequency of decelerations increases and the ability to correct the pattern diminishes, the probability of cord problems increases. Kubli et al. (93) have classified the severity of variable decelerations according to their duration and amplitude without consideration of baseline variability. Such a classification may be misleading because it does not take into account the variability of the baseline. As previously discussed with late decelerations, the impact of a deceleration on the acid-base status of the fetus may be estimated from the effect of the deceleration on variability and baseline rate (Fig. 11). For a given amplitude of decelerations, the pH will be significantly higher if variability is preserved than when it is absent (123). Thus, we pay relatively little attention to the amplitude or duration of the deceleration compared to the changes in baseline variability (24,49).

Two other features of the variable deceleration deserve comment. In many instances, decelerations are preceded and followed by brief, erratic accelerations of FHR. These accelerations, associated with normal baseline variability (and referred to as ''shoulders'') signify fetal resiliency. They may result from isolated umbilical vein occlusion or sympathetic responses (79). These anticipatory accelerations are blunted or lost if the baseline FHR is elevated or when profound hypoxia has reduced the sympathetic response. With absent baseline variability,

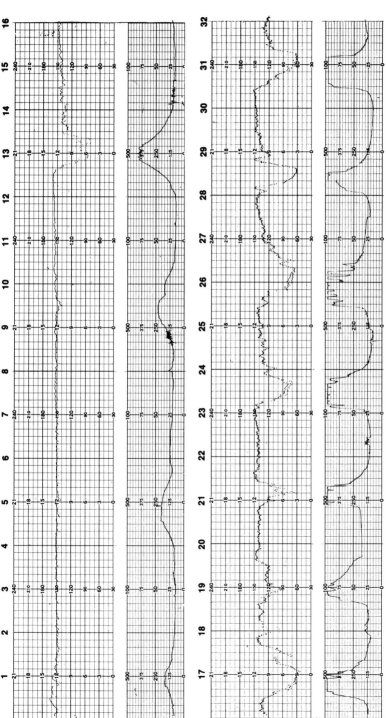

FIG. 9. Clinical: normal pregnancy on epidural; weeks: term; baseline rate: 150; short-term variability: decreased/average; long-term variability: decreased/average; decelerations: variable; accelerations: variable ("shoulders"); uterine contraction: regular—on oxytocin **(upper)**, late labor, pushing **(lower)**; outcome: normal. Comment: Posterior position, typical pattern above showing onset of descent (transition) with sudden appearance of variable decelerations. Note characteristic differences in shape, onset, duration, and amplitude of various decelerations. Note also the differences in angle of deceleration as it returns to the baseline. Decelerations with "slow return to baseline" (a term that should not be used) generally associated with more variability than those in which return is more abrupt. Duration of return is of little consequence. Determine impact of deceleration by looking at changes in baseline rate and variability that follow it. Note several presentations of junctional fetal cardiac rhythms at base of variable decelerations toward end of lower panel.

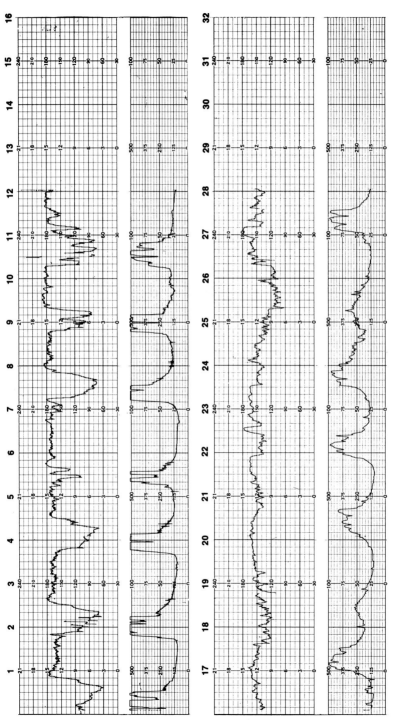

FIG. 10. Clinical: normal, occiput posterior **(upper)**, occiput anterior **(lower)**; weeks: term fetuses (2); baseline rate: 180 top, 150 to 160 bottom; short-term variability: average; long-term variability: average; accelerations: variable; decelerations: variable ("shoulders"); uterine contraction: late labor with pushing; outcome: normal Apgar scores. Comment: In addition to the many obvious features of variable decelerations and the frequent correspondence of changes in the heart rate associated with expulsive efforts, the top pattern is consistent with second stage with the head in the occiput posterior position. The occiput anterior position tends to have a much less well-defined pattern of decelerations.

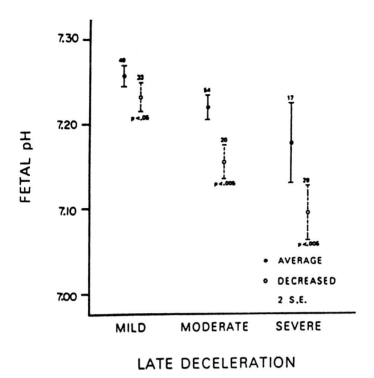

LATE DECELERATION

FIG. 11. Relationship between fetal blood pH and severity of late decelerations at time of blood sampling. Each fetal heart rate (FHR) classification is further divided into average (>5 beats/min) of decreased (<5 beats/min) FHR variability. (From ref. 123.)

smooth accelerations following variable decelerations are a potentially ominous feature (see below) (44).

Threatening FHR patterns warrant corrective measures as outlined in Table 10. Therapy is directed toward correction of the underlying disturbance in fetal or placental blood flow (73). In the vast majority of cases, these maneuvers suffice and recovery may be anticipated. It is axiomatic that prevention is more important than therapeutic intervention. Thus, placing the mother on her side and properly regulating oxytocin infusion are considered appropriate measures in all pregnancies. Beta-sympathomimetics (tocolytics) are gaining popularity as a temporizing measure in the treatment of fetal distress. However, bicarbonate and glucose infusions are not of demonstrable value (7,127).

The response of variable decelerations to corrective measures is less predictable than is the response of late decelerations. Often, variable decelerations may be corrected by maneuvers that alter the geometry of fetus, cord, and uterine wall. Thus, altering the mother's position between lateral, supine, and Trendelenburg positions will frequently improve the pattern. When such maneuvers fail, placing the patient in knee-chest position may be helpful (25). If there is still no response

TABLE 10. *Methods of treatment for fetal distress*

Improve uterine blood flow
Avoid supine position
Reduce uterine contraction
Decrease oxytocin
(Uterine relaxants)
Improve umbilical blood flow
Alter maternal position
(Elevate vertex)
Enhance maternal substrate
Oxygen
(Glucose)
(Bicarbonate)

and if baseline changes become superimposed on the variable decelerations, elevation of the vertex may be therapeutic. Elevation of the vertex, however, should be attempted only in the delivery room in case a prolapse of the cord is precipitated by this maneuver.

Severe variable decelerations may occasionally be accompanied by brief episodes of cardiac asystole (heart block) (Fig. 12). These episodes appear to relate to excessive vagal response in an otherwise healthy fetus. They are associated invariably with average or increased baseline variability following the deceleration, and the outcome has been uniformly good (82). Irrespective of associated asystole, in some instances, the baseline of the decelerations may demonstrate absent variability with FHR of 60 bpm. This pattern represents nodal rhythm and, like the occasional episode of asystole, should be treated as any other severe variable deceleration. The variability at the trough of a variable deceleration reflects the pacing mechanism rather than the oxygenation of the fetus, i.e., sinus (with variability) or nodal (without variability).

Although variable decelerations occur more commonly in the second stage of labor, the interpretation of the tracing and the treatment of the decelerations are similar during both the first and second stages of labor. Except when the head is crowning and delivery imminent, therapy should be governed by the conservative principles elaborated above, with emphasis on intrauterine resuscitation whenever possible. Cesarean section is warranted only if the FHR pattern deteriorates or prolonged decelerations recur. Deterioration of variable decelerations (i.e., progressive hypoxia, hypercarbia, and acidosis) is revealed by rising baseline FHR, smoothing of the deceleration, and overshoot. "Slow return of the baseline," which is usually associated with normal variability and no increase in baseline rate or loss of variability, does not represent deterioration.

Although there is a natural tendency to attempt to correct variable decelerations by changing the patient's position, this maneuver will have limited success during the second stage of labor. Furthermore, there is no evidence that the condition of the fetus will deteriorate as long as there is recovery of FHR and variability be-

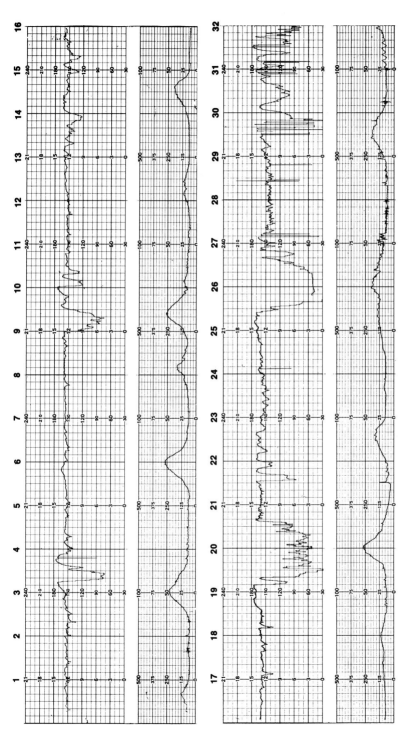

FIG. 12. Clinical: normal pregnancy; weeks: 40; baseline rate: 150 bpm; short-term variability: average; long-term variability: average, increased; decelerations: variable; accelerations: variable ("shoulders"); uterine contraction: spontaneous active labor; outcome: normal. Comment: This tracing illustrates a number of features about variable decelerations including their intermittent nature, variable pattern, and coassociation with variable accelerations ("shoulders"). Exaggerated long-term variability (saltatory) pattern (17) is especially likely at the end of the deceleration. Most decelerations are anticipated by a variable acceleration followed by a rather abrupt downslope, occasionally culminating (20,26 M) in a brief episode of asystole (heart block). Note the dramatic difference between the bases of these two variable decelerations (please do not call them "severe"). In one the recovery is more than 60 bpm and the variability at the base of the deceleration is exaggerated. In the other, the recovery is less than 60 bpm and reveals the characteristic pattern of nodal rhythm with its brief deceleration and subtle warmup. In both instances, the return to baseline is prompt although erratic, but the baseline rate and variability after the decelerations are quite similar. It seems unreasonable to argue that the pattern at the base of the deceleration carries any prognostic value. Rather the appearance of the base of the variable deceleration in the reactive fetus is simply a reflection of the mechanism of cardiac pacing (nodal or sinus), which in turn reflects the level to which the rate descends.

tween decelerations (43). With recurrent decelerations that occur especially in early labor and are not associated with change in baseline FHR, amnio-infusion may prove helpful (108). When cesarean section has been decided on, cessation of pushing is an important palliative maneuver.

Prolonged decelerations characteristically last longer than 2 min and are associated with decreased FHR of more than 30 bpm (Fig. 13). The causes of prolonged decelerations include manipulation of the patient, maternal voiding, vaginal examination, fetal scalp sampling, uterine hypertonus, maternal seizures, hypoxemia, and hypotension (12,13,142). Prolonged decelerations generally occur in a previously healthy fetus with normal variability. They may be preceded by an acceleration, but the descent in FHR is usually precipitous. If the lowest FHR is less than 60 bpm, conduction defects, i.e., nodal or junctional rhythms, are common and are associated with a flat FHR. Recovery is usually associated with prompt resumption of variability, although there may be a transient late deceleration during the period of recovery. Unless the deceleration has been brief, the return to baseline will be associated with decreased variability and relative tachycardia. The extent and duration of the reactive tachycardia following the deceleration is a function of the severity of the hypoxemia that has developed during the bradycardia. That is, the more rapid the recovery of FHR and variability, the more limited has been the hypoxic insult during the deceleration. Sustained tachycardia, out of proportion to the duration or severity of the deceleration, may indicate intracranial hemorrhage.

Regional anesthetic blocks (PCB or epidural) may also precipitate prolonged decelerations related to uterine hypertonicity. The deceleration usually begins between 5 and 15 min after the block (occasionally sooner) and may last as long as 20 to 30 min. The typical duration is less than 4 to 8 min. Direct fetal toxicity from the drug is an unlikely mechanism for the production of prolonged bradycardia (45). Spasm of the uterine arteries in association with excessive uterine stimulation appears to be a more probable explanation (45,59). Except in large dosages, injection of local anesthetics directly into the fetus does not produce bradycardia (45). Because of their potential adverse effects, epidural and paracervical blocks should not be administered to the potentially compromised fetus.

Prolonged decelerations/bradycardia may develop in the fetus just before death. These findings are often preceded by repetitive decelerations and loss of variability. Under these circumstances, bradycardia is a very late sign of fetal distress and the fetus is rarely salvageable. A prolonged deceleration in a previously normal fetus, however, may evolve into a serious asphyxial emergency. In this situation, the FHR will appear flat after several minutes and then continue to decrease. Prolonged decelerations may also occur in association with rupture of a placental vessel or fetal exsanguination.

During the second stage of labor, prolonged decelerations occur most commonly in association with pushing, especially if the fetus is in an occiput-posterior position (75). Corrective maneuvers advocated previously for treatment of variable decelerations are also appropriate in this situation. Scalp sampling should not be performed during the deceleration. Although atropine will minimize the extent and

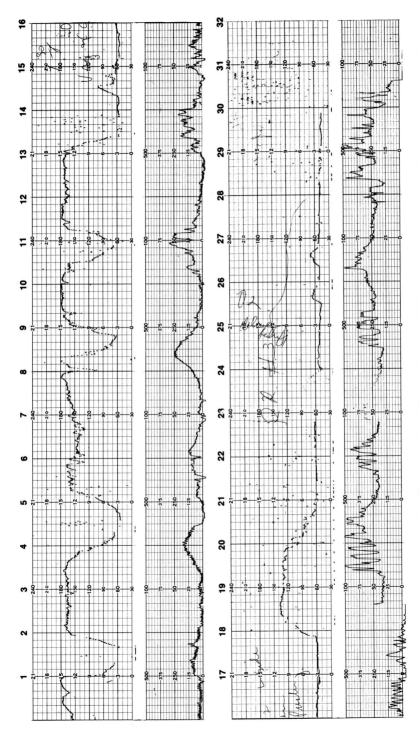

FIG. 13. Clinical: normal labor; weeks: 38; baseline rate: 160 to 170; short-term variability: average; long-term variability: average; decelerations: recurrent variable; accelerations: none; uterine contraction: late labor, pushing with contractions; outcome: Apgar 1, 6, and 8. Comment: Acute fetal distress with recurrent variable decelerations evolving into a prolonged deceleration. The sequence is more common when the occiput is posterior. Its frequency can be minimized by reducing the patient's expulsive efforts until the fetal heart rate decelerations have recovered.

duration of these decelerations, it is not clear whether this medication has a role in fetal resuscitation (105,115,118). The required dosages are substantial and will produce abnormal FHR patterns with diminished variability, increased baseline rate, and variable decelerations with overshoot.

Ominous Patterns

Ominous patterns contain a combination of pathologic decelerations and abnormalities of the baseline. These patterns strongly suggest severe and progressive fetal compromise. The underlying mechanisms have been discussed previously. Rebound accelerations (''overshoot'') represent uniform accelerations following variable decelerations and are accompanied by absent baseline variability (Fig. 14). Relative baseline tachycardia is common. Uniform accelerations rarely precede variable decelerations. When present, this pattern indicates autonomic imbalance. It may be seen with chronic hypoxic stress, following administration of atropine in premature fetuses or in fetuses who are neurologically abnormal.

An unstable FHR that may appear ''sinusoidal'' with absent short-term variability suggests that compensatory mechanisms have been exhausted (10), although sinusoidal patterns are not necessarily ominous. They may be observed consistently following narcotic administration and occasionally in association with infection (Fig. 15) (51,55,80,161). Such patterns have been reported in dying fetuses (22) and those severely affected with Rh-isoimmunization. In some of these fetuses, only the ominous baseline changes may be present, and late or variable decelerations may be absent (Fig. 7) (22). Although bradycardia is common in the severely compromised fetus, the rate may occasionally be in the normal range (146). Cardiac arrest may occur, but unlike those associated with variable decelerations, these episodes are predictable, associated with sinus rhythm, and invariably fatal (82,158).

Although the same conservative measures advocated earlier for treatment of threatening patterns may be applied to the patient with ominous FHR patterns, preparations should also be made for expeditious delivery because recovery is unlikely with conservative measures alone.

Chronic Pattern

We have recently recognized a variant of the ominous pattern in which absent variability accompanies small variable decelerations with overshoot, with absence of late decelerations (44,91,137). Although some of these fetuses are terminally ill from asphyxia, many survive with residual neurologic handicap (86). The baseline FHR is stable, in the normal range or slightly elevated, and there may be accelerations associated with fetal movement. The pH is usually normal and intervention appears to be of little benefit.

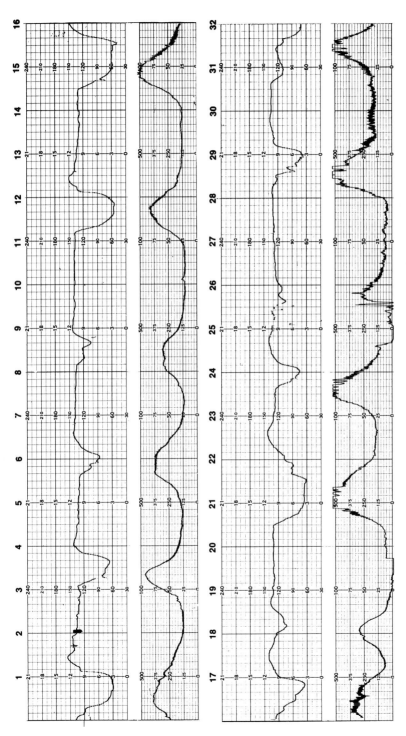

FIG. 14. Clinical: meconium staining, oligohydramnios; weeks: 41; baseline rate: 140; short-term variability: absent; long-term variability: absent; decelerations: recurrent variable; accelerations: overshoot; uterine contraction: late spontaneous labor, pushing with contractions toward end of record; outcome: low Apgar, dysmature. Comment: Recurrent variable decelerations with overshoot. Note relatively leisurely descent of most decelerations, the occasional step function during descent (at 6 and 29 M) and episodes of nodal rhythm when the nadir of the deceleration reaches 60–70 bpm (12, 15, and 21 M). This pattern represents moderate acute asphyxia superimposed on chronic distress. Delivery ought to be undertaken but the damage may have already taken place.

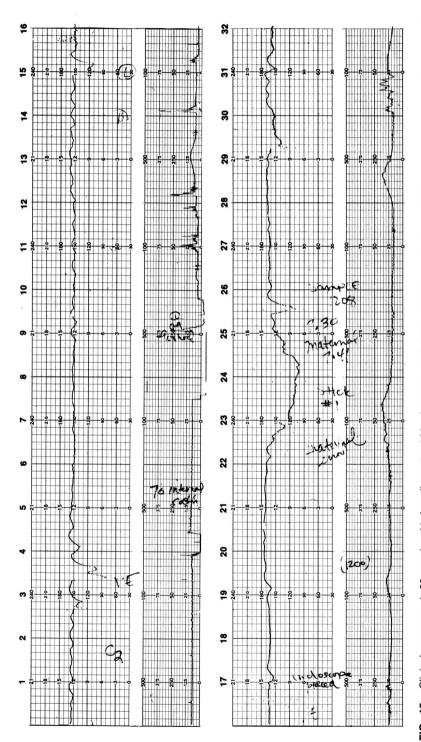

FIG. 15. Clinical: same as 1–29; weeks: 41; baseline rate: 160; short-term variability: absent; long-term variability: decreased; decelerations: variable, prolonged; accelerations: overshoot; uterine contraction: irregular, early labor; outcome: neurologic handicap. Pattern reflects long-standing compromise. Note "sinusoidal" type pattern (1–2, 9–15 M) and normal pH. Intervention unlikely to be of any benefit.

FETAL ACID-BASE BALANCE

The feasibility of FBS was demonstrated by Saling in 1962 (133). This technique enabled the obstetrician to document the impact of obstetrical procedures on the acid-base status of the fetus. It has been known for some time that maternal blood has a higher pH and is more highly oxygenated than fetal blood (133). Previously, these biochemical differences were thought to reflect a state of chronic acidosis and hypoxia in the fetus ("Mt. Everest *in utero*"). This notion has been discarded because of evidence that the gradients for hydrogen ions and carbon dioxide across the placenta are small. Furthermore, there is a close correlation between maternal and fetal blood gas values (3,78,133). Adequate oxygenation of the fetal tissues is maintained by the high fetal cardiac output and hemoglobin content, as well as the favorable oxygen-dissociation curve of fetal hemoglobin.

The fetal acid-base balance is regulated closely. In the adult, the pH is adjusted by both pulmonary and renal mechanisms. However, the fetus must rely entirely on placental function for oxygen uptake, nutrition, and the elimination of wastes. Under ordinary circumstances, the major nutrient for energy in the fetus is supplied by the transplacental passage of glucose from the mother. The fetus has limited capability to use ketones as an energy source and anaerobic metabolism is usually unnecessary (33). In the presence of oxygen, glucose is metabolized to carbon dioxide and water to yield 39 moles of adenosinetriphosphate (ATP) for every mole of glucose oxidized. Under anaerobic conditions, glucose can be metabolized only to pyruvic and lactic acid, a process that yields only 2 moles of ATP per mole of glucose and that is accompanied by a fall in pH. Thus, pH may be used as an indirect measure of oxygen availability to the fetus. In fact, in combination with pCO_2, pH is a better determinant of fetal oxygenation than pO_2. In addition, hypoxic-ischemic insults in the fetus usually occur intermittently. Because the pO_2 "has no memory" for the previous insults, it will improve between contractions. However, such insults will be accompanied by a progressive fall in pH.

Although fetal asphyxia may result from many factors (Table 11), the most common cause is interruption of either uterine or umbilical blood flow. Irrespective of etiology, the results of fetal asphyxia include rising pCO_2, falling pH, and development of base excess. These metabolic abnormalities reflect a combined respiratory and metabolic acidosis. The problem is further compounded by a fall in the affinity of hemoglobin for oxygen as the pH decreases and as glycolysis becomes impaired progressively. If the fetal asphyxia is brief, only the pCO_2 will rise, resulting in a respiratory acidosis.

FETAL BLOOD SAMPLING

Fetal blood sampling (FBS) requires experienced personnel and specialized equipment. Application of the technique requires that the membranes must be rup-

TABLE 11. *Causes of fetal asphyxia*

Maternal factors
   Hypotension
      Blood loss
      Medication
      Regional anesthesia
   Sedation
   Anesthesia
   Laryngospasm
   Aspiration
   Breathing low O_2 mixtures
   High altitude
   Anemia
   Methemoglobinemia
   Chronic pulmonary disease
   Congenital or acquired heart disease
   Exercise

Uterine blood flow
   Supine position—compression of vena cava and aorta
   ? Vasopressors for relief of hypotension
   Preeclampsia, chronic hypertension, diabetes
   ? Ruptured membranes

Placental factors
   Decreased area of exchange—abruptio
      ? Inflammation
      ? Edema
      ? Increased thickness (erythroblastosis or lues)
   Placental infarcts
   Chronic placental insufficiency (postmaturity)

Fetal factors
   Cord compression—1/3 of all deliveries (vaginal)
   ? Fetal hypotension—Blood pressure normally increases with gestation
      Effect of hypotensive agents to mother
   Hydropic infants are always acidotic during labor

Questions
   Does the functional capacity of the placenta as an organ of transfer keep pace with the
      needs of the fetus as gestation advances or does it fall behind?
   Can babies suffer marked nutritional deprivation without significant compromise in O_2
      and CO_2 transport?

tured and the cervix dilated at least 2 cm. The presenting part of the fetus first is visualized with an amnioscope (Fig. 16). The scalp then is dried with a cotton swab and silicone applied over the anticipated puncture site. When FBS was first introduced, ethyl chloride was sprayed on the scalp to promote hyperemia. More recently, this step has been abandoned. The incision is made with a shielded blade, which prevents penetration of the skin beyond 2 mm. A second incision, parallel and adjacent to the first, may facilitate blood flow. For optimal blood flow the incision should be made just before a UC and sampling should be completed before the peak of the UC. The globule of blood is collected in a heparinized capillary tube, and its acid-base composition determined by suitable micromethod.

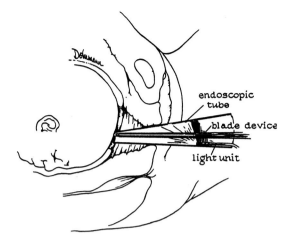

FIG. 16. Technique of obtaining fetal blood from scalp during labor. (From ref. 31.)

After the blood sample is obtained, it is important to stop the bleeding by maintaining pressure on the incision through the next UC.

The normal range of scalp blood pH is 7.25 to 7.40 (Table 12). This pH tends to remain stable during the first stage of labor but may decrease during the expulsive second phase (78). The fall in pH may be prevented or minimized by avoidance of the supine position during the second stage of labor and by proper attention to the FHR response to the mother's expulsive efforts (72). There is significant variation in the range of normal pH as well as in the interpretation of blood pH levels (99). Nevertheless, most authors consider values less than 7.20 to be low. Values less than 7.24 are generally considered to require further evaluation (133,155). If low or borderline values are obtained, the sample is immediately repeated and maternal acid-base balance simultaneously determined (131). If fetal acidosis is confirmed or if the pH is falling progressively, immediate delivery is considered appropriate, provided that the mother is not acidemic. If the mother is found to have a simultaneously low pH, primary attention should be directed to-

TABLE 12. *Normal arterial acid-base values*

| | Adult | | | |
	Nonpregnant	Pregnant	Before labor	Fetal 2nd stage
pH		7.4	7.4	7.37	7.3
CO_2 (mm Hg)		40	34	38	43
HCO_3 (mm/liter)		24	21	21	21
Base excess (mmole/liter)		0	−4	−3	−5

ward correction of her acidemia with hydration and bicarbonate if necessary. The fetal scalp sample should be repeated subsequently. Obtaining a baseline scalp sample in a high-risk pregnancy with normal or only suspicious FHR pattern is probably of little value, in that fetuses who deteriorate later usually have normal pH values at the onset of labor. On the other hand, uncorrectable, ominous FHR patterns do not require confirmation by scalp sampling, and rapid delivery is the most appropriate response.

Fetal scalp sampling is of limited value in the analysis of variable or profound decelerations. Because even inconsequential variable decelerations will affect the pH transiently, blood sampling performed immediately following the onset of the deceleration may yield a low pH. The optimal timing for pH analysis is just before the next deceleration. In practical terms, if there is stable baseline FHR and if variability is maintained or if the fetus responds to the manipulation of the scalp sampling procedure with an acceleration, there is no need for either intervention or scalp sampling, irrespective of the frequency, amplitude, or duration of the decelerations.

In general, fetal outcome is related to the severity and type of acidosis, whether metabolic or respiratory acidosis. Approximately one-third of fetuses with pH less than 7.25 are born with low Apgar scores (68). When the pH is less than 7.10, almost 90% of fetuses are depressed. Thus, fetal acidosis is associated with significantly increased risk of subsequent neurological handicap (15,133,155).

CORRELATIONS

There is a clear relationship between abnormal FHR patterns, low pH, and neonatal compromise in both humans and experimental animals (141,156,159,160) (Table 13). In addition, preliminary evidence suggests an increased risk of seizures in unmonitored fetuses as well as a relationship between abnormal FHR patterns and subsequent neurological abnormalities (37,100,113).

A number of reports demonstrate a correlation between FHR patterns and scalp blood pH (116). Innocuous FHR patterns are invariably associated with normal pH values and normal fetal outcome. However, abnormal FHR patterns or modestly low pH values do not often correlate with compromised neonatal outcome. On the

TABLE 13. *Relationship between fetal blood pH and FHR deceleration patterns in preceding 20 min*

Deceleration pattern	Blood pH[a]
Early, mild variable, or absent	7.30 ± 0.04
Moderate variable	7.26 ± 0.04
Mild or moderate late	7.22 ± 0.06
Severe late or variable	7.14 ± 0.07

[a]Approximate mean ± standard deviation.

other hand, virtually all fetuses who are compromised at birth as a result of as-phyxia may be anticipated on the basis of abnormal FHR patterns or low pH. If mean values are considered, the pH declines progressively with increasing severity of the late or variable decelerations. The specificity of the prediction improves if variability and decelerations are considered in combination (123). Tracings with poor variability and no decelerations are associated almost invariably (>97%) with normal pH values (162).

Furthermore, patterns of development of fetal acidosis have corroborated the proposed mechanisms for FHR decelerations. Transient umbilical cord compression is accompanied by a rapid but short-lived fall in pH and rise in pCO_2, i.e., respiratory acidosis. More prolonged cord compression results in a combined respiratory and metabolic acidosis. In addition, the respiratory acidosis of transient cord compression recovers much more rapidly than the combined acidosis.

Many of the fetal monitoring tracings that are illustrated in this chapter demonstrate unequivocal fetal distress. Nevertheless, intervention was only rarely considered necessary in these cases. The fetal indication for intervention is *nonremedial fetal distress*. This requires knowledge about the capability of the maternal placental unit to sustain the fetus. If placental function and fetal blood flow are intact, operative delivery does not appear warranted. The intact placenta is a faster, safer, and more efficient apparatus for resuscitating the fetus than is any man-made apparatus for resuscitating the newborn. If patterns of distress are not remediable, intervention should be undertaken as quickly as is consistent with maternal and fetal safety. Nevertheless, with this approach, an appropriate interval between onset of distress and time of delivery cannot be defined, nor is it possible to determine the degree of intermittent hypoxia that may be tolerated without compromise (24).

PITFALLS, FALSE RESULTS, AND COMPLICATIONS
OF MONITORING

The complications of monitoring and scalp sampling are uncommon and rarely of clinical significance (30,42,47,50,94,145). In general, the misinterpretation of monitor tracings and results of fetal pH appear to be responsible for more complications in both mother and baby. Overreaction to abnormal values may lead to ill-advised operative delivery, whereas underreaction results in unjustified delay with resultant increased perinatal mortality and morbidity. At the present time, there is no way of quantifying the frequency of these problems. The reported reliability of fetal monitoring varies with the monitoring method and the endpoint chosen for outcome.

FBS is associated with several technical and physiological pitfalls (Table 14). It is self-evident that the apparatus must be properly maintained and calibrated. In addition, it is essential that only one machine be used for sequential samples in a single patient. Each institution must establish its own range of normal values and reproducibility of results. The literature suggests that values may vary by almost 0.1 pH units under clinical (not research) conditions. A slow rate of collection

TABLE 14. *Variables confounding interpretation of fetal blood pH values*

Relationship to maternal pH blood gases
Accuracy of sampling and measurement
    (e.g., caput, air contamination, machine calibration)
Type of acidosis (respiratory or metabolic)
Stage of labor
Duration of asphyxial insult
Impact of conservative treatment
Relationship to uterine contractions
Relationship to FHR pattern and clinical situation

may also influence pH values. In this instance, a lower pH will be found in the blood collected initially in the tube (155).

FBS is performed most easily with the patient in the dorsal lithotomy position. This position may diminish the pH because of supine hypotension. A more physiologic approach, involving only minimal adjustments in technique, involves sampling the patient in the lateral position. Severe fetal asphyxia with marked vasoconstriction may prevent successful sampling. Furthermore, caput succedaneum and cephalhematoma as well as excessive pressure on the amnioscope may compromise local scalp blood flow.

There are several explanations for false results with both EFM and pH. During labor, the majority of fetuses who demonstrate late decelerations are not seriously asphyxiated nor do they require immediate delivery. Thus, one study of more than 250 patients demonstrated a prohibitively high incidence of late decelerations following administration of oxytocin, epidural anesthesia, or both (135). Nevertheless, the outcome of these fetuses was comparable to those without late decelerations. In fact, the insult was usually short lived and the FHR abnormalities responded rapidly to positional changes and diminution in oxytocin infusion rate. Only ominous FHR patterns and fetal acidosis reflect fetal asphyxia. Thus, FBS and EFM can only be expected to predict low Apgar score in those fetuses compromised as a result of asphyxia, which constitutes approximately 50% of babies with low Apgar scores (97).

IMPACT OF MONITORING

It has been reported that EFM improves perinatal outcome, with reduction of the incidence of intrapartum stillbirth and of low Apgar score (6,68,88,92, 109,122,136). The sudden, unexpected death of a fetus with a normal FHR pattern has not been reported (124). Furthermore, EFM has been reported to be beneficial in both high- and low-risk patients (152). Definitive analysis of the benefits of EFM is complicated because the increasing utilization of EFM has coincided with changing obstetrical and neonatal practices, declining perinatal and maternal mortality rates, and a rising cesarean section rate. The problem is compounded because both controlled and noncontrolled studies are available for statistical analysis. The noncontrolled studies either compare survival in epochs before and after EFM or compare outcome of monitored patients to that of patients who were not monitored. These studies, which involve more than 100,000 patients (117), readily support but do not prove the hypothesis that monitoring is beneficial. In contrast, several randomized controlled trials have concluded that monitoring offers no benefit over auscultation (66,84,157). These trials, which involve limited numbers of patients and significant methodological flaws, have served only to confuse the issue (117).

Several recent studies suggest that EFM should be used routinely in obstetrical practice. Ingemarsson (75) studied the longitudinal effect of increasing utilization of EFM on subsequent neurological handicap. During the first 2 years of the 6-year study only selected high-risk patients were monitored. Their data indicate that 35.2 of 1,000 such patients displayed signs of neurological handicap after 14 months. During the next 2 years, *all* high-risk patients were monitored, and the incidence of neurological handicap dropped to 9.2 per 1,000 patients. Finally, during the last 2 years of the study, when 90% of all patients were monitored, the incidence of handicap decreased to 4.6 per 1,000 patients.

Similarly, in a study of more than 30,000 deliveries during a 12-year period, Erkkola et al. (40) found an 80% reduction in intrapartum fetal death and a 40% to 50% reduction in overall perinatal mortality as utilization of EFM increased from 9% of patients to almost 100%.

In both studies, EFM appeared to be effective for decreasing the risk of poor outcome in high-risk pregnancies and appeared to have an even greater impact on low-risk pregnancies. Erkkola et al. (40) found EFM particularly effective for decreasing the consequences of cord complications and placental abruptions—complications that are not limited to high-risk patients. Evaluation of patient outcome may be considered more correctly to evaluate the overall pattern of obstetrical care, of which EFM is only one component. Thus, the impact of monitoring cannot be determined by examining the relationship between individual patterns and outcome but only by considering total perinatal outcome in all patients monitored.

CORRELATION BETWEEN FHR PATTERNS AND NEUROLOGICAL HANDICAP

The pathogenesis of cerebral palsy (CP) is considered multifactorial (62,112). Few risk factors predict its development, and a number of different mechanisms are known or believed to contribute toward its development. Much of what is known about predisposing factors comes from relatively small data bases; the largest one is the Collaborative Project (112). These data, derived from more than 50,000 deliveries between 1959 and 1964, confirm that perinatal asphyxia is an important antecedent of CP. However, because CP apparently develops in association with a number of other predisposing factors, its absolute role has not been defined. These studies, obtained before the availability of EFM, were compromised by the absence of reliable fetal markers of distress and acidosis. The definition of asphyxia used for the study, i.e., an Apgar score less than 3, fetal bradycardia, and prolonged time to first cry, would not be considered acceptable markers today. Indeed, delayed time to cry and seizures in the neonatal period proved better predictors of CP than the other primitive markers of asphyxia (112). More recent studies with EFM yield conflicting results. In the study of Painter et al. (113,114), prolonged abnormal FHR pattern correlated with neurological signs early in the neonatal period but failed to do so in long-term follow-up. In the large controlled study of EFM conducted in Dublin, those fetuses assigned to monitoring had fewer seizures as newborns than did fetuses who were monitored by auscultation (100). On the other hand, Keegan and Quilligan (83) studied infants who exhibited seizures during the neonatal period and found significant deviations in the FHR pattern in those with seizures compared to those without seizures. Low and colleagues (98) have shown a definite correlation between asphyxia, FHR patterns, and neonatal encephalopathy, including seizures. In none of these studies was there a relationship defined between specific FHR patterns and specific neurological outcomes. It has been demonstrated that there may be five distinct patterns of brain injury associated with acute and intermittent asphyxia (16,111).

Schifrin and Shields (137) sought to investigate the relationship of certain perinatal events, including specific FHR patterns, to the subsequent development of CP and other neurological handicaps. These authors classified the etiology of 54 selected cases of CP according to the FHR pattern, the nature of the delivery, neonatal resuscitation, and findings in the newborn period (137). *Acute fetal distress* was defined as the evolution of repetitive late or severe variable decelerations in a previously normal tracing. *Potentially traumatic delivery* was defined only in the presence of obvious physical findings such as bruising, hematomas, fractures, intracranial hemorrhage, or nerve damage. *Chronic fetal distress* was defined according to unique FHR tracings as described above. The various patterns of FHR were detailed in Table 8. The late FHR pattern, defined as the pattern during the 1 hr preceding delivery, revealed acute fetal distress in 29% of the cases. Most cases were of low birth weight but were not premature; 10% involved macrosomic babies. The incidence of thick nonterminal meconium and, by inference, oligohydramnios was approximately 70%. The incidence of meconium aspiration, however, was 14%. A number of these fetuses were postmature by clinical characteristics, although only about one-third were 42 weeks of gestation or beyond.

The authors concluded that the chronic FHR pattern is an important predictor of CP. This pattern develops in association with such clinical features as meconium staining, dysmaturity, oligohydramnios, fetal dehydration, and polycythemia. This constellation of features, plus the absence of demonstrable acidosis during labor in a significant percentage of these patients, implies a chronic rather than acute form of *nutritional* placental insufficiency. The finding of normal, reactive FHR patterns before the occurrence of the chronic pattern suggested that this syndrome may evolve in a previously normal fetus. They concluded from these and other data that in the presence of oligohydramnios, intermittent umbilical cord compression may lead to repetitive, transient, ischemic episodes in the fetal brain. These ischemic episodes, in turn, may be responsible for subsequent neurological handicap.

MEDICOLEGAL CONSIDERATIONS (138)

The diagnosis of asphyxia around the time of labor and delivery is frequently offered to explain subsequent neonatal handicap. In this respect and for reasons elaborated above, FHR patterns and pH data play crucial roles. A normal pH value or FHR patterns containing adequate baseline variability, a stable baseline FHR of about 110 to 150 bpm, and absent or infrequent decelerations are inconsistent with an acute injury. Periodic accelerations in the FHR are considered a reassuring sign of fetal well-being (95). Given such a tracing, it is within reasonable medical probability that any damage must either be unrelated to asphyxia or represent a problem unrelated to the period of monitoring. Similarly, umbilical cord gases in the normal range preclude acute asphyxia as a cause of neonatal depression. On the other hand, a strip in which a period of normal tracing is followed by persistent late or variable decelerations, a rising baseline, and decreasing variability is consistent with an acute asphyxial insult and will usually be corroborated by results of blood gas sampling.

The FHR pattern may also be consistent with chronic insult only. In such instances, the tracing reveals decreased or absent variability and small variable decelerations with overshoot. Other decelerations, if present, are rarely prolonged or severe and usually do not modify the baseline rate. Accelerations are absent and the baseline rate may be normal or elevated; the pH is usually normal. Occasionally one may find evidence of both chronic and acute insult. In this circumstance, decreased variability and significant, recurrent late or variable decelerations may coexist. Current understanding of FHR patterns does not permit the reviewer to apportion the contribution of chronic and acute factors to the ultimate outcome.

Thus, the most experienced reviewer is limited in the conclusions he or she may reach. The normal FHR tracing is conclusive evidence of the absence of significant fetal asphyxia. However, abnormal tracings often do not correlate with poor outcome and, therefore, must not be used to infer fetal asphyxia (distress) or inevitable brain damage. The reviewer cannot determine, on the basis of the pattern alone, except by exclusion, either the cause or timing of nonasphyxial injury. Similarly, either because the pattern shows no abnormality or a chronic one, the reviewer may conclude with reasonable medical probability that the period of labor did not contribute to the poor outcome.

REFERENCES

1. Adams, R.D., Prod'hom, L.S., and Rabinowicz, T.H. (1977): Intrauterine brain death. *Acta Neuropathol.*, 40:41–49.

2. Adamsons, K., and Myers, R.E. (1977): Late decelerations and brain tolerance of the fetal monkey to intrapartum asphyxia. *Am. J. Obstet. Gynecol.*, 128:893–900.

3. Adamsons, K., Beard, R.W., and Myers, R.E. (1970): Comparison of the composition of arterial venous and capillary blood of the fetal monkey during labor. *Am. J. Obstet. Gynecol.*, 107:435–440.

4. Afriat, C., and Schifrin, B.S. (1976): Sources of error in fetal heart rate monitoring. *J. Obstet. Gynecol. Neonat. Nurs.*, 12:11–15.

5. Aladjem, S., Feria, A., Rest J., and Stojanovic, J. (1977): Fetal heart rate responses to fetal movements. *Br. J. Obstet. Gynaecol.*, 84:487–491.

6. Amato, J. (1977): Fetal monitoring in a community hospital. *Obstet. Gynecol.*, 50:269–274.

7. Arias, F. (1978): Intrauterine resuscitation with terbutaline: A method for the management of acute intrapartum fetal distress. *Am. J. Obstet. Gynecol.*, 131:39–43.

8. Barcroft, J. (1947): *Researches on Prenatal Life.* Charles C. Thomas, Springfield, IL.

9. Barham, K.A. (1969): Amnioscopy, meconium, and fetal well-being. *J. Obstet. Gynecol. Br. Commonw.*, 76:412–418.

10. Baskett, T.F., and Koh, K.S. (1974): Sinusoidal fetal heart rate pattern: A sign of fetal hypoxia. *Obstet Gynecol,* 44:379–382.

11. Benson, R.C., Shubeck, F., Deutschberger, J., et al. (1968): Fetal heart rate as a predictor of fetal distress. A report from the collaborative project. *Obstet. Gynecol.*, 32:259–266.

12. Boehm, F., and Growdon, J. (1974): The effect of eclamptic convulsions on the fetal heart rate. *Am. J. Obstet. Gynecol.*, 120:851–852.

13. Boehm, F.H. (1975): Prolonged end stage fetal heart rate deceleration. *Obstet. Gynecol.*, 45:579–582.

14. Boehm, F.H. (1977): FHR variability, key to fetal well-being. *Contemp. Obstet. Gynecol.*, 9:57–65.

15. Bowe, E.T., Beard, R.W., Finster, M., Poppers, P.J., Adamsons, K., and James, L.S. (1970): Reliability of fetal blood sampling, maternal-fetal relationships. *Am. J. Obstet. Gynecol.*, 107:279–287.

16. Brann, A.W., and Myers, R.E. (1975): Central nervous system findings in the newborn monkey following severe *in utero* partial asphyxia. *Neurology,* 25:327–338.

17. Bronatek, V., and Scheffs, J. (1973): The pathogenesis and significance of saltatory patterns in the fetal heart rate. *Int. J. Gynecol. Obstet.*, 11:223.

18. Bruce, S.L., James, L.S., Bowe, E.T., Rey, H., and Shamsi, H. (1978): Umbilical cord complication as a cause of perinatal morbidity and mortality. *J. Perinatol. Med.*, 6:89–94.

19. Cabal, L.A. Siassi, B., Zanini, B., et al. (1980): Factors affecting heart rate variability in preterm infants. *Pediatrics,* 65:50–56.

20. Caldeyro-Barcia, R., Mendez-Bauer, C., Poseiro, J.J., et al. (1966): Control of human fetal heart rate during labor. In: *The Heart and Circulation in the Newborn and Infant,* edited by D.E. Cassels, pp. 7–36. Grune and Stratton, New York.

21. Carson, B.S., Losey, R.W., Bowes, W.A., and Simmons, M.A. (1976): Combined obstetric and pediatric approach to prevent meconium aspiration syndrome. *Am. J. Obstet. Gynecol.*, 126:712–715.

22. Cetrulo, C.L., and Schifrin, B.S. (1976): Fetal heart rate patterns preceding death *in utero.* *Obstet. Gynecol.*, 48:521–527.

23. Cibils, L.A. (1975): Clinical significance of fetal heart rate patterns during labor. Variable decelerations. *Am. J. Obstet. Gynecol.*, 132:791–805.

24. Cohen, W.R., and Schifrin, B.S. (1982): Diagnosis and treatment of fetal distress. In: *Perinatal Medicine,* 2nd ed., edited by R.J. Bolognese, R.H. Schwarz, and J. Schneider, pp. 223–243. Williams and Wilkins Co., Baltimore.

25. Cohen, W.R., Schifrin, B.S., and Doctor, G. (1975): Elevation of the fetal presenting part: A method of intrauterine resuscitation. *Am. J. Obstet. Gynecol.*, 123:646–649.

26. Cohn, H.E., Piasecki, G.J., and Jackson, B.T. (1976): Effect of atropine blockade on the fetal cardiovascular response to hypoxemia. *Gynecol. Invest.*, 7:57.

27. Cohn, H.E., Piasecki, G.J., and Jackson, B.J. (1980): The effect of fetal heart rate on cardiovascular function during hypoxemia. *Am. J. Obstet. Gynecol.*, 138:1190–1199.

28. Cohn, H.E., Sacks, E.J., Heymann, M.A., and Rudolph, A.M. (1974): Cardiovascular responses to hypoxemia and acidemia in fetal lambs. *Am. J. Obstet. Gynecol.*, 120:817–824.

29. Comline, R.S., and Silver, M. (1966): Developmeent of activity in the adrenal medulla of the fetus and new-born animal. *Br. Med. Bull.*, 22:16–20.

30. Cordero, L., Jr., and Hon, E.G. (1971): Scalp abscess: A rare complication of fetal monitoring. *J. Pediatr.,* 78:533–536.
31. Creasy, R.K., and Parer, J.T. (1977): Prenatal care and diagnosis. In: *Pediatrics,* 16th ed., edited by A.M. Rudolph. Appleton-Century-Crofts, Englewood Cliffs, NJ.
32. Dalton, K.J., Dawes, G.S., Patrick, J.E., et al. (1983): The autonomic nervous system and fetal heart-rate variability. *Am. J. Obstet. Gynecol.,* 146:456–462.
33. Dawes, G. (1968): *Fetal and Neonatal Physiology.* Year Book Medical Publishers, Inc, Chicago.
34. Dawes, G.S., Gardner, W.N., Johnston, B.M., et al. (1983): Breathing in fetal lambs: The effects of brain stem section. *J. Physiol.,* 335:535–553.
35. Day, E., Maddern, C., Wood, C. (1968): Auscultation of fetal heart rate: An assessment of its error and significance. *Br. Med. J.,* 4:422–424.
36. De Haan, J., van Bemmel, J.H., Stolte, L.A.M., et al. (1971): Quantitative evaluation of the fixed heart-rate during pregnancy and labor. *Eur. J. Obstet. Gynecol.,* 3:103.
37. De Souza, S.W., and Richards, B. (1978): Neurological sequelae in newborn babies after perinatal asphyxia. *Arch. Dis. Child.,* 53:564–569.
38. Divon, M.Y., Muskat, Y., Platt, L.D., and Paldi, E. (1984): Increased beat-to-beat variability during uterine contractions: A common association in uncomplicated labor. *Am. J. Obstet. Gynecol.,* 149:893–896.
39. Divon, M.Y., Yeh, S.Y., Zimmer, E.Z., Platt, L.D., Paldi, E., and Paul, R.H. (1985): Respiratory sinus arrhythmia in the human fetus. *Am. J. Obstet. Gynecol.,* 151:425–428.
40. Erkkola, R., Gronroos, M., Punnonen, R., Kikku, P. (1984): Analysis of intrapartum fetal deaths: Their decline with increasing electronic fetal monitoring. *Acta Obstet. Gynecol. Scand.,* 63:459–462.
41. Fenton, A.N., and Steer, C.M. (1962): Fetal distress. *Am. J. Obstet. Gynecol.,* 83:354–362.
42. Fernandez-Rocha, L., and Oulette, R. (1976): Fetal bleeding: An unusual complication of fetal monitoring. *Am. J. Obstet. Gynecol.,* 125:1153–1155.
43. Fleischer, A., Schulman, H., Jagani, N., Mitchell, J., and Randolph, G. (1982): The development of fetal acidosis in the presence of an abnormal fetal heart rate tracing. I. The average for gestational age fetus. *Am. J. Obstet. Gynecol.,* 144:55–60.
44. Freeman, R.K., and James, J. (1975): Clinical experience with the oxytocin challenge test. II. An ominous atypical pattern. *Obstet. Gynecol.,* 46:255–259.
45. Freeman, R.K., and Schifrin, B.S. (1973): Wither paracervical block? *Int. Anesthesiol. Clin.,* 11:69–91.
46. Gabbe, S., Ettinger, B., Freeman, R., and Martin, C. (1976): Umbilical cord compression associated with amniotomy: Laboratory observations. *Am. J. Obstet. Gynecol.,* 126:353–355.
47. Gal, D., Jacobson, L.M., Ser H., et al. (1978): Sinusoidal pattern: An alarming sign of fetal distress. *Am. J. Obstet. Gynecol.,* 132:903–905.
48. Garite, T.J., Linzey, E.M., Freeman, R.K., and Dorchester, W. (1979): Fetal heart rate patterns and fetal distress in fetuses with congenital anomalies. *Obstet. Gynecol.,* 53:716–720.
49. Gaziano, E.P. (1979): A study of variable decelerations in association with other heart-rate patterns during monitored labor. *Am. J. Obstet. Gynecol.,* 135:360–363.
50. Gibbs, R.S., Jones, P.M., and Wilder, C.J.Y. (1978): Internal fetal monitoring and maternal infection following cesarean section. A prospective study. *Obstet. Gynecol.,* 53:193–197.
51. Gleicher, N., Runowicz, C.D., and Brown, B.L. (1980): Sinusoidal fetal heart rate pattern in association with amnionitis. *Obstet. Gynecol.,* 56:109–111.
52. Glick, G., and Braunwald, E. (1965): Relative roles of the sympathetic and parasympathetic nervous systems in the control of heart rate. *Circ. Res.,* 16:363–375.
53. Goodlin, R.C., and Lowe, E.W. (1974): A functional umbilical cord occlusion heart-rate pattern: The significance of overshoot. *Obstet. Gynecol.,* 43:22–30.
54. Goodlin, R.C., and Schmidt, W. (1972): Human fetal arousal levels as indicated by heart rate recordings. *Am. J. Obstet. Gynecol.,* 114:613–621.
55. Gray, J.H., Cudmore, D.W., Luther, E.R., et al. (1978): Sinusoidal fetal heart rate pattern associated with alphaprodine administration. *Obstet. Gynecol.,* 52:678–681.
56. Green, J.N., and Paul, R.H. (1978): The value of amniocentesis in prolonged pregnancy. *Obstet. Gynecol.,* 51:293–298.
57. Greenfield, A.D.M., and Shepherd, J.T. (1953): Cardiovascular responses to asphyxia in the fetal guinea pig. *Physiology,* 120:538–549.
58. Gregory, G.., Gooding, C.A., Phibbs, R.H., and Tooley, W.H. (1974): Meconium aspiration in infants—A prospective study. *J. Pediatr.,* 85:848–852.

59. Greiss, F.C., Still, G.J., and Anderson, S.G. (1976): Effects of local anesthetic agents on the uterine vasculatures and myometrium. *Am. J. Obstet. Gynecol.,* 124:889–899.
60. Greiss, F.C.H. (1973): Concepts of uterine blood flow. In: *Obstetrics & Gynecology Annual,* edited by R. Wynn, p. 55. Appleton-Century Crofts, New York.
61. Griffin, R.L., Caron, F.J.M., and Van Geijn, H.P. (1985): Behavioral states in the human fetus during labor. *Am. J. Obstet. Gynecol.,* 152:828–833.
62. Hagberg, B., Hagberg, G., and Olow, I. (1975): The changing panorama of cerebral palsy in Sweden 1954–70. *Acta Pediatr. Scand.,* 64:187–200.
63. Hammacher, K. (1969): The clinical significance of cardiotocography. In: *Perinatal Medicine,* edited by P.S. Huntingford, E.A. Huter, and E. Saling, pp. 80–93. Georg Thieme Verlag, K.G., Stuttgart.
64. Hammacher, K., Huter, K.A., Bokelmann, J., and Werners, P.H. (1968): Fetal heart frequency and condition of the fetus and newborn. *Gynecologia,* 166:349–360.
65. Harris, J.L., Krueger, T.R., and Parer, J.T. (1982): Mechanisms of late decelerations of the fetal heart rate during hypoxia. *Am. J. Obstet. Gynecol.,* 144:491–496.
66. Haverkamp, A.D., Orleans, M., Langendoerfer, S., et al. (1979): A controlled trial of the differential effect of intrapartum monitoring. *Am. J. Obstet. Gynecol.,* 134:399–412.
67. Herbert, C.M., and Boehm, F.H. (1981): Prolonged end-stage fetal heart-rate deceleration: A reanalysis. *Obstet. Gynecol.,* 57:589–593.
68. Hobbins, J.C., Grannum, P.A.T., Romero, R., Reece, E.A., and Mahoney, J.J. (1988): Percutaneous umbilical blood sampling. *Am. J. Obstet. Gynecol. (in press).*
69. Hon, E.H., Bradfield, A.H., and Hess, O.W. (1961): The electronic evaluation of the fetal heart rate. V. The vagal factor in fetal bradycardia. *Am. J. Obstet. Gynecol.,* 82:291–300.
70. Hon, E.H., Khazin, A.F., and Paul, R.H. (1969): Biochemical studies of the fetus. II. Fetal pH and Apgar scores. *Obstet. Gynecol.,* 33:237–255.
71. Hon, E.H., and Quilligan, E.J. (1967): The classification of fetal heart rate. II. A revised working classification. *Conn. Med.,* 31:779–784.
72. Humphrey, M.D., Chang, A., and Wood, E.C. (1974): A decrease in fetal pH during the second stage of labor when conducted in the dorsal position. *J. Obstet. Gynecol. Br. Commonw.,* 81:600–602.
73. Hutson, J.M., and Mueller-Heubach, E. (1982): Diagnosis and management of intrapartum reflex fetal heart rate changes. *Clin. Perinatol.,* 9:325–337.
74. Ibarra-Polo, A.A., Guiloff, F.E., and Gomez-Rogers, C. (1972): Fetal heart rate throughout pregnancy. *Am. J. Obstet. Gynecol.,* 113:814–818.
75. Ingemarsson, E. (1981): Routine electronic fetal monitoring during labor. *Acta Obstet. Gynecol. Scand. [Suppl.],* 99.
76. Itskovitz, J., LaGamma, E.F., and Rudolph, A.M. (1983): Heart-rate and blood pressure responses to umbilical cord compression in fetal lambs with special reference to the mechanism of variable deceleration. *Am. J. Obstet. Gyencol.,* 147:451–457.
77. Iwamoto, H.S., Rudolph, A.M., Keil, L.C., and Heymann, M.A. (1979): Hemodynamic responses of the sheep fetus to vasopressin infusion. *Circ. Res.,* 44:430–436.
78. Jacobson, L., and Rooth, G. (1971): Interpretative aspects of the acid base composition and its variation in fetal scalp blood and maternal blood during labor. *J. Obstet. Gynecol. Br. Commonw.,* 78:971–980.
79. James, L.S., Yeh, M.N., Morishima, H.O., et al. (1976): Umbilical vein occlusion and transient acceleration of the fetal heart rate. *Am. J. Obstet. Gynecol.,* 126:276–283.
80. Johnson, T.R.B., Compton, A.A., Rotmensch, J., et al. (1981): Significance of the sinusoidal fetal heart rate pattern. *Am. J. Obstet. Gynecol.,* 139:446–453.
81. Kariniemi, V., Lehtovirta, P., Rauramo, I., and Forss, M. (1984): Effects of smoking on fetal heart-rate variability during gestational weeks 27 to 32. *Am. J. Obstet. Gynecol.,* 149:575–576.
82. Kates, R.B., and Schifrin, B.S. (1986): Fetal cardiac asystole during labor. *Obstet. Gynecol.,* 67:549–555.
83. Keegan, K.A., Waffarn, F., and Quilligan, E.J. (1986): Obstetric characteristics and fetal heart rate patterns of infants who convulse during the newborn period. *Am. J. Obstet. Gynecol.,* 153:732–737.
84. Kelso, I.M., Parson, R.J., Lawrence, G.F., et al. (1978): An assessment of continuous fetal heart-rate monitoring in labor. *Am. J. Obstet. Gynecol.,* 131:526–532.
85. Kero, P., Antila, K., Ylitalo, V., et al. (1978): Decreased heart rate variation in decerebration syndrome: Quantitative clinical criterion of brain death? *Pediatrics,* 62:307–311.
86. Knuppel, R.A., and Cetrulo, C.L. (1978): Fetal acidosis and a low Apgar in the presence of

meconium staining and a normal fetal heart rate pattern: A case report. *J. Reprod. Med.*, 21:241–243.

87. Krebs, H.B., Petres, R.E., Dunn, L.J., Jordann, H.V., and Segreti, A. (1979): Intrapartum fetal heart rate monitoring. I. Classification and prognosis of fetal heart rate patterns. *Am. J. Obstet. Gynecol.*, 133:762–772.

88. Krebs, H.B., Petres, R.E., and Dunn, L.J. (1980): Intrapartum fetal heart rate monitoring. IV. Observations on elective and non-elective fetal heart-rate monitoring. *Am. J. Obstet. Gynecol.*, 138:213–219.

89. Krebs, H.B., Petres, R.E., Dunn, L.J., et al. (1979): Intrapartum fetal heart rate monitoring. II. Multifactorial analysis of intrapartum fetal heart-rate tracings. *Am. J. Obstet. Gynecol.*, 133:773–780.

90. Krebs, H.B., Petres, R.E., Dunn, L.J., et al. (1982): Intrapartum fetal heart-rate monitoring. VI. Prognostic significance of accelerations. *Am. J. Obstet. Gynecol.*, 142:297–305.

91. Krebs, H.B., Petres, R.E., and Dunn, L.J. (1983): Intrapartum fetal heart-rate monitoring. VII. Atypical variable decelerations. *Am. J. Obstet. Gynecol.*, 145:297–305.

92. Kubli, F. (1969): Impact of intrapartum monitoring on perinatal mortality and morbidity. *Contraception Gynecol.*, 104:1190.

93. Kubli, F.W., Hon, E.H., Khazin, A.F., et al. (1979): Observations on heart rate and pH in the human fetus during labor. *Am. J. Obstet. Gynecol.*, 133:779.

94. Ledger, W.J. (1978): Complications associated with invasive monitoring. *Semin. Perinatol.*, 2:187–194.

95. Lee, C.Y., Di Loreto, R.C., and O'Lane, J.M. (1975): A study of fetal heart rate acceleration patterns. *Obstet. Gynecol.*, 45:142–146.

96. Leveno, K.J., Quirk, J.G., Cunningham, F.G., et al. (1984): Prolonged pregnancy. I. Observations concerning the causes of fetal distress. *Am. J. Obstet. Gynecol.*, 150:465–473.

97. Low, J.A. Cox, M.J., Karchmar, E.J., McGrath, M.J., Pancham, S.R., and Piercy, W.N. (1981): The prediction of intrapartum fetal metabolic acidosis by fetal heart-rate monitoring. *Am. J. Obstet. Gynecol.*, 139:299–305.

98. Low, J.A., Galbraith, R.S., Muir, D.W., Killen, H.L., Pater, E.A., and Karchmar, E.J. (1985): The relationship between perinatal hypoxia and newborn encephalopathy. *Am. J. Obstet. Gynecol.*, 152:256–260.

99. Lumley, J., McKinnon, L., and Wood, C. (1971): Lack of agreement of normal values for fetal scalp blood. *J. Obstet. Gynecol. Br. Commonw.*, 78:13–21.

100. MacDonald, D., Grant, A., Sheridan-Pereira, M., Boylan, P., and Chalmers, I. (1985): The Dublin randomized controlled trial of intrapartum fetal heart rate monitoring. *Am. J. Obstet. Gynecol.*, 152:524–539.

101. Martin, C.B. (1978): Regulation of the fetal heart-rate and genesis of FHR patterns. *Semin. Perinatol.*, 2:131.

102. Martin, C.B. (1982): Physiology and clinical use of fetal heart-rate variability. *Clin. Perinatol.*, 9:339–352.

103. Martin, C.B., de Haan, J., van der Wildt, B., Jomgsma, H.W., Dieleman, A., and Arts, T.H.M. (1979): Mechanisms of late decelerations in the fetal heart rate. A study with autonomic blocking agents in fetal lambs. *Eur. J. Obstet. Gynecol. Reprod. Biol.*, 9:361.

104. Martin, C.B., Jr. (1981): Behavioral states in the human fetus. *J. Reprod. Med.*, 26:425–432.

105. Mendez-Bauer, C., Poseirio, J.J., Arellano-Hernandez, G., et al. (1963): Effects of atropine on the heart-rate of the human fetus during labor. *Am. J. Obstet. Gynecol.*, 85:1033–1053.

106. Mendez-Bauer, C., Ruiz Canseco, A., Andujar, R., et al. (1978): Early deceleration of the fetal heart-rate from occlusion of the umbilical cord. *J. Perinat. Med.*, 6:69–79.

107. Miller, F.C., Sacks, D.A., Yeh, S.Y., et al. (1975): Significance of meconium during labor. *Am. J. Obstet. Gynecol.*, 122:573–580.

108. Miyazaki, F.S., and Nevarez, F. (1985): Saline amnioinfusion for relief of repetitive variable decelerations: A prospective randomized study. *Am. J. Obstet. Gynecol.*, 153:301–306.

109. Mueller-Heubach, E., MacDonald, H.M., Joret, D., et al. (1980): Effects of electronic fetal heart-rate monitoring on perinatal outcome and obstetric practices. *Am. J. Obstet. Gynecol.*, 137:758–763.

110. Myers, R.E. (1972): Two patterns of perinatal brain damage and their conditions of occurrence. *Am. J. Obstet. Gynecol.*, 112:245–276.

111. Myers, R.E., Mueller-Heubach, E., and Adamsons, K. (1973): Predictability of the state of fetal oxygenation from a quantitative analysis of the components of late deceleration. *Am. J. Obstet. Gynecol.*, 115:1083–1094.

112. Nelson, K.B., Ellenburg, J.H. (1979): Epidemiology of cerebral palsy. In: *Advances in Neurology*, vol. 19, edited by B.L. Schomberg, p. 421. Raven Press, New York.

113. Painter, M.J., Depp, R., O'Donoghue, P.D. (1979): Fetal heart-rate patterns and development in the first year of life. *Am. J. Obstet. Gynecol.*, 132:271–277.

114. Painter, M.J., Scott, M., and Deep, R. (1985): Neurological and developmental follow-up of children at six to nine years relative to intrapartum fetal heart-rate patterns. In: *Fifth Annual Clinical, Scientific, and The Society of Perinatal Obstetricians*, Las Vegas.

115. Parer, J.T. (1977): Effects of atropine on heart-rate and oxygen consumption of the hypoxic fetus. *Gynecol. Invest.*, 8:50.

116. Parer, J.T. (1980): The current role of intrapartum fetal scalp sampling. *Clin. Obstet. Gynecol.*, 23:565–582.

117. Parer, J.T. (1981): FHR monitoring: Answering the critics. *Contemp. Obstet. Gynecol.*, 17:163–174.

118. Parer, J.T. (1984): The effect of atropine on heart-rate and oxygen consumption of the hypoxic fetus. *Am. J. Obstet. Gynecol.*, 148:1118–1122.

119. Parer, J.T., Krueger, T.R., and Harris, J.L. (1980): Fetal oxygen consumption and mechanisms of heart-rate response during artificially produced late decelerations of fetal heart rate in sheep. *Am. J. Obstet. Gynecol.*, 136:478–482.

120. Patrick, J., Carmichael, L., Chess, L., Probert, C., and Staples, C. (1985): The distribution of accelerations of the human fetal heart-rate at 38 to 40 weeks' gestational age. *Am. J. Obstet. Gynecol.*, 151:283–287.

121. Patrick, J., Carmichael, L., Chess, L., and Staples, C. (1984): Accelerations of the human fetal heart rate at 38 to 40 weeks' gestational age. *Am. J. Obstet. Gynecol.*, 148:35–45.

122. Paul, R., and Hon, E. (1974): Clinical fetal monitoring. V. Effect on perinatal outcome. *Am. J. Obstet. Gynecol.*, 118:529–533.

123. Paul, R.H., Suidan, A.K., Yeh, S., Schifrin, B.S., and Hon, E.H. (1975): Clinical fetal monitoring. VII. The evaluation and significance of intrapartum baseline FHR variability. *Am. J. Obstet. Gynecol.*, 123:206–210.

124. Perkins, R.P. (1980): Sudden fetal death in labor. The significance of antecedent monitoring characteristics and clinical circumstances. *J. Reprod. Med.*, 25:309–314.

125. Petrie, R.H., Yeh, S., Murata, Y., et al. (1978): The effects of drugs on fetal heart-rate variability. *Am. J. Obstet. Gynecol.*, 130:294–299.

126. Pinkerton, J. (1969): Kergaradec, friend of Laennec and pioneer of fetal auscultation. *Proc. R. Soc. Med.*, 62:477–483.

127. Reece, E.A., Chervenak, F.A., Romero, R., and Hobbins, J.C. (1984): Magnesium sulfate in the management of acute intrapartum distress. *Am. J. Obstet. Gynecol.*, 148:104–106.

128. Renou, P., Chang, A., Anderson, I., et al. (1976): Controlled trial of fetal heart rate. *Am. J. Obstet. Gynecol.*, 126:470–476.

129. Renou, P., Newman, W., and Wood, C. (1969): Autonomic control of fetal heart rate. *Am. J. Obstet. Gynecol.*, 105:949–953.

130. Ron, M., Adoni, A., Hochner, D., Celnikier, A., and Palto, Z. (1980): The significance of baseline tachycardia in the postterm fetus. *Int. J. Gynecol. Obstet.*, 18:76–77.

131. Roversi, G.D., Cannussio, V., and Spennacchio, M. (1975): Recognition and significance of maternogenic fetal acidosis during intensive monitoring of labor. *J. Perinat. Med.*, 3:53–63.

132. Sadovsky, E., Rabinowitz, R., Freeman, A., and Yarkoni, S. (1984): The relationships between fetal heart-rate accelerations, fetal movements, and uterine contractions. *Am. J. Obstet. Gynecol.*, 149:187–189.

133. Saling, E. (1981): Fetal scalp blood analysis. *J. Perinat. Med.*, 9:165–177.

134. Schifferili, P.Y., and Caldeyro-Barcia, R. (1973): Effects of atropine and beta-autonomic drugs on the heart-rate of the human fetus. In: *Fetal Pharmacology*, edited by L. Boreus. Raven, New York.

135. Schifrin, B.S. (1972): Fetal heart rate patterns following epidural anesthesia and oxytocin infusion during labor. *J. Obstet. Gynecol. Br. Commonw.*, 79:332–339.

136. Schifrin, B.S., and Dame, L. (1972): Fetal heart-rate patterns, prediction of Apgar score. *JAMA*, 219:1322–1325.

137. Shields, J.R., and Schifrin, B.S. (1988): Perinatal antecedents of cerebral palsy. *Obstet. Gynecol.*, 71:899–905.

138. Schifrin, B.S., Weissman, H., and Wiley, J. (1985): Electronic fetal monitoring and obstetrical malpractice in proceedings of obstetrical malpractice. In: *Law, Medicine and Health Care*, vol. 13, pp. 100–105. Academic Press, New York.

139. Shenker, L. (1979): Fetal cardiac arrhythmias. *Obstet. Gynecol. Surv.,* 34:561–572.
140. Siassi, B., Blanco, C., and Martin, C.B. (1979): Baroreceptor and chemoreceptor responses to umbilical cord occlusion in fetal lambs. *Biol. Neonat.,* 35:66.
141. Tejani, N., Mann, L., Bhakthavathsalan, A., and Weiss, R. (1975): Correlation of fetal heart rate—Uterine contraction patterns with fetal scalp blood pH. *Obstet. Gynecol.,* 46:392–396.
142. Tejani, N., Mann, L., Bhakthavathsalan, A., and Weiss, R. (1975): Prolonged fetal bradycardia with recovery: Its significance and outcome. *Am. J. Obstet. Gynecol.,* 122:975–978.
143. Tejani, N., Schulman, H., Fleischer, A., et al. (1983): The value of quantitative analysis of fetal heart-rate tracings. *Perinat-Neonat.,* 7:55.
144. Teroa, T., Kawashima, Y., Noto, H., et al. (1984): Neurological control of fetal heart rate in 20 cases of anencephalic fetuses. *Am. J. Obstet. Gynecol.,* 149:201–208.
145. Turbeville, D.F., and McCaffree, M.A. (1979): Fetal scalp electrode complications: Cerebrospinal fluid leak. *Obstet. Gynecol.,* 54:469–470.
146. Tushuizen, P.B.T., Stoot, J.E.G.M., and Ubachs, J.M.H. (1974): Fetal heart rate monitoring of the dying fetus. *Am. J. Obstet. Gynecol.,* 120:922–931.
147. van der Moer, P.E., Gerretsen, G., and Visser, G.H.A. (1985): Fixed fetal heart-rate pattern after intrauterine accidental decerebration. *Obstet. Gynecol.,* 65:125–127.
148. Vintzileos, A.M., Campbell, W., Dreiss, R.J., Neckles, S., and Nochimson, D.J. (1985): Intrapartum fetal heart rate monitoring of the extremely premature fetus. *Am. J. Obstet. Gynecol.,* 151:744–745.
149. Visser, G.H.A., Goodman, J.D.S., Levine, D.H., et al. (1982): Diurnal and other cyclic variations in human fetal heart-rate near term. *Am. J. Obstet. Gynecol.,* 142:535–544.
150. Visser, G.H.A., Zeelenberg, H.J., De Vries, J.I.P., and Dawes, G.S. (1983): External physical stimulation of the human fetus during episodes of low heart rate variation. *Am. J. Obstet. Gynecol.,* 145:579–584.
151. Walker, N.F. (1975): Reliability of the signs of fetal distress. *S. Afr. Med. J.,* 49:1732–1736.
152. Westgren, M., Ingemarsson, E., Ingemarsson, I., and Solum, T. (1980): Intrapartum electronic fetal monitoring in low-risk pregnancies. *Obstet. Gynecol.,* 56:301–304.
153. Wolf, S. (1969): Central autonomic influences on cardiac rate and rhythm. *Mod. Concepts Cardiovasc. Dis.,* 38:29–34.
154. Wolfson, R.N., Sorokin, Y., and Rosen, M.G. (1982): Autonomic control of fetal cardiac activity. In: *Cardiac Problems in Pregnancy. Diagnosis and Management of Maternal and Fetal Disease,* edited by U. Elkayam and N. Gleicher, p. 365. Alan R. Liss, New York.
155. Wood, C. (1979): Fetal scalp sampling: Its place in management. *Semin. Perinatol.,* 2:169–179.
156. Wood, C., Ferguson, R., Leeton, J., Newman, W., and Walker, A. (1967): Fetal heart-rate in relation to fetal scalp blood measurements in the assessment of fetal hypoxia. *Am. J. Obstet. Gynecol.,* 98:62–70.
157. Wood, C., Renou, P., and Oats, J. (1981): A controlled trial of fetal heart-rate monitoring in a low risk obstetric population. *Am. J. Obstet. Gynecol.,* 141:527–534.
158. Yeh, S.Y., Zanini, B., Petrie, R.H., and Hon, E.H. (1977): Intrapartum fetal cardiac arrest: A preliminary observation. *Obstet. Gynecol.,* 50:571–577.
159. Katz, M., Wilson, S.J., and Young, B.K. (1980): Sinusoidal fetal heart rate. II. Continuous tissue pH studies. *Am. J. Obstet. Gynecol.,* 136:594–596.
160. Young, B.K., Katz, M., Klein, S.A., and Silverman, F. (1979): Fetal blood and tissue pH with moderate bradycardia. *Am. J. Obstet. Gynecol.,* 135:45–47.
161. Young, B.K., Katz, M., and Wilson, S.J. (1980): Sinusoidal fetal heart rate. I. Clinical significance. *Am. J. Obstet. Gynecol.,* 136:587–593.
162. Zalar, R.W., and Quilligan, E.J. (1979): The influence of fetal scalp sampling on the cesarean section rate for fetal distress. *Am. J. Obstet. Gynecol.,* 135:239–246.
163. Zanini, B., Paul, R.H., and Huey, J.R. (1980): Intrapartum fetal heart-rate: Correlation with scalp pH in the preterm fetus. *Am. J. Obstet. Gynecol.,* 136:43–47.

Fetal Neurology, edited by
A. Hill and J.J. Volpe.
Raven Press, New York © 1989.

Commentary on Chapter 8

*Alan Hill and **Joseph J. Volpe

*Division of Neurology, Department of Paediatrics, University of British Columbia,
British Columbia's Children's Hospital, Vancouver, British Columbia, Canada V6H 3V4;
and **Division of Pediatric Neurology, Washington University School of Medicine,
St. Louis, Missouri 63110

In the preceding chapter, Dr. Schifrin described the parameters that have been used for the identification of intrapartum fetal distress. In addition, he addressed some of the ambiguities surrounding the relationship between perinatal asphyxia and neurologic outcome. Although it is clear from experimental animal data that perinatal asphyxia may result in cerebral injury (1,4,7), the precise significance of this relationship in the human infant has recently been called into question (6).

Although the severity and duration of the asphyxia are obviously critical, it has been suggested that the relationship between hypoxia-ischemia and outcome is not a simple direct correlation, in that a small amount of an adverse factor causes a small amount of damage and larger amounts cause more severe damage. Rather, thresholds have been proposed, beyond which irreversible brain injury occurs, i.e., milder degrees and/or durations of hypoxia are tolerated without subsequent untoward effects on mental or motor functions, whereas when the duration or severity of hypoxia-ischemia exceeds a certain threshold, neurologic abnormalities result.

To complicate the situation further, there is confusion related to the use of the terms *fetal distress, fetal asphyxia,* and *asphyxial trauma,* which are not interchangeable. Thus, although the term *distress* implies a degree of increased risk to the fetus, *asphyxia* refers to a biochemical constellation caused by an impairment in exchange of respiratory gases and characterized by hypoxemia, hypercarbia, and acidosis. Neither term implies irreversible cellular death that results in fetal morbidity or mortality, and neither fetal asphyxia nor fetal distress necessarily correlates closely with clinical outcome.

Prevention of neurologic injury requires early identification of the asphyxiated infant, before or during labor, as well as quantification of the severity and duration of intrauterine asphyxia. In this context, Apgar scores have been used to predict subsequent neurologic deficit. However, Apgar scores are influenced by factors other than asphyxia, e.g., observer errors, gestational age, use of medications in the mother, and other disease states. Recent studies of the use of Apgar scores demonstrate that only when the Apgar score is low (<3) for at least 10 to 15 min is there a high risk of cerebral palsy and mental retardation. Even in such infants, at least 50% do not develop significant neurologic sequelae (5,9). It is appropriate to suggest that the *duration* of intrapartum asphyxia is the critical factor rather than simply its presence just before delivery. In addition, the substrate upon which asphyxia is superimposed is crucial. Thus, the infant who is small-for-gestational age and/or postmature appears to have less tolerance to an additional intrauterine insult, e.g., acute asphyxia.

Additional indicators of prior fetal distress include the presence of early and heavy meconium staining of the amniotic fluid, abnormalities of electronic fetal monitoring, and acidosis, measured by fetal blood sampling. Fetal acid-base assessment is discussed in detail in the chapter by Low. The major focus of the chapter by Schifrin is the role of electronic fetal heart rate monitoring in intrapartum fetal assessment and the relationship of this assessment to neurologic outcome. Major aspects of fetal heart rate monitoring include fetal heart rate, beat-to-beat variability, and accelerations or decelerations in relation to uterine contractions. Abnormalities of each of these factors have been documented to be associated with fetal acidosis, increased incidence of intrauterine fetal death, and low Apgar scores. However, the necessity and relative merits of electronic fetal heart rate monitoring when applied to all patients are still considered controversial (2,3,8,10). Despite these controversies, such monitoring during labor has become standard obstetrical practice in the management of the high-risk pregnancy.

The primary importance of the techniques for intrapartum fetal assessment, i.e., heart rate monitoring and acid-base measurements, rests in the fact that identification of subtle alterations in heart rate and acid-base balance may enable immediate institution of preventive measures that, in turn, may eliminate the need for more drastic operative intervention (e.g., cesarean section). In this context, as discussed by Schifrin, the fetoplacental unit should be considered generally a far more efficient tool for fetal resuscitation than urgent surgical delivery followed by artificial resuscitation. On the other hand, in some instances, careful intrapartum surveillance may indicate the need for urgent surgical intervention. In virtually all such infants, compromise at birth as a result of asphyxia will have been anticipated on the basis of a combination of abnormal fetal heart rate patterns or low pH. However, the major limitation of each of these techniques, both electronic fetal heart rate monitoring and fetal blood sampling, is that they reflect fetal condition at single points in time only, rather than the duration of hypoxic-ischemic stress.

In summary, although the techniques for identification of intrapartum risk factors for neurologic injury are improving, most infants with clearly identifiable risk factors have a favorable neurologic outcome. It should be emphasized that neurologic sequelae in infants who have sustained hypoxic-ischemic insult are not observed unless there has been an identifiable hypoxic-ischemic encephalopathy in the neonatal period. Clearly, future studies must focus on combinations of risk factors that warrant obstetric intervention.

REFERENCES

1. Brann, A.W., and Myers, R.E. (1975): Central nervous system findings in the newborn monkey following severe *in utero* partial asphyxia. *Neurology,* 25:327–338.
2. Haverkamp, A.D., Orleans, M., Langendoefer, S., et al. (1979): A controlled trial of the differential effects of intrapartum fetal monitoring. *Am. J. Obstet. Gynecol.,* 134:399–412.
3. Hobbins, J.C., Freeman, R., and Queenan, J.T. (1980): Reply (Letter). *Pediatrics,* 65:367.
4. Myers, R.E. (1975): Four patterns of perinatal brain damage and their conditions of occurrence in primates. *Adv. Neurol.,* 10:223–234.
5. Nelson, K.B., and Ellenberg, J.H. (1981): Apgar scores as predictors of chronic neurologic disability. *Pediatrics,* 68:36–44.
6. Nelson, K.B., and Ellenberg, J.H. (1986): Antecedents of cerebral palsy. *N. Engl. J. Med.,* 315:81–86.
7. Rice, J.E., III, Vannucci, R.C., and Brierley, J.B. (1981): The influence of immaturity on hypoxic ischemic brain damage in the rat. *Ann. Neurol.,* 9:131–141.
8. Schifrin, B.S. (1982): The fetal monitoring polemic. *Clin. Perinatol.,* 9:399–408.
9. Thomson, A.J., Searle, M., and Russell G. (1977): Quality of survival after severe birth asphyxia. *Arch. Dis. Child.,* 52:620–626.
10. Zuspan, F.P., Quilligan, E.J., Iams, J.D., and Van Geijn, H.P. (1979): NICHD consensus development task force report: Predictors of intrapartum fetal distress—The role of electronic fetal monitoring. *J. Pediatr.,* 95:1026–1030.

Fetal Neurology, edited by
A. Hill and J.J. Volpe.
Raven Press, New York © 1989.

9

Fetal Acid-Base Status and Outcome

J.A. Low

*Department of Obstetrics and Gynecology, Queen's University,
Kingston, Ontario, Canada K7L 3N6*

The significance of fetal asphyxia in regard to mortality and subsequent handicaps in surviving children has been of interest since 1862, when Little (33) observed that cerebral palsy was associated with perinatal problems such as abnormal parturition, difficult labor, premature birth, and asphyxia neonatorum. Despite extensive research, the clinical significance of fetal asphyxia has not been clearly defined. "Although intrapartum fetal asphyxia is established as an important cause of perinatal loss, there is little consensus as to how much of the burden of neurologic handicap in the community is attributable to intrapartum and neonatal asphyxia as measured clinically" (57). Much of this continuing dilemma is owing to two factors. Firstly, most clinical epidemiological studies lack a specific diagnosis for fetal asphyxia, and secondly, many prospective follow-up studies have used different measures for assessment of outcome of motor and cognitive development.

Two questions will be addressed in this chapter: What is the contribution of fetal asphyxia to mortality and to motor and cognitive deficits in surviving children? What is the frequency of such morbidity in infants following an asphyxic insult?

DIAGNOSIS OF ASPHYXIA IN THE HUMAN FETUS

Normal Blood Gas and Acid-Base Measures

A definitive diagnosis of fetal asphyxia requires the determination of fetal acid-base status from assessment of blood gases. Fetal blood gases may be obtained during labor by fetal scalp sampling and at the time of delivery by sampling blood from the umbilical vein and artery. The interpretation of blood gases and fetal acid-base status requires knowledge of normal values, and extensive research has provided reliable normal values for blood gases obtained from the umbilical vein or artery (35) (Table 1).

TABLE 1. *Normal fetal blood gas and acid-base measures*

	Umbilical vein	Umbilical artery
O_2 tension (mm)	28	15
O_2 saturation (%)	65	25
O_2 capacity (vol%)	22	
O_2 content (vol%)	13	5
CO_2 tension (mm)	40	48
pH	7.34	7.26
Buffer base (mmole/liter)	43	41
Base excess (mmole/liter)	−3	−5
Lactate (mmole/liter)	1.7	
Pyruvate (mmole/liter)	0.14	

Fetal umbilical venous and arterial oxygen tensions are significantly lower than the corresponding maternal values. This maternal-fetal gradient of oxygenation is important for the transfer of oxygen from the mother to the fetus. However, the oxygen content in the umbilical vein is within the normal adult range because fetal blood has a greater oxygen affinity and a higher oxygen-carrying capacity. Similarly, fetal umbilical venous and arterial carbon dioxide tensions are of the same order as adult values because of a fetal-maternal gradient related to maternal hyperventilation and hypocapnia. Fetal blood pH values from samples obtained from the umbilical vein and artery are lower than pH values of maternal arterial and venous blood. However, fetal blood buffer base or base deficit in the umbilical vein and artery parallel closely the corresponding maternal values. The best estimations of resting fetal blood lactate and pyruvate levels obtained following elective cesarean section indicate that the normal fetus depends primarily on aerobic metabolism with no accumulation of fixed acids.

Measures of Fetal Asphyxia

The identification of fetal metabolic acidosis confirms that an episode of fetal hypoxia has occurred. An umbilical artery buffer base less than 34 mmole/liter is generally considered to represent significant metabolic acidosis caused by fetal hypoxia (Table 2). Although a buffer base of 36 mmole/liter represents two standard deviations below the mean in a normal population (44), approximately one-third of the lactic acid responsible for the metabolic acidosis results from an increase of pyruvic acid rather than from a primary tissue oxygen debt (42). Therefore, the adjusted umbilical artery buffer base attributable to tissue hypoxia is approximately 34 mmole/liter. The related umbilical artery pH will vary with the degree of respiratory acidosis at the time of sampling. The average equivalent arterial pH is 7.150. Corresponding capillary blood pH (e.g., from fetal scalp) is somewhat higher, i.e., a pH less than 7.200 is generally considered abnormal. The criteria for significant metabolic acidosis caused by hypoxia are summarized in Table 2.

TABLE 2. *Measures of a significant metabolic acidosis caused by fetal hypoxia*

	Umbilical artery	Capillary
pH	<7.150	<7.200
Buffer base (mmole/liter)	<34.0	<36.0

Clinical Indicators of Fetal Asphyxia

Many studies of outcome following fetal asphyxia lack data on fetal blood gas values and acid-base status. The diagnosis of fetal asphyxia in these studies is based primarily on clinical criteria such as abnormal fetal heart rate patterns, the presence of meconium in the amniotic fluid during labor, and low Apgar scores with delayed onset of respiration at delivery.

It has been demonstrated that baseline fetal heart rate and fetal heart rate accelerations are not predictive of intrapartum fetal hypoxia with metabolic acidosis (36). In contrast, fetal heart rate decelerations are predictive but not diagnostic of fetal asphyxia. Thus, even with late decelerations, the probability of fetal hypoxia and significant metabolic acidosis is less than 50% (43).

The relationship between fetal hypoxia with significant metabolic acidosis, as determined by umbilical vein and artery blood gas and acid-base determinations, meconium in amniotic fluid, and Apgar scores at 1 and 5 min following delivery, has been examined in 1,773 obstetric patients (Table 3). Moderate and severe meconium was observed in 262 patients (15%). Of these, 12 fetuses (32%) had significant metabolic acidosis at delivery. On the other hand, 250 fetuses with moderate or severe meconium had blood gas and acid-base measures within the normal range, i.e., a false positive rate of 95%.

An Apgar score of 0 to 3 at 1 min was recorded in 115 newborns (6%) and at 5 min in 11 newborns (1%). Of the infants with a low Apgar score of 0 to 3 at 1 min, 18 (46%) had significant metabolic acidosis at delivery. A low Apgar score of 0 to 3 at 5 min was recorded in three (8%) of the newborns with a significant metabolic acidosis at delivery. On the other hand, the majority of newborns with low Apgar scores did not have evidence of fetal hypoxia with metabolic acidosis. An Apgar score of 0 to 3 at 1 min was observed in 97 newborns with normal blood gas and acid-base values, indicating a false positive rate of 84%. Similarly, an Apgar score of 0 to 3 at 5 min was recorded in eight newborns with normal blood gas and acid-base values, indicating a false positive rate of 73%.

The presence of acute, clinical hypoxic-ischemic encephalopathy in the newborn, particularly seizures and recurrent apnea, has been introduced in order to improve the predictive power of the variables discussed earlier (71) and represents an important predictor of subsequent motor and cognitive deficits (39,54). A direct relationship between severity of perinatal hypoxic insult and severity of encepha-

TABLE 3. *The relationship between meconium and Apgar scores at 1 and 5 min and umbilical artery buffer base*

	Umbilical artery buffer base		
	≥34	<34	
Meconium			
None/minimal	1,464	26	
Moderate/severe	250	12	
Total			1,752
Apgar score 1 min			
7–10	1,459	13	
4–6	178	8	
0–3	97	18	
Total			1,773
Apgar score 5 min			
7–10	1,348	31	
4–6	12	3	
0–3	3	3	
Total			1,405

lopathy in the newborn has been identified in several studies. Clinical studies of birth asphyxia (62) have demonstrated that most children who survive with neuro-developmental sequelae had recognizable encephalopathy during the neonatal period. Studies of term infants with clinical markers of intrapartum hypoxia and subsequent encephalopathy have demonstrated neurological deficits in 25% to 50% of survivors (24). The relationship between fetal hypoxia, confirmed by blood gas and acid-base assessments, and newborn encephalopathy has been examined in 303 high risk children. There was evidence of fetal asphyxia with significant metabolic acidosis in 12% of newborns with mild to moderate encephalopathy and in 22% of newborns with severe encephalopathy (41).

Thus, an association exists between clinical markers of hypoxia, e.g., meconium in amniotic fluid, late decelerations of the fetal heart rate, low Apgar scores at 1 and 5 min, newborn encephalopathy, and intrapartum fetal hypoxia as identified by blood gas and acid-base assessment. However, fetal hypoxia with severe metabolic acidosis may occur in the absence of some or all of these clinical markers. Furthermore, these clinical markers are also observed frequently in the absence of fetal hypoxia, i.e., there is a high incidence of false positive results (Table 4).

Summary

An accurate diagnosis of fetal asphyxia may be made on the basis of blood gas and acid-base assessment of fetal blood. The clinical criteria that are commonly used may be indicative but are not diagnostic of fetal asphyxia. Their greatest limitations are related to their relatively low sensitivity and high false positive rates.

TABLE 4. *The sensitivity and frequency of false positives in clinical markers of fetal asphyxia*

| Clinical markers | Fetal asphyxia | |
	Sensitivity (%)	False positives (%)
Late decelerations	50	>50
Moderate/severe meconium	32	95
Apgar score		
0–3 at 1 min	46	84
0–3 at 5 min	8	73
Newborn encephalopathy—severe	22	78

PERINATAL MORTALITY WITH FETAL ASPHYXIA

A summary of perinatal mortality in our center between 1979 and 1984 is presented in Table 5. There were 12,339 births. The perinatal mortality for all births of more than 500 g was 16.2 per 1,000 total births. There were 68 fetal deaths caused by asphyxia. In relation to the steady decrease of perinatal mortality in recent years, fetal asphyxia remains the single most important cause of mortality.

Eighty percent of perinatal deaths occur in patients with one or more antepartum or intrapartum risk factors. Approximately 40% of deaths occur in fetuses of low birth weight, i.e., between 500 and 1,000 g. The significance of these figures relates to the fact that 60% of deaths occur in otherwise normal fetuses of more than 1,000 g. Such deaths theoretically are preventable if the responsible disorders are identified early and managed with appropriate intervention.

Although it is reasonable to conclude that fetal asphyxia is an important cause of mortality, the diagnosis is confirmed only rarely by blood gas or acid-base assessment. More commonly, the diagnosis is made on the basis of the absence of other complications and on autopsy findings of pulmonary aspiration and extensive petechial hemorrhages over serosal surfaces. It is possible that some perinatal deaths that are presumed to be caused by asphyxia may prove in the future to be caused by other mechanisms.

SIGNIFICANCE OF FETAL ASPHYXIA IN EXPERIMENTAL ANIMALS

Total Asphyxia

Between 1957 and 1963, Windle and colleagues performed a series of controlled experiments in approximately 100 rhesus monkeys to determine the effects of an acute asphyxial insult. The principal findings were reported in the first publication (59). In this study, five pregnant monkeys and two controls were subjected to an acute asphyxial insult of 11 to 16 min. Subsequently, the fetus was intubated

TABLE 5. *The classification of perinatal mortality (1979–1984)*[a]

Fetal asphyxia	68
Fetal growth retardation	18
Newborn respiratory failure	53
Congenital anomalies	45
Infants of diabetic mothers	2
Intracranial hemorrhage	6
Infection	3
Other	6

[a]The perinatal mortality rate during this period for all births >500 g was 16.2 per 1,000 total births.

and resuscitated by means of positive pressure ventilation. The neuropathology was examined 2 to 9 days following delivery. The acute neuropathological findings consisted of nonhemorrhagic bilateral focal lesions, located principally in relay nuclei of the somesthetic, auditory, and vestibular systems and extrapyramidal cell groups. Certain nuclei were involved consistently. The most striking lesion observed was necrosis of the inferior colliculi. In addition, severe damage was seen in the gracile and cuneate nuclei, superior olivary nucleus, putamen, globus pallidus, and the ventral lateral group of the thalamic nuclei. Cytolysis of neurons and, to a lesser extent, neuroglia was evident within 2 days. The intensity of the phagocytic reaction, which was observed initially between 24 and 60 hr following the injury, was related to the degree of cell damage. Reactive changes involving astrocytes and microglia were evident in 7 to 10 days. The uniform and bilateral symmetric involvement of the individual nuclei suggested specific regional susceptibility. These initial findings were confirmed in approximately 50 subsequent studies in which the neuropathology was examined within 3 months of the insult. In many instances, the major respiratory complications of the asphyxiated newborn appeared to increase the severity of the cerebral lesions.

The long-term neuropathological findings following acute fetal asphyxia were described (13) in 12 animals that survived between 10 months and 9 years following the initial insult. The findings were compared with those of five nonasphyxiated controls. Abnormalities included atrophy and gliosis, as well as evidence of secondary degeneration with widespread depletion of nerve cell populations, without associated gliosis, in regions remote from the initial site of injury. These secondary changes were seen most clearly in the regions of cerebral cortex supplied by thalamocortical radiations, as well as in the reticular formation of the brainstem and in the dorsal columns of the spinal cord.

The neurological sequelae of asphyxia observed in 16 monkeys that survived for at least 3 years or more have been reported (72). The monkeys appeared to adapt to their environment despite initial evidence of severe brain damage and subsequent transneuronal atrophy. Neurological abnormalities observed initially either disappeared or improved for 3 to 4 years following the insult. At this stage the animals often appeared overtly normal clinically but were hypoactive and lacked manual dexterity.

Windle (72) concluded that an acute asphyxial insult of less than 8-min duration that does not require active resuscitation of the newborn may not cause brain injury. Asphyxia of more than 8-min duration invariably produced at least transient neurological signs. Asphyxia of more than 10-min duration resulted in neuropathological abnormalities the severity of which correlated with the duration of asphyxia.

Partial Asphyxia

Myers and colleagues (50) noted that the brainstem abnormalities that were observed in monkeys following acute asphyxia did not correspond to the neuropathological findings in humans following perinatal injury, i.e., ulegyria, diffuse white matter sclerosis, and status marmoratus (45). The concept of prolonged partial asphyxia emerged from observations of cerebral cortical necrosis with status marmoratus in several instances in the studies of acute asphyxia (48).

Studies of the effect of prolonged partial hypoxia, induced by either oxytocin stimulation or maternal hypotension in term fetal monkeys for periods of 3 to 5 hr, demonstrated that the severity of brain injury depended on the degree and duration of the hypoxic insult. Many newborns in whom the hypoxic insult was brief and the metabolic acidosis less severe (pH ≥7.0–7.1) did not develop permanent neuropathological abnormalities. Permanent lesions were observed with more prolonged tissue hypoxia, i.e., 30 to 120 min in duration and with severe metabolic acidosis (pH ≤6.9–7.0) (49,50) (Table 6).

In severe cases, neuropathological abnormalities included both generalized and focal cerebral necrosis, which involved principally the parasagittal regions and the junctional zone between the parietal and occipital lobes. Furthermore, there was involvement of basal ganglia, including the caudate nucleus, putamen, and occasionally the globus pallidus. Atrophic cortical necrosis, with varying degrees of white matter injury, was observed in animals examined 6 months following the initial insult. These findings are similar to those reported in children with cerebral palsy.

The importance of both systemic hypotension with decreased cerebral blood flow and the degree of lactic acidosis in the pathogenesis of central nervous system injury was supported by subsequent studies in the fetal monkey and fetal lamb. Thus, there was a correlation between moderate hypotension, serum and brain lactate levels, and brain injury in hypoxic fetal monkeys (51). Similarly, in 28 midgestational fetal lambs, subjected to a 2-hr hypoxic insult and examined 3 days after the insult, neuropathological abnormalities were not observed in 21 lambs, whereas seven lambs exhibited well-demarcated areas of cortical necrosis, with extensive damage to white matter and basal ganglia. The fetuses with neuropathological lesions also had more severe metabolic acidosis, higher lactate

TABLE 6. *The fetal blood gas and acid-base measures of animals with and without evidence of neuropathology*

	Neuropathology	
	None	Present
pH	≥ 7.0–7.1	≤ 6.9–7.0
Base deficit (mmole/liter)	13–18	< 10–13
pCO_2 (mm Hg)	< 70	80–90
O_2 sat (%) n	> 30	< 30

concentrations, and more severe hypotension than those without neuropathological findings (69). A similar relationship between cardiovascular instability and neuropathological sequelae has been reported in the fetal lamb by Mann and colleagues (6). These observations support the concept that systemic hypotension with reduced cerebral blood flow is an important factor in the pathogenesis of hypoxic-ischemic cerebral injury.

Summary

These studies confirm the relationship between fetal asphyxia and central nervous system injury. Furthermore, they demonstrate that the common mechanism most probably involves a degree of relative hypoxia of more than 1 hr in duration and with a progressive metabolic acidosis.

EPIDEMIOLOGIC STUDIES OF MOTOR AND COGNITIVE DEFICITS

Motor Deficits

Most studies of motor handicap following fetal asphyxia describe cerebral palsy as the principal feature (30). Kiely has reviewed the trend in incidences of cerebral palsy in recent years from countries with comparable health care facilities, including Bristol, England (73); Birmingham, England (17); Iceland (18); Sweden (22); Denmark (16); the United States (53); Ireland (8); and Australia (63). No uniform trend is apparent. Thus, the occurrence of cerebral palsy showed a mixed pattern, with declining, stable, fluctuating, or rising trends. The encouraging decline reported in Sweden between 1959 to 1970 has not persisted. Thus, the prevalence rate of cerebral palsy has increased in the 1970s because of an increase in the incidence of spastic diplegia, perhaps related to improved survival of low birth weight infants who require ventilation (23).

The prevalence rates for cerebral palsy between countries are not strictly comparable because the definitions and methods of assessment were not uniform. However, when congenital nervous system anomalies are excluded, prevalence rates for cerebral palsy ranging between 2.0 and 2.5 cases per 1,000 live births are reported.

Abnormal events that cause cerebral palsy are assumed to occur primarily in the prenatal and perinatal periods, with a minor contribution from postnatal factors. The relative significance of various factors has been examined in detail in two major studies, i.e., the National Collaborative Perinatal Project, a large prospective project in the United States, and an epidemiological study from Gothenberg, Sweden, which includes the total population in a western region of Sweden.

The majority of the 202 children with cerebral palsy reported in the National Collaborative Perinatal Project were of normal birth weight and gestational age. However, the importance of fetal asphyxia is implied by the fact that the most significant predictors of cerebral palsy were (1) Apgar scores of 0 to 3 at 10 min or later, and (2) the occurrence of neonatal seizures (54). The Swedish study reported the clinical data of approximately 600 patients with cerebral palsy born between 1954 and 1969 (22). The complications observed in these pregnancies were classified as either prenatal, perinatal, postnatal, or untraceable. Perinatal problems included obvious complications during delivery and during the first 28 days of life in normally grown newborns and low birth weight newborns ($\leq$2,500 g). Sixty-five percent of the children were judged to have had perinatal problems, which presumably included fetal asphyxia.

The Swedish study examined the significance of fetal asphyxia in the context of different types of cerebral palsy. Thus, the birth records were reviewed of 110 children with dyskinetic cerebral palsy, of whom 34 were classified as hyperkinetic and 76 as primarily dystonic. Fetal asphyxia was defined as moderate (Apgar score $\leq$7) or severe (Apgar score $\leq$3 during the first 10 min of life). On the basis of these criteria, fetal asphyxia was significant in the pathogenesis of dyskinetic cerebral palsy and occurred in 35% of the hyperkinetic and 54% of the dystonic children (31). In 93 children with spastic diplegia, of whom 49 were born at term and 44 were preterm, the term newborns appeared to be affected more severely. The criteria for fetal asphyxia included the presence of meconium in the amniotic fluid, fetal heart rate $\leq$100 or $\geq$160, or delayed onset of respiration $\geq$1 min and requiring active resuscitation. Spastic diplegia in term infants was associated frequently with growth retardation and asphyxia. Birth asphyxia was identified in 31%. It was concluded in this study that prolonged asphyxia correlated significantly with more severe handicap (70).

Cognitive Deficits

Epidemiological studies of mental retardation are based principally on IQ scores. Because "severe" mental retardation (IQ <50) and "mild" mental retardation (IQ 50–69) differ with regard to etiologic factors, they will be discussed separately.

The expected prevalence rate for "severe" mental retardation is 3.5 to 4 per 1,000 children of school age (65). In 122 children with "severe" mental retardation born in Sweden between 1959 and 1970 (19), chromosomal anomalies, congenital malformations, and inborn errors of metabolism were observed in 63% (19). In the remaining cases, apparent causes were classified as prenatal (8%), perinatal (8%), infectious (6%), and miscellaneous (15%). These observations suggest that fetal asphyxia, which would be considered a perinatal complication, plays a minor role in the pathogenesis of "severe" mental retardation.

"Mild" mental retardation may be observed frequently as an isolated disturbance in children of lower socioeconomic status. The predicted prevalence rate is approximately 10 to 30 per 1,000 school age children. Mild mental retardation is stated to result primarily from environmental deprivation (57). An exception to this general statement was reported in a study of 91 children with "mild" mental retardation who were born between 1966 and 1970 in Sweden (20). The prevalence of "mild" mental retardation of 4 per 1,000 was much lower than the expected rate, and this lower rate was attributed to the relatively high socioeconomic level of this particular population. The mental retardation was associated in 43% of children with other neurological abnormalities, which included cerebral palsy (9%), clumsiness (23%), and epilepsy (12%). "Mild" mental retardation was an isolated finding in 55% of the children. However, prenatal complications were identified in 23%, and perinatal complications, principally fetal asphyxia, occurred in 18% (21). These observations suggest that fetal asphyxia may play a modest role in the pathogenesis of "mild" mental retardation, particularly if social, environmental, and economic circumstances are otherwise favorable.

The relationship between perinatal hypoxia and cognitive development in infancy and childhood was examined also in the National Collaborative Perinatal Project (3). The criteria for asphyxia in this study included fetal tachycardia in the first stage of labor, low Apgar scores at 1 and 5 min, the presence of meconium at delivery, primary apnea, single or multiple apneic spells, resuscitation during and after the first 5 min, and respiratory difficulties in the nursery. Asphyxiated infants, particularly those with respiratory difficulties, had relatively lower cognitive scores subsequently during infancy and at the age of 7 years. This association appeared to be independent of socioeconomic factors.

Summary

Because accurate diagnosis of fetal asphyxia is difficult to establish with certainty on clinical criteria alone, it is not possible to determine precisely the significance of fetal asphyxia for subsequent neurological abnormalities from epidemiological studies. However, data from such studies suggest that asphyxia in the human fetus may account for a moderate proportion of cerebral palsy and a minor proportion of mental retardation.

SIGNIFICANCE OF CLINICAL INDICATORS OF FETAL ASPHYXIA

Apgar Scores

Newborn depression, as expressed by low Apgar scores and delayed onset of respiration, has been used most frequently as an indicator of fetal asphyxia in studies of neurological outcome. A relationship between Apgar scores and neurological outcome has been demonstrated in the National Collaborative Perinatal Project (10). Low Apgar scores at 1 min are related only weakly to subsequent motor and cognitive development (4). Therefore, attention has been directed primarily toward low Apgar scores at 5 min or later following delivery. Low Apgar scores at 5 min are associated with an increased incidence of severe motor and cognitive deficits (52). The significance of prolonged low Apgar scores was demonstrated in 128 children with moderate and severe cerebral palsy (54) (Table 7). This association of prolonged low Apgar scores with subsequent neurological abnormalities occurs principally in term newborns, reflecting in part the low survival rate of preterm newborns with prolonged low Apgar scores (55). The association between low Apgar scores and poor neurological outcome has been reported in pregnancies both with and without definable obstetric complications (56).

Although there is clearly an association between low Apgar scores and poor neurological outcome, the majority of children with low Apgar scores have normal outcome. This has been emphasized in several studies. Thus, Steiner and Neligan (66) reported the outcome of 22 newborns who experienced perinatal cardiac arrest, with recovery of heart rate within 5 min and spontaneous respirations within 30 min. Major handicaps were observed in four children (20%). Scott (62) reported the outcome of 23 newborns who had either an Apgar score of zero or a delay in onset of spontaneous respiration greater than 20 min. Major handicaps were observed in six children (25%). It should be recognized that in both of these studies only surviving newborns were studied and that approximately an equal number of infants died in the immediate postdelivery period. Thomson et al. (67)

TABLE 7. *The relationship between low Apgar scores (0–3) and mortality or deficits in survivors in the National Collaborative Perinatal Project*

Apgar scores 0–3 (min)	n	Mortality (%)	Deficits in survivors (%)
5	788	44	5
10	362	68	13
15	232	81	23
20	181	87	38

Modified from ref. 54.

reported on the outcome of 31 children with an Apgar score of 0 to 3 at 5 min. The interval of time to sustained respiration ranged from 5 to 60 min. Major abnormalities were observed in only two children (7%). Mulligan et al. (47) reported the outcome of 65 children with delayed onset of spontaneous respiration between 2 and >20 min. Major handicaps were observed in 12 children (18%). Furthermore, Ergander and Erikson (12) reported on 81 children with an Apgar score of 0 to 3 at 5 min. Major handicaps were observed in 16 children (20%). Significant neurological abnormalities were associated frequently with a delay in the onset of spontaneous respiration of >20 min.

Newborn Encephalopathy

The significance of neonatal seizures as a predictor of poor outcome has been well documented (1,68). Thus in a study of 137 term newborns with seizures, Rose and Lombroso (61) reported a mortality of 20%. A further 30% of these infants survived with serious neurological deficits. Holden et al. (25) identified deficits in 30% of 181 survivors of neonatal seizures followed to 7 years of age as part of the National Collaborative Perinatal Project.

Brown et al. (5), in a study of 94 asphyxiated newborn infants, emphasized the importance of abnormal tone in the prediction of poor outcome. The criteria of asphyxia included meconium-stained amniotic fluid and/or abnormal fetal heart rate, Apgar scores <3 at 1 min and/or <5 at 5 min, and resuscitation requiring positive pressure ventilation. Abnormal neurological signs in the newborn included apnea, apathy, seizures, hypothermia, "cerebral" cry, persistent vomiting, and abnormal muscle tone. Twenty asphyxiated newborns with abnormal neurological signs died. Of the 74 asphyxiated infants who survived, 24 had significant handicap, 15 had minor deficits. and 34 were normal.

Fitzhardinge et al. (14) reported the outcome of 62 term infants with postasphyxial encephalopathy. The criteria of asphyxia included the presence of meconium-stained amniotic fluid and/or abnormal fetal heart rate, Apgar score <6 at 5 min, or resuscitation requiring ventilation for longer than 2 min. Clinical features of encephalopathy in the newborn included seizures, increased intracranial pressure, and abnormal tone. Major abnormalities were identified subsequently in 29 infants (47%) and minor abnormalities in five infants (8%).

Robertson and Finer (60) reported the outcome of 167 term newborns with evidence of hypoxic-ischemic encephalopathy who were followed until 3 to 5 years of age. The criteria of asphyxia included abnormal fetal heart rate, Apgar score <5 at 1 min and/or Apgar score <5 at 5 min, and newborn resuscitation with ventilation >5 min. Encephalopathy in the infants was classified according to the staging system of Sarnat, which is based on assessment of alterations in consciousness, alterations of muscle tone, and abnormal neonatal reflexes. Neurological sequelae occurred in 27 children, and these correlated with the severity of the acute encephalopathy (Table 8). Moderate encephalopathy was more likely to be associated with deficits when accompanied by seizures. All newborns with severe encephalopathy either died or survived with severe neurological abnormalities.

TABLE 8. *The relationship between the severity of newborn encephalopathy and the frequency of handicap*

Newborn encephalopathy	n	Handicap	
		n	%
Mild	66	0	
Moderate	74	20	27
Severe	7	7	100

Modified from ref. 60.

Summary

The aforementioned studies cannot lead to entirely accurate determination of the incidence of poor outcome following asphyxia in the human fetus because fetal asphyxia accounts for only a limited proportion of the patients with low Apgar scores at 5 min and with clinical encephalopathy. Nevertheless, the frequency of motor and cognitive deficits reported in children with these features ranges from 5% to 50%. Although these clinical markers are not pathognomonic of fetal asphyxia, they provide valuable adjunctive information to blood gas and acid-base assessments in that they indicate the biological impact of asphyxic episodes. The severity of acute encephalopathy in the newborn is of particular importance in this regard.

SIGNIFICANCE OF FETAL ASPHYXIA IN THE HUMAN

Significance of Fetal Asphyxia

Although it is clear that fetal or newborn complications may affect the central nervous system and result in motor and cognitive deficits, the relative importance of individual complications has not yet been determined. Because these complications often occur concurrently, it is difficult to determine the significance of individual ones.

A study by Low et al. (37) of 364 unselected preterm and term infants with one or more fetal or newborn complications examined these issues. Motor and/or cognitive deficits were identified in 24% of the children at 1 year of age. Complications that were independently associated with neurological sequelae included fetal hypoxia, newborn respiratory complications, and infection. These complications also had an independent association with newborn encephalopathy. These observations support the concept that fetal hypoxia, newborn respiratory complications, and infections may cause central nervous system dysfunction and injury. Acute encephalopathy in the newborn reflects the immediate injury and is an important predictor of outcome.

A review of the 86 children with identified abnormalities at 1 year of age demonstrated that the importance of individual complications differed in preterm and term children. Thus, 29 preterm infants (58%) experienced primarily respiratory complications. Infection and fetal hypoxia were of minor significance in this group. In contrast, in 11 term infants (30%) the principal problem was fetal hypoxia. Infection and respiratory complications were less important. Thus, there is a stronger correlation between intrapartum fetal hypoxia with metabolic acidosis and poor outcome in term than in preterm pregnancies.

Significance of Severity and Duration of Asphyxia

The relationship between fetal hypoxia as defined by blood gas and acid-base assessments and outcome has been examined in several studies. In a prospective study (38), 37 children who experienced an episode of fetal hypoxia before delivery and a control group of 59 children with no evidence of fetal hypoxia were followed to 6 years of age. All infants were full term and of appropriate birth weight for gestation. The infants in the hypoxic group did *not* display evidence of encephalopathy during the newborn period. There was no significant difference in physical growth or in the incidence of motor and cognitive deficits in the children of the hypoxic group compared to the children of the control group. These data indicate that a fetus may experience a terminal episode of fetal hypoxia with significant metabolic acidosis without developing apparent subsequent motor or cognitive deficit. It is noteworthy that in such infants, no neonatal signs of central nervous system disturbance were observed.

A second study (40) analyzed the outcome of 60 children with biochemical evidence of intrapartum fetal hypoxia in an attempt to determine the degree and duration of fetal hypoxia required to cause central nervous system injury. The objective was to establish the distinguishing features of children with deficits at 1 year of age. Eight children (13%) had major neurological abnormalities and 10 children (16%) had minor abnormalities at 1 year of age. Children with deficits had generally experienced more severe, prolonged hypoxia and had a greater incidence of respiratory complications, apnea, and newborn encephalopathy following delivery. These findings suggest that an episode of hypoxia *in excess of 1 hr* may be followed by a higher incidence of motor and cognitive deficits. This study also demonstrated that the relationship between fetal hypoxia and outcome varies with gestational age. Twelve of the 18 asphyxiated children (67%) who developed neurological sequelae were born at term. Six of the 18 children (33%) with fetal hypoxia who developed sequelae were born prematurely. Thus, although there was an increased incidence of neurological abnormalities in preterm and particularly in very low birth weight infants, fetal hypoxia appears to play only a limited contributory role in this context. The majority of problems in infants born prematurely appears to be related to respiratory complications following delivery.

The nature of the deficits following fetal hypoxia has been studied in 36 term newborns, with 76 normal term infants employed as controls. The incidence of

TABLE 9. *The frequency of motor and/or cognitive deficits in infants with and without evidence of fetal hypoxia and significant metabolic acidosis at delivery*

Motor and cognitive development	Controls (n = 76)		Hypoxia (n = 36)	
	n	%	n	%
Normal	70	93	22	61
Minor deficit	5	6	9	25
Major deficit	1	1	5	14

deficits in the hypoxic and control groups is outlined in Table 9. These data suggest that there is an increased incidence of both minor and major deficits in the children who experienced fetal hypoxia. The minor abnormalities observed following fetal hypoxia included principally motor developmental delays, with a Bayley Psychomotor Developmental Index in the borderline range (70–84). There was no evidence of cognitive developmental delay. The five children with major sequelae had motor abnormalities. Thus, two children had hemiplegia, one had spastic diplegia, and two had severe hypotonia. Cognitive development was in the normal range in two children, one had a minor deficit, and two other children had severe cognitive abnormalities.

Summary

These observations support the notion that prolonged fetal asphyxia defined by blood gas and acid-base assessments may result in long-term motor and cognitive deficits. On the other hand, these observations emphasize that the majority of infants who experience a central nervous system asphyxic insult will not develop neurological sequelae that are recognizable by 1 year of age. Neurological abnormalities in the newborn period are important features of brain injury caused by fetal asphyxia.

DISCUSSION

The significance of fetal asphyxia in the pathogenesis of brain injury has not been established fully because of the complexity of the multiple factors that may contribute to such injury. Thus, in a summary statement in a recent review of the prenatal and perinatal causes of mental retardation, cerebral palsy, and epilepsy, Freeman (15) emphasized "how little we know of the factors controlling, modifying, or altering brain development."

Nevertheless, significant progress has been made in the understanding of the contribution of fetal asphyxia to subsequent neurological outcome. In spite of their limitations, epidemiological studies have provided valuable information in this regard. Thus, these studies have demonstrated prevalence rates of 2 per 1,000 live births for cerebral palsy, 4 per 1,000 live births for ''severe'' mental retardation, and 10 to 30 per 1,000 live births for ''mild'' mental retardation. There is compelling evidence to suggest that the risk factors differ for different abnormalities. Socioeconomic and environmental variables appear to be particularly important concerning ''mild'' mental retardation. The pathogenesis of cognitive deficits associated with cerebral palsy may be significantly different from that of isolated intellectual deficit.

It is evident from these studies that major abnormalities are principally caused by mechanisms other than fetal asphyxia. Thus, many cases of cerebral palsy are owing to central nervous system anomalies, metabolic disturbances, infection, and postnatal complications. Moreover, 50% to 60% of children with severe mental retardation have conditions that are genetically determined. Recent data suggest that the principal factors associated with mild mental retardation are genetic defects and environmental deprivation.

Studies of fetal asphyxia in experimental animals have confirmed the relationship between fetal asphyxia and specific patterns of central nervous system injury. Acute total asphyxia for periods in excess of 10 min consistently results in lesions that are located principally in the brainstem, with limited involvement of the cerebral hemispheres. In contrast, prolonged partial hypoxia with progressive metabolic acidosis over 30 to 120 min and a pH ≤6.9 to 7.0 may result in lesions that characteristically involve the cerebral cortex and white matter and the basal ganglia.

Recent observations in the human fetus indicate the importance of the *duration* as well as the *severity* of the metabolic acidosis, as identified by blood gas and acid-base assessment, in the determination of asphyxial injury. A terminal episode of fetal asphyxia may occur in the term newborn without recognizable neurological sequelae. However, if the hypoxic episode lasts longer than 1 hr, permanent brain injury commonly occurs.

The importance of gestational age in the occurrence of fetal asphyxial injury is also apparent. Thus, fetal asphyxia appears to be a more important cause of poor outcome in the term newborn than in the preterm infant. The current data suggest that fetal asphyxia is only one of many factors that may result in major or minor motor or cognitive abnormalities. A better understanding of the significance of fetal asphyxia will require accurate determination of the degree and duration of fetal asphyxia in a prospective assessment of a large population.

A fetal blood gas and acid-base assessment provides an accurate measure of the severity of hypoxemia at a single point in time. Metabolic acidosis in the fetus may reflect a severe hypoxic episode of short duration or partial intermittent hypoxia of longer duration. This observation relates to the relatively slow resolution of fixed acids by the placenta or fetal kidneys (42). There is no single measurement that will indicate the precise duration of the hypoxic episode in the fetus.

Such information may be provided by serial blood gas and acid-base measurements or by continuous reliable recording of pH. Unfortunately, at the present time, serial scalp sampling is used rarely, and a pH electrode for continuous monitoring is not yet available.

Furthermore, in order to determine the frequency of neurological sequelae following fetal asphyxia, it is essential to define the criteria of fetal asphyxia. The criteria of fetal asphyxia used in our center, i.e., umbilical artery buffer base of less than 34 mmole/liter, occurs in approximately 2% of newborns. The frequency of major and/or minor neurological abnormalities at 1 year of age in these infants is approximately 20%.

In this context, it is important not to overlook the fact that 80% of children who experience a significant hypoxic-ischemic insult do not develop neurological abnormalities. This may relate to factors such as growth retardation or, more importantly, to the fetal cardiovascular response to acute asphyxia. The principal response involves an increase of arterial pressure, caused by increased systemic vascular resistance (with reduced blood flow to the pulmonary, renal, gastrointestinal, and skeletal muscle circulations) with a resulting simultaneous increase in blood flow to vital organs such as the brain, heart, and adrenals (7,58). In addition, there is evidence that during acute hypoxia, there is a loss of autoregulation in the cerebral circulation with a pressure-passive relationship resulting (34). The increased cerebral blood flow, which is dependent on arterial pressure and correlates directly with it (29), occurs preferentially in critical brainstem regions (58). Following prolonged partial hypoxia, the increased cerebral blood flow returns to baseline values within at least 24 hr without apparent impairment of the microcirculation (2). Thus, this response of increase in cerebral blood flow is vital for the preservation of the integrity of the central nervous system in the context of hypoxic-ischemic insult. Such hypoxic insults may be caused by maternal hypoxemia, reduced uteroplacental blood flow, or compromised fetal blood flow through the umbilical cord (11,26,34).

Several mechanisms account for this systemic vascular response of the fetus to hypoxia. The alpha-adrenergic receptors of the autonomic nervous system cause redistribution of cardiac output during acute hypoxia. Alpha-adrenergic blockade during hypoxia will abolish the increased systemic vascular resistance with a resultant decrease of arterial pressure. Recent evidence suggests that this alpha-adrenergic response to hypoxia may be initiated through the arterial chemoreceptors (27) and possibly by circulating endogenous opiates (32). Other factors that may contribute to the increased systemic vascular resistance during acute hypoxia include increased angiotension activity (28,46) and the release of vasopressin (9,64). The preferential shunting of blood flow to brainstem also may be mediated by endogenous opiates. Although the relationship between fetal asphyxia and neurological abnormalities has not been clearly defined, this is an area of research that is of great interest at the present time. Future progress will depend on well-designed clinical studies with accurate assessment of the degree and duration of asphyxia and follow-up into later childhood.

REFERENCES

1. Amiel-Tison, C. (1969): Cerebral damage in full term newborn. Aetiological factors, neonatal status and long-term follow-up. *Biologia Neonatorum,* 14:234–250.
2. Ashwal, S., Majcher, J.P., and Longo, L.D. (1981): Patterns of fetal lamb regional cerebral blood flow during and after prolonged hypoxia studies during the post hypoxic recovery period. *Am. J. Obstet. Gynecol.,* 139:365–372.
3. Broman, S. (1979): Perinatal anoxia and cognitive development in early childhood. In: *Infants Born at Risk,* edited by T. Field, A.M. Sostek, and S. Goldberg, pp. 29–52. S.P. Medical and Scientific Books, New York.
4. Broman, S.H., Nicholas, P.L., Kennedy, W.A. (1975): *Preschool IQ: Prenatal and Early Developmental Correlates.* Erlbaum, Hillsdale, NJ.
5. Brown, J.K., Purvis, R.J., Forfar, J.O., and Cockburn, F. (1974): Neurological aspects of perinatal asphyxia. *Dev. Med. Child Neurol.,* 16:567–580.
6. Clapp, J.F., Mann, L.I., Peress, N.S., and Szeto, H.H. (1981): Neuropathology in the chronic fetal lamb preparation: Structure-function correlates under different environmental conditions. *Am. J. Obstet. Gynecol.,* 141:973–986.
7. Cohn, H.E., Sacks, E.T., Heymann, M.A., and Rudolph, A.M. (1974): Cardiovascular responses to hypoxemia and acidemia in fetal lambs. *Am. J. Obstet. Gynecol.,* 120:817–824.
8. Cussen, G.H., Barey, J.E., Maloney, A.M., Buckley, N.M., Crowley, M., and Daly, C. (1978): Cerebral palsy: A regional study. *Ir. Med. J.,* 71:568–572.
9. DeVane, G.W., Noden, R.P., Porter, J.C., and Rosenfeld, C.R. (1982): Mechanism of arginine vasopressin release in the sheep fetus. *Pediatr. Res.,* 16:504–507.
10. Drage, J.S., Kennedy, C., Berendes, H., Schwarz, B.K., and Weiss, W. (1966): The Apgar score as index of infant morbidity. A report from the Collaborative Study of Cerebral Palsy. *Dev. Med. Child Neurol.,* 8:141–148.
11. Edelston, D.I. (1980): Regulation of blood flow through the ductus venosus. *J. Dev. Physiol.,* 2:219–238.
12. Ergander, V., and Erikson, H. (1980): Severe neonatal asphyxia. *Acta Paediatr. Scand.,* 72:321–325.
13. Faro, M.G., and Windle, W.F. (1969): Transneuronal degeneration in brain of monkeys asphyxiated at birth. *Exp. Neurol.,* 24:38–53.
14. Fitzhardinge, P.M., Flodmark, O., Fitz, C.R., and Ashby, S. (1981): The prognostic value of computed tomography as an adjunct to assessment of the term infant with post asphyxial encephalopathy. *J. Pediatr.,* 99:777–781.
15. Freeman, J.M. (ed.) (1985): *Prenatal and Perinatal Factors Associated with Brain Disorders.* U.S. Dept. of Health and Human Services Public Health Services, N.I.H. Publication No. 85-1149, p. 111.
16. Glenting, P. (1976): Variations in the population of congenital (pre and perinatal) cases of cerebral palsy in Danish countries east of the Little Belt during the years 1950–1969. *Ugeskr. Laeger,* 138:1356–1361.
17. Griffiths, M.I., and Barrett, N.M. (1967): Cerebral palsy in Birmingham. *Dev. Med. Child Neurol.,* 9:33–46.
18. Gudmundsson, G. (1967): Cerebral palsy in Iceland. *Acta Neurol. Scand. [Suppl.],* 34.
19. Gustavson, K.H., Hagberg, B., Hagberg, G., and Sars, K. (1977): Severe mental retardation in a Swedish country. I. Epidemiology, gestational age, birth weight and associated CNS handicaps in children born 1959–70. *Acta Paediatr. Scand.,* 66:373–379.
20. Hagberg, B., Hagberg, G., Lewerth, A., and Landberg, U. (1981): Mild mental retardation in Swedish school children. I. Prevalence. *Acta Paediatr. Scand.,* 70:441–444.
21. Hagberg, B., Hagberg, G., Lewerth, A., and Landberg, U. (1981): Mild mental retardation in Swedish school children. II. Etiologic and pathogenetic aspects. *Acta Paediatr. Scand.,* 70:445–452.
22. Hagberg, B., Hagberg, G., and Olow, I. (1975): The changing panorama of cerebral palsy in Sweden 1954–1970. I. Analysis of general changes. *Acta Paediatr. Scand.,* 64:187–192.
23. Hagberg, B., Hagberg, G., and Olow, I. (1982): Gains and hazards of intensive neonatal care: An analysis from Swedish cerebral palsy epidemiology. *Dev. Med. Child Neurol.,* 24:13–19.
24. Hill, A., and Volpe, J.J. (1981): Seizures, hypoxic-ischemic brain injury and intraventricular hemorrhage in the newborn. *Ann. Neurol.,* 10:109–121.

25. Holden, K.R., Mellits, E.D., and Freeman, J.M. (1982): Neonatal seizures. I. Correlation of prenatal and perinatal events with outcomes. *Pediatrics,* 70:165–176.
26. Itskovitz, J., Goetzman, B.W., and Rudolph, A.M. (1982): Effects of hemorrhage on umbilical venous return and oxygen delivery in fetal lambs. *Am. J. Physiol.,* 242:543–548.
27. Itskovitz, J., LaGamma, E.F., and Rudolph, A.M. (1983): The effect of reducing umbilical blood flow in fetal oxygenation. *Am. J. Obstet. Gynecol.,* 145:813–818.
28. Iwammato, H.L., and Rudolph, A.M. (1981): Effects of angiotensin II on the blood flow and its distribution in fetal lambs. *Circ. Res.,* 48:183–189.
29. Johnson, G.N., Palahnick, R.J., Tweed, W.A., Jones, M.V., and Wade, J.G. (1979): Regional cerebral blood flow changes during severe fetal asphyxia produced by slow partial umbilical cord compression. *Am. J. Obstet. Gynecol.,* 135:48–52.
30. Kiely, J., Paneth, N., Stein, Z.A., and Susser, M.N. (1981): Cerebral palsy and newborn care. I. Secular trends in cerebral palsy. *Dev. Med. Child Neurol.,* 23:533–538.
31. Kyllerman, M. (1982): Diskinetic cerebral palsy. II. Pathogenetic risk factors and intrauterine growth. *Acta Paediatr. Scand.,* 71:551–558.
32. LaGamma, E.F., Itskovitz, J., and Rudolph, A.M. (1982): Effects of naloxone on fetal circulatory responses to hypoxemia. *Am. J. Obstet. Gynecol.,* 143:933–940.
33. Little, W.J. (1862): On the influence of abnormal parturition, difficult labor, premature birth and asphyxia neonatorum on the mental and physical condition of the child, especially in relation to deformities. *Trans. Lond. Obstet. Soc.,* 3:293–294.
34. Lou, H.C., Lassen, N.A., Tweed, W.A., Johnson, G., Jones, M., and Palahnick, R.J. (1979): Pressure passive cerebral blood flow and breakdown of the blood brain barrier in experimental fetal asphyxia. *Acta Paediatr. Scand.,* 68:57–63.
35. Low, J.A. (1986): Maternal and fetal blood gas and acid-base metabolism. In: *Scientific Foundations of Obstetrics and Gynecology,* edited by J. Barnes, M. Newton, and E.E. Phillipp, p. 254. Hinemann, London.
36. Low, J.A., Cox, M.J., Karchmar, E.J., McGrath, M.J., Pancham, S.R., and Piercy, W.N. (1981): The prediction of intrapartum fetal metabolic acidosis by fetal heart rate monitoring. *Am. J. Obstet. Gynecol.,* 139:299–305.
37. Low, J.A., Galbraith, R.S., Muir, D.W., Broekhoven, L.H., Wilkinson, J.W., and Karchmar, E.J. (1985): The contribution of fetal-newborn complications to motor and cognitive deficits. *Dev. Med. Child Neurol.,* 27:578–587.
38. Low, J.A., Galbraith, R.S., Muir, D.W., Killen, H.L., Pater, E.A., and Karchmar, E.J. (1983): Intrapartum fetal hypoxia: A study of long term morbidity. *Am. J. Obstet. Gynecol.,* 145:129–134.
39. Low, J.A., Galbraith, R.S., Muir, D.W., Killen, H.L., Pater, E.A., and Karchmar, E.J. (1983): The predictive significance of biological risk factors for deficits in children of a high risk population. *Am. J. Obstet. Gynecol.,* 145:1059–1068.
40. Low, J.A., Galbraith, R.S., Muir, D.W., Killen, H.L., Pater, E.A., and Karchmar, E.J. (1984): Factors associated with motor and cognitive deficits in children after intrapartum fetal hypoxia. *Am. J. Obstet. Gynecol.,* 148:533–539.
41. Low, J.A., Galbraith, R.S., Muir, D.W., Killen, H.L., Pater, E.A., and Karchmar, E.J. (1985): The relationship between perinatal hypoxia and newborn encephalopathy. *Am. J. Obstet. Gynecol.,* 152:256–260.
42. Low, J.A., Pancham, S.R., Piercy, W.N., Worthington, D., and Karchmar, J. (1978): Maternal and fetal lactate characteristics during labor and delivery. In: *Lactate in Acute Conditions,* edited by H. Bressart and C. Karger, pp. 257–265. Karger, Basel.
43. Low, J.A., Pancham, S.R., and Worthington, G. (1977): Intrapartum fetal heart rate profiles with and without fetal asphyxia. *Am. J. Obstet. Gynecol.,* 127:729–737.
44. Low, J.A., Pancham, S.R., Worthington, G., and Boston, R.W. (1974): Acid-base, lactate and pyruvate characteristics of the normal obstetric patient and fetus during the intrapartum period. *Am. J. Obstet. Gynecol.,* 120:862–867.
45. Malamud, N. (1959): Sequelae of perinatal trauma. *J. Neuropathol. Exp. Neurol.,* 18:141–155.
46. Montquin, J.M., and Liggins, G.C. (1981): Effects of partial lower aortic obstruction in the pregnant ewe on fetal arterial pressure, heart rate, plasma renin activity and prostaglandin E concentration. *J. Dev. Physiol.,* 3:75–84.
47. Mulligan, J.C., Painter, M.J., O'Donoghue, P.A., MacDonald, H.M., Allen, A.C., and Taylor, I.M. (1980): Neonatal asphyxia. II. Neonatal mortality and long-term sequelae. *J. Pediatr.,* 96:903–907.

49. Myers, R.E. (1969): *Fetal Asphyxia and Perinatal Brain Damage Affecting Human Development,* Publ. No. 185, pp. 205–214. Pan American Health Organization, Washington.
50. Myers, R.E., Beard, R., and Adamson, K. (1969): Brain swelling in the newborn rhesus monkey following prolonged partial asphyxia. *Neurology,* 19:1012–1018.
51. Myers, R.E., Wagner, K.R., and De Courten, G.M. (1981): Lactic acid accumulation in tissue as cause of brain injury and death in cardiogenic shock from asphyxia. In: *Clinical Perinatal Biochemical Monitoring,* edited by N.H. Lauersen and H.M. Hochberg, p. 11–34. Williams & Wilkins Co., Baltimore.
52. Nelson, K.B., and Broman, S.H. (1977): Perinatal risk factors in children with serious motor and mental handicaps. *Ann. Neurol.,* 2:371–377.
53. Nelson, K.B., and Ellenberg, J.H. (1978): Epidemiology of cerebral palsy. In: *Advances in Neurology,* vol. 19, edited by B.L. Schomberg, p. 421. Raven Press, New York.
54. Nelson, K.B., and Ellenberg, J.H. (1979): Neonatal signs as predictors of cerebral palsy. *Pediatrics,* 64:225–232.
55. Nelson, K.B., and Ellenberg, J.H., (1981): Apgar scores as predictors of chronic neurologic disability. *Pediatrics,* 68:36–44.
56. Nelson, K.B., and Ellenberg, J.H. (1984): Obstetric complications as risk factors for cerebral palsy or seizure disorders. *JAMA,* 251:1843–1848.
57. Paneth, N., and Stark, R.I. (1983): Cerebral palsy and mental retardation in relation to indicators of perinatal asphyxia. An epidemiologic overview. *Am. J. Obstet. Gynecol.,* 147:960–966.
58. Peeters, L.L., Sheldon, R.D., Jones, M.D., Makowski, E.L., and Meschia, G. (1979): Blood flow to fetal organs as a function of arterial oxygen content. *Am. J. Obstet. Gynecol.,* 135:637–646.
59. Ranck, J.B., and Windle, W.F. (1959): Brain damage in the monkey, *Maccaca mulatta,* by asphyxia neonatorum. *Exp. Neurol.,* 1:130–154.
60. Robertson, C., and Finer, N. (1985): Term infants with hypoxic-ischemic encephalopathy: Outcome at 3–5 years. *Dev. Med. Child Neurol.,* 27:473–484.
61. Rose, A.L., and Lombroso, C.T. (1970): Neonatal seizure states. A study of clinical pathological and electroencephalographic features in 137 full-term babies with a long-term follow-up. *Pediatrics,* 45:404–425.
62. Scott, H. (1976): Outcome of very severe birth asphyxia. *Arch. Dis. Child.,* 51:712–716.
63. Stanley, F.J. (1979): An epidemiology study of cerebral palsy in Western Australia 1956–1975. I. Changes in total cerebral palsy incidence and associated factors. *Dev. Med. Child Neurol.,* 21:701–713.
64. Stark, R.I., Wardlaw, S.L., Daniel, S.S., et al. (1982): Vasopressin secretion induced by hypoxia in sheep: Developmental changes and relationship to beta-endorphin release. *Am. J. Obstet. Gynecol.,* 143:204–215.
65. Stein, Z.A., and Susser, M.W. (1980): Mental retardation. In: *Public Health and Preventive Medicine,* 2nd ed., edited by J.M. Last. Appleton-Century-Crofts, New York.
66. Steiner, H., and Neligan, G. (1975): Perinatal cardiac arrest. *Arch. Dis. Child.,* 50:696–702.
67. Thomson, A.J., Searle, M., and Russell, G. (1977): Quality of survival after severe birth asphyxia. *Arch. Dis. Child.,* 52:620–626.
68. Thorn, I. Cerebral symptoms in the newborn. Diagnostic and prognostic significance of symptoms of presumed cerebral origin. *Acta Paediatr. Scand. [Suppl.],* 1950–1969.
69. Ting, P., Yamaguchi, S., Bacher, J.G., Killens, R.H., and Myers, R.E. (1983): Hypoxic-ischemic cerebral necrosis in midgestational sheep fetuses: Physiopathologic correlations. *Exp. Neurol.,* 80:227–245.
70. Veelken, N., Hagberg, B., Hagberg, G., and Olow, I. (1983): Diplegic cerebral palsy in Swedish term and preterm children. Differences in reduced optimality, relations to neurology and pathogenetic factors. *Neuropediatrics,* 14:20–28.
71. Volpe, J.J. (1987): *Neurology of the Newborn.* W.B. Saunders, Philadelphia.
72. Windle, W.F. (1968): Brain damage at birth: Functional and structural modifications with time. *JAMA,* 106:1967–1972.
73. Woods, G.E. (1963): A lower incidence of infantile cerebral palsy. *Dev. Med. Child Neurol.,* 5:449–450.

Fetal Neurology, edited by
A. Hill and J.J. Volpe.
Raven Press, New York © 1989.

Commentary on Chapter 9

*Alan Hill and **Joseph J. Volpe

*Division of Neurology, Department of Paediatrics, University of British Columbia,
British Columbia's Children's Hospital, Vancouver, British Columbia, Canada V6H 3V4;
and **Division of Pediatric Neurology, Washington University School of Medicine,
St. Louis, Missouri 63110*

In the current era of legal hostility toward the obstetrician, there has been increasing interest in our profession in the definition of causes of cerebral palsy *other than* intrapartum asphyxia. As with any other reactive response, there results a danger that certain truths become overlooked or ignored. Low's review of neurological injury caused by fetal asphyxia emphasized the importance of intrapartum hypoxic-ischemic insults in the causation of a considerable proportion of examples of subsequent motor and cognitive deficits, particularly in term infants. The importance of *duration* as well as *severity* of insult is appropriately emphasized, and Low's work provided definitive data on the former (as well as the latter) issue for the first time.

In other chapters, techniques available for the assessment of fetal well-being during pregnancy and before the onset of labor have been discussed. These techniques included the nonstress test (Smith and Phelan), the contraction stress test (Phelan and Smith), the fetal biophysical profile (Brar and Platt), and the measurement of umbilical artery blood flow (FitzGerald and Stuart). Until relatively recently, the diagnosis of *intrapartum* asphyxia principally depended on the recognition of the passage of meconium and/or fetal bradycardia. More recently, intrapartum assessment of the fetus has been refined to include detailed electronic monitoring of fetal heart rate and fetal blood sampling to assess acid-base status. The relationship of fetal heart rate monitoring to fetal outcome is discussed in detail in the chapter by Schifrin. The chapter by Low discussed the value of fetal acid-base measurements as a critical adjunct to fetal heart rate monitoring in the intrapartum assessment of fetal well-being.

Abnormalities of fetal heart rate patterns in combination with fetal acid-base measurements are excellent predictors of the condition of the infant at birth, assessed in terms of Apgar scores and clinical signs of central nervous dysfunction, e.g., seizures, abnormalities of tone (5). In general, studies have demonstrated excellent correlation between the severity of variable and late fetal heart rate decelerations and the occurrence of fetal acidosis (7,10,13,15,16,18,21).

It must be remembered that the technique of fetal scalp sampling to assess fetal blood gas status and pH is somewhat limited for general use because the approach requires trained technicians and support resources to be available in close proximity to the labor room. Furthermore, because data from a single sample of scalp blood document the acid-base status at only a single point in time during the course of labor, repeated sampling may be required.

Despite the difficulties associated with the technique, recent studies of outcome at 1 year of age support the value of fetal acid-base assessment (14,17). In one study of 60 children with intrapartum hypoxia documented by fetal acid-base studies, 29% exhibited neurological abnormalities at 1 year of age. Of these, approximately one-half were severely affected. The severity of deficits correlated with the severity of intrapartum hypoxia as judged by the associated acidosis (14). Interestingly, if acidosis developed over a period "in excess of 1 hour" before birth, there was a high probability of major neurological deficits at follow-up. Conversely, if acidosis developed within the hour before delivery, the children were usually normal (14). Thus, observations of fetal acid-base status provide major insight into the severity of intrapartum asphyxia as well as the determination of a critical threshold for the duration of hypoxic insult, which will probably result in at least some degree of cerebral injury. These observations in the human fetus are supported by data from experimental animals (3).

More recent advances in technology have improved the technique for intermittent sampling of scalp blood and for continuous assessment of acid-base status by transcutaneous measurement of fetal pH, pO_2, and pCO_2. Transcutaneous measurement of pH in the fetus may be the most reliable of these three measurements and in some units correlates well with pH values obtained by fetal blood sampling (1,4,11,19). Thus, clinical studies have shown distinct decreases in pH within minutes following late decelerations of the fetal heart rate. Transcutaneous measurement of fetal pO_2 has been achieved with a modified Clark electrode, which may be inserted into the scalp (2,8,9,12,20). Transcutaneous assessment of fetal pCO_2 is possible using a carbon dioxide electrode attached to the scalp by a suction device (6). If these technologies become consistently reliable and convenient enough for general use, a major advance in monitoring of the fetus during a critical and dangerous time will have been achieved.

REFERENCES

1. Antoine, C., Silverman, F., and Young, B.K. (1982): Current status of continuous fetal pH monitoring. *Clin. Perinatol.*, 9:409–422.
2. Baxi, L.V. (1982): Current status of fetal oxygen monitoring. *Clin. Perinatol.*, 9:423–431.
3. Brann, A.W., Jr., and Myers, R.E. (1975): Central nervous system findings in the newborn monkey following severe *in utero* partial asphyxia. *Neurology*, 25:327–338.
4. Flynn, A.M., and Kelly, J. (1978): An evaluation of the continuous tissue pH electrode (+pH) during labor in the human fetus. *Arch. Gynecol.*, 226:105–113.
5. Gimovsky, M.L., and Caritis, S.N. (1982): Diagnosis and management of hypoxic fetal heart rate patterns. *Clin. Perinatol.*, 9:313–324.
6. Hansen, P.K., Thomsen, S.G., Secher, N.J., and Weber, T. (1984): Transcutaneous carbon dioxide measurements in the fetus during labor. *Am. J. Obstet. Gynecol.*, 150:47–51.

7. Hon, E.H., and Khazin, A.F. (1969): Observations on fetal heart rate and fetal biochemistry. I. Base deficit. *Obstet. Gynecol.,* 105:721–729.
8. Huch, A., and Huch, R. (1976): Transcutaneous, noninvasive monitoring of pO_2. *Hosp. Pract.,* 11:43–52.
9. Huch, R., Lucey, J.F., and Huch, A. (1978): Oxygen: Noninvasive monitoring. *Perinatal Care,* 2:18.
10. Kubli, F.W., Hon, E.H., Khazin, A.F., and Takemura, H. (1969): Observations on heart rate and pH in the human fetus during labor. *Am. J. Obstet. Gynecol.,* 104:1190–1206.
11. Lauersen, N.H., Miller, F.C., and Paul, R.H. (1979): Continuous intrapartum monitoring of fetal scalp pH. *Am. J. Obstet. Gynecol.,* 133:44–50.
12. Lofgren, O. (1981): Continuous transcutaneous oxygen monitoring in fetal surveillance during labor. *Am. J. Obstet. Gynecol.,* 141:729–734.
13. Low, J.A., Cox, M.J., Karchmar, E.J., et al. (1981): The prediction of intrapartum fetal metabolic acidosis by fetal heart rate monitoring. *Am. J. Obstet. Gynecol.,* 139:299–305.
14. Low, J.A., Galbraith, R.S., Muir, D.W., et al. (1984): Factors associated with motor and cognitive deficits in children after intrapartum fetal hypoxia. *Am. J. Obstet. Gynecol.,*148:533–539.
15. Low, J.A., Phancham, S.R., Piercy, W.N., et al. (1977): Intrapartum fetal asphyxia: Clinical characteristics, diagnosis and significance in relation to pattern of development. *Am. J. Obstet. Gynecol.,* 129:857–872.
16. Miller, F.C. (1982): Prediction of acid-base values from intrapartum fetal heart rate data and their correlation with scalp and funic values. *Clin. Perinatol.,* 9:353–361.
17. Painter, M.J., Depp, R., and O'Donoghue, P.D. (1978): Fetal heart rate patterns and development in the first year of life. *Am. J. Obstet. Gynecol.,* 132:271–277.
18. Schifrin, B.S. (1982): The fetal monitoring polemic. *Clin. Perinatol.,* 9:399–408.
19. Weber, T. (1983): pH-Monitoring during labor with special reference to continuous fetal scalp tissue pH. *Dan. Med. Bull.,* 30:215–229.
20. Weber, T., and Secher, N.J. (1979): Continuous measurement of transcutaneous fetal oxygen tension during labour. *Br. J. Obstet. Gynaecol.,* 86:954–958.
21. Westgren, M., Hormquist, P., Ingemarsson, I., and Svenningsen, N. (1984): Intrapartum fetal acidosis in preterm infants: Fetal monitoring and longterm morbidity. *Obstet. Gynecol.,* 63:355–359.

Fetal Neurology, edited by
A. Hill and J.J. Volpe.
Raven Press, New York © 1989.

10

Neurosurgery of the Fetus

Kim H. Manwaring

Division of Pediatric Neurosurgery, Phoenix Children's Hospital, Phoenix, Arizona 85066

Congenital anomalies of the nervous system frequently cause severe emotional, economic, and physical hardship for both child and family. Spina bifida may result in varying degrees of paralysis of the extremities as well as incontinence of bowel and bladder. Congenital hydrocephalus may result in neonatal death or mental and motor disability. Craniofacial and developmental abnormalities may cause social unacceptability. Frequent hospitalizations or prolonged institutionalization may be necessary for the many surviving patients.

Experimental studies suggest that earlier (i.e., fetal) intervention may diminish these problems. With the advent of the diagnostic techniques of amniocentesis, direct fetoscopy, real-time ultrasound, computerized tomography, and magnetic resonance imaging, improved accuracy in the diagnosis of the fetal abnormalities and in determination of prognosis is possible in many instances. When confronted with the diagnosis of a fetal anomaly, there are essentially five options for management: (a) no intervention; (b) termination of the pregnancy, which is often appropriate when the condition is uniformly fatal, e.g., anencephaly; (c) allowing pregnancy to proceed to term; (d) induction of preterm delivery followed by postnatal intervention; and (e) intrauterine surgical intervention.

This chapter will focus on the last option. Decisions concerning direct fetal neurosurgical intervention are determined in large part by the accuracy of antenatal diagnosis, recognition of other anomalies, a clear concept of what the modified outcome might be, and an understanding of potential risks or complications to both the fetus and the mother. If a corrective procedure can be carried out sufficiently early in fetal life, the abnormality of development may be ameliorated or corrected.

The technology involved in surgical repair of fetal anomalies has evolved rapidly during the last decade, both in experimental animals and humans. Indeed, it would appear that the neurosurgical capability to undertake prolonged, complex craniotomies has developed to a sufficient extent that there is only a small risk to the mother and an acceptable risk to the fetus, at least in the subhuman primate. In regard to human fetal neurosurgical procedures, a major concern, based on current experience, is whether the intervention significantly alters the developmental outcome. Assessment is complicated by factors such as inaccuracy of diagnosis, variable timing of surgical intervention, and the so-called surgical learning curve (i.e., the improvement in outcome that occurs with refinement of surgical technique and experience).

Finally, the option of intrauterine surgical intervention should, in time, evolve from its present "experimental" status to a routine procedure for specific, treatable conditions. The ethical issues of the rights of both mother and unborn child should become clearer as the indications for surgical intervention become more apparent and as the results improve (44).

In an effort to amplify these considerations, this chapter will review the history of mammalian fetal intervention, review the results of human fetal procedures to date, and outline present therapeutic controversies.

SURGERY OF THE MAMMALIAN FETUS

The understanding of development of the nervous system and its pathophysiology in relation to surgical intervention has been impeded primarily by the inaccessibility of the fetus within the uterus. Initial efforts were directed toward simple ablations of various parts of the central nervous system with the observation of subsequent development. More recently, models for human disease have been developed, some of which are reviewed below:

1925—The first reported successful fetal procedure was performed by Bors in 1925 (5). He created a small incision in the uterus and amputated the limbs of guinea pig fetuses. After closure of the incision, viable offspring were eventually delivered.

1925—Nicholas reported ablation of an eye, leg, or tail in fetal rats (38).

1930—Hooker and Nicholas performed transection of spinal cord in the rat fetus (23).

1949—Foote and Foote performed decapitation of the hamster fetus to study the effect of the pituitary gland on subsequent development (16).

1950—Barron and colleagues performed resections of cortex in the fetal lamb (2).

1969, 1972—Myers investigated long-term effects of fetal vascular occlusion on brain development in primates (35,36).

1974—Taub et al. described a technique for spinal cord surgery in the primate fetus (46).

1978—Goldman et al. reported complex ablation procedures by craniotomy in the monkey and examined neurologic function postdelivery (20,42).

1981—Michejda et al. developed a pharmacologically induced model of fetal hydrocephalus in monkeys and demonstrated the efficacy of ventriculo-amniotic cerebrospinal fluid (CSF) diversion in reversing its anatomic and physiological effects (30,32).

1982—Michejda and Hodgen developed a model in the fetal monkey of a neural tube defect and its *in utero* repair (29,31).

1983—Harrison et al. developed a fetal lamb model of hydrocephalus by injecting kaolin into the cisterna magna; CSF shunting was shown to be effective in improving the resultant ventriculomegaly (18,21,37).

1984—Michejda developed a model of *in utero* repair of occipital encephalocele with subsequent normal development of visual cortex (29).

Techniques of Primate Fetal Surgery

Rakic and Goldman-Rakic (42) have reported the technical operative features of a series of over 100 surgical interventions in fetal primates involving exteriorization of the fetus from the uterus. These procedures were undertaken to study mechanisms of formation of neuronal connections or to manipulate the developmental processes in order to gain insight into fetal brain development and the functional consequences of fetal brain injury. The surgical manipulations included enucleation, injection of radioactive tracers into selected brain regions, and complex craniotomies with ablation of specific cortical areas. Although this type of experimental neurosurgery is considered more extensive than the correctional or diagnostic procedures presently contemplated for the human fetus, the principles involved illustrate their potential technical feasibility.

The authors have emphasized several aspects of surgical technique to optimize success and long-term survival of the fetus. These include assurance of adequate oxygenation of both mother and fetus, rigorous enforcement of sterile procedure, careful selection of incision, preservation of amniotic fluid, appropriate suturing of fetal membranes, and the use of both systemic and locally applied relaxants of uterine musculature. Most of the surgery on monkeys was carried out between days 90 and 120 of gestation (term is 165 days). The survival rates varied according to the procedure performed. Eye injection, requiring a 1-day survival, had a 90% to 95% success rate. Eye enucleation at mid-gestation was associated with a success rate of approximately 75% to 80%. Fetuses in whom the cortex was removed during the first half of gestation had a 60% chance of survival.

Overall, there was a 65% to 70% survival in more than 100 procedures. None of the mothers died from fetal surgery, some having been operated on in as many as five consecutive pregnancies. The most probable cause of death of the fetus was damage to the fetal environment, including disruption of placental perfusion, loss of amniotic fluid, detachment or bleeding of the placenta, and, in particular, irritability and contraction of the uterine muscles with possible compression and asphyxiation of the fetus.

Three observations, made by Rakic and Goldman-Rakic, as well as other investigators of fetal surgical technique, emphasize features of histologic response that are unique to this period of development (6,22,32,42). First, the rapidly growing epithelium of the skin and other fetal tissues results in rapid healing and minimal scar formation, even when compared to the neonatal period. Second, injuries in the fetal brain may show remarkable sparing of the capacity for delayed recovery when compared with animals that have sustained similar injury in the neonatal or young adult period. Finally, ablations of portions of the fetal nervous system may extensively and permanently alter the adult cellular organization of synaptic connectivity. These responses may provide a critical window of opportunity to alter the course of some fetal neuropathological processes.

Fetal Hydrocephalus

Models of human fetal hydrocephalus have been developed in an effort to determine whether intrauterine surgical intervention can reverse the neural damage caused by hydrocephalus (7,18,30,32,37). Michejda and Hodgen (30,32) successfully induced hydrocephalus in fetal monkeys with a success rate of greater than 90% by injection of triamcinolone acetonide intramuscularly in the mother on days 21, 23, and 25 of gestation. The progressive ventriculomegaly was followed with ultrasonography and fetoscopy. Unfortunately, the hydrocephalus was accompanied by other malformations including porencephaly, cranium bifidum, and encephalocele. The investigators developed an intrauterine ventriculoamniotic shunt, similar in appearance to a Richmond intracranial pressure monitoring screw, which contained a spring-loaded, pressure-sensitive mechanism to allow drainage of CSF when the intracranial pressure exceeded 60 mm CSF. Hysterotomy was performed in these monkeys at the beginning of the third trimester with measurement of intracranial pressure. Normal fetal intracranial pressure was noted to be in the range of 45 to 55 mm CSF. Hydrocephalus was associated with intracranial pressures in excess of 100 mm CSF. The hydrocephalic fetuses that were treated by a ventriculoamniotic vent [hydrocephalic antenatal vent for intrauterine treatment (HAVIT)] were delivered by cesarean section at term. Monkeys that were not treated with the shunt had severe and progressive ventricular enlargement. At delivery, the latter were noted to be growth retarded with deficiency of motor skills and coordination. The majority of untreated monkeys died within 2 weeks of birth. In contrast, most monkeys who had been treated with the shunt did not die but demonstrated progressive physical dexterity and grew at near normal rates. Furthermore, the incidence of porencephaly was minimal. In instances where encephalocele formation had occurred by mid-gestation, intrauterine shunting appeared to arrest the process and restore a more normal developmental course. The study demonstrated a remarkable reversibility of hypertensive ventriculomegaly when treated with the HAVIT device.

In an effort to determine the efficacy of treatment in a model of isolated hydrocephalus without other malformations, Harrison and co-workers (18,37) developed a fetal lamb and monkey model of hypertensive ventriculomegaly by injection of kaolin into the cisterna magna during the third trimester. All animals developed ventriculomegaly and massive cranial enlargement with fibrosis of the leptomeninges and subarachnoid spaces around the fourth ventricle. Approximately 3 weeks after the injection, shunting was performed by ventriculoamniotic, ventriculoatrial, or ventriculopleural routes. Most shunted lambs improved with reduction of head circumference and restoration of normal ventricular size and had improved survival. However, in most of the shunted monkeys, little anatomic improvement occurred. All had significant inflammatory ventriculitis, consistent with the previously described effects of the kaolin model. Again, the concept that fetal shunting may improve the appearance of the hydrocephalic brain as well as the ability to survive was demonstrated.

Spina Bifida

Two surgically created models of fetal spina bifida have been described, both with varying degrees of spinal and cephalic dysrhaphism (6,22,28,29). Brunelli and Brunelli (6) induced disruption of vertebral bony elements and dura, as well as partial destruction of the lumbosacral spinal cord in fetal rabbits. Assessment following delivery at term was remarkable in that there was healing without scar formation or adhesions of the spinal cord, suggesting that the accompanying hydrocephalus and Chiari malformation may relate to scar formation and consequent stretching of the spinal cord. It was suggested that prenatal surgery may minimize these anatomic effects.

Finally, Michejda (28,29) and Hodgen (22) have described an intrauterine technique of bony closure over dysrhaphic anomalies utilizing crushed bone particles in an agar-based medium to sculpt and overlay the region of noninduced bone.

HUMAN FETAL SURGERY

Just as experimental mammalian fetal surgery began with simple destructive lesions (5,16,23,38), human fetal surgery in its broadest historical sense began with intentional destructive lesions to facilitate delivery. Celsus, a first-century Roman physician, recommended decapitation for transverse lie (34,40). Such destructive lesions continue to play a role in obstetrics in developing countries (14,41). Similarly, a technique for selective fetal termination in multiple pregnancy has been developed recently to allow the demise of a fetus with a major congenital anomaly, e.g., myelomeningocele, while leaving the normal fetus undisturbed (13,43). The fetocide is conventionally performed by intracardiac air embolism guided by fetoscopy or real-time ultrasound.

Therapeutic human fetal surgery began with the work of Liley (24) in Auckland, New Zealand, with the successful transperitoneal transfusion of red blood cells in severe Rh incompatibility, and erythroblastosis fetalis, using an impaling technique. In the same year, Freda and Adamsons (17) performed an open uterine cannulation of the fetal femoral vein. Subsequently, because of the difficulty in maintaining effective vascular cannulation, a technique of open peritoneal transfusion was developed for treatment of erythroblastosis fetalis (1). Because of the diminished risk of complications, the percutaneous needling technique became the prevalent practice. However, use of this early fetal surgery decreased over the ensuing years because the incidence of erythroblastosis fetalis diminished (40). Pringle (40) has observed that fetal surgical corrective techniques may have evolved significantly further if it had not been for Liley's less invasive and successful percutaneous approach.

The implementation of therapeutic fetal neurosurgical procedures has been influenced by the development of an effective technique for antenatal diagnosis of congenital anomalies of the nervous system. With the advent of improvements in the resolution of real-time ultrasound scanners, over 190 congenital abnormalities have been recognized in the antenatal period (45). In most instances, fetal hydrocephalus is associated with a constellation of other abnormalities, especially myelomeningocele (15,39). It occurs also in association with other entities, e.g., holoprosencephaly, infection, chromosomal abnormalities (e.g., trisomy 13 and 18), Dandy-Walker malformation, vein of Galen aneurysm, tumor, achondroplasia. In some instances there is no known cause. Fetal ventriculomegaly without elevated pressure has been reported to be idiopathic or to result from infarction, infection, or previous hemorrhage (39). The more unusual finding of isolated progressive ventricular dilatation, which may be diagnosed in the second trimester, has been identified as a lesion possibly amenable to intrauterine CSF diversion (21). The rationale for CSF diversion was that the persistent elevation of fetal intracranial pressure caused such severe brain damage that shunting after delivery was of little benefit except to facilitate custodial care (10). It was considered that early intrauterine ventricular drainage might improve the chance for normal development.

Birnholz and Frigoletto (3) have published the results of serial transperitoneal cephalocenteses in an effort to ameliorate progressive ventriculomegaly in a hydrocephalic fetus. From 40 to 180 ml of CSF was aspirated on six separate occasions between the 25th and 32nd weeks of gestation. In the later weeks, cranial puncture became more difficult because of ossification. The infant was delivered at 35 weeks and subsequently underwent placement of a ventriculoperitoneal shunt. At 16 months of age the child was severely retarded and had seizures.

Because serial ventricular aspiration is usually not effective for long-term control of neonatal hydrocephalus (10,26,49), Clewell and his co-workers (10) at the University of Colorado in Denver undertook the first ventriculoamniotic shunting procedure in 1982. Under ultrasound control, a valved silicone catheter was placed in the left parietal region through a percutaneous approach using a 13-gauge needle at 24 weeks of gestation. The fetus had progressive ventriculomegaly, which had begun at 16 weeks of gestation. A sibling had X-linked aqueductal stenosis and there was further positive family history. After shunt placement, the head grew normally and the ventriculomegaly decreased until the 32nd week of gestation. At this time, the shunt was considered to have failed because of recurrent ventriculomegaly. The child was delivered by cesarean section at 34 weeks of gestation. The shunt was obstructed by ingrown tissue. A subsequent ventriculoperitoneal shunting procedure was performed. The child is now moderately retarded (41).

A number of infants with intrauterine hydrocephalus have been treated with a ventriculoamniotic shunting procedure. The International Fetal Treatment Registry was established in 1982 for documentation and assessment of procedures that have been performed to correct congenital defects in the fetus (21). The primary diagnosis and details of survival of 41 fetuses treated by ventriculoamniotic shunting (22) or serial ventriculocentesis (5) as reported to the registry from 1982 to the end of 1985 (27) are displayed in Table 1.

In 34 of 39 fetuses, the ventriculoamniotic shunt was a valved silicone tube similar to that used by Clewell et al. (10). In all cases progressive ventriculomegaly was defined by monitoring of absolute ventricular size and the ratio of ventricular to hemispheric size. The mean gestational age at diagnosis was 25 ± 2.7 weeks (range 18–31 weeks). The mean age at initial treatment was 27 ± 2.7 weeks (range 23–33 weeks).

The outcome of the 41 fetuses is displayed in Table 2. Seven of the 41 fetuses died (17%), one before and six after birth. The stillbirth was a direct result of needle trauma to the brainstem. Three of the six postnatal deaths were attributed to premature labor, which occurred within 48 hr of shunt placement. In one case of premature labor, chorioamnionitis was diagnosed. The calculated procedure-related mortality rate was therefore 9.75% (4/41). The other three deaths were related to the following associated lethal anomalies: holoprosencephaly (1 infant), craniofacial abnormalities and pulmonary hypoplasia (1 infant), and multiple arthrogryposis (1 infant).

The 34 surviving infants were followed for 8.2 ± 5.8 months (range 1–18). Twelve with aqueductal stenosis were normal at follow-up. The remaining 22 survivors had varying degrees of neurologic handicap. All 18 infants with severe handicaps had gross delay in developmental milestones. Five had cortical blindness, three seizures, and two spastic diplegia. The developmental quotient in infants of this group who were tested was less than 60. Two of the four infants in the group with mild to moderate impairment had developmental quotients less than 80. Aqueductal stenosis of uncertain origin was the most common cause of obstructive hydrocephalus; the only normal survivors were those with this disorder.

TABLE 1. *Primary diagnosis and survival of 41 fetuses treated for hydrocephalus*

Primary diagnosis (postnatal)	No. of fetuses (%)	No. of deaths (%)	No. of survivors (%)
Aqueductal stenosis	32 (76.9)	4 (13)	28 (87)
Associated anomalies	5 (12.7)	2 (40)	3 (60)
Holoprosencephaly	1 (2.6)	1 (100)	0 (0)
Dandy-Walker malformation	1 (2.6)	0 (0)	1 (100)
Porencephalic cyst	1 (2.6)	0 (0)	1 (100)
Chiari malformation	1 (2.6)	0 (0)	1 (100)
Total	41 (100)	7 (17)	34 (83)

TABLE 2. *Outcome of treatment in 34 surviving infants with fetal hydrocephalus*

Primary diagnosis (postnatal)	No. of infants	No. normal (%)	No. with mild/moderate handicaps (%)	No. with severe handicaps (%)
Aqueductal stenosis	28	12 (42.8)	2 (7.2)	14 (50)
Associated anomalies	3	0 (0)	0 (0)	3 (100)
Dandy-Walker malformation	1	0 (0)	1 (100)	0 (0)
Porencephalic cyst	1	0 (0)	0 (0)	1 (100)
Chiari malformation	1	0 (0)	1 (100)	0 (0)
Total	34	12 (35.3)	4 (11.8)	18 (52.9)

In addition to the complications of shunt failure, other problems contributed to the morbidity, e.g., shunt migration, accidental instrumentation of the brain, and meningitis caused by *N. gonorrhoeae,* probably secondary to premature rupture of membranes (4).

As a direct response to the increased interest of an international body of pediatric surgeons, neurosurgeons, obstetricians, radiologists, and medical ethicists, for the diagnosis and management of the fetus with correctable congenital defects, the Fetal Medicine and Surgery Society was organized in Aspen, Colorado, in 1983. In April 1986, the first issue of the journal *Fetal Therapy* was published. The purpose of the publication was to provide a rapid exchange of information and the development of new strategies of fetal treatment as well as to promote this newly emerging field of medicine (33).

PRESENT THERAPEUTIC CONTROVERSIES

Although the sophisticated techniques of intrauterine craniotomy and laminectomy have provided significant advances in our understanding of mammalian developmental neuroanatomy, these procedures presently have an uncertain role in the clinical arena. Until satisfactory fetal animal models of human dysrhaphic conditions, craniostenosis, and other primary developmental anomalies are developed and until fetal surgery is shown to change the recognized natural history of such disorders in a clearly beneficial manner, human fetal neurosurgery will remain limited to the management of highly selected cases of progressive ventriculomegaly.

A uniform plan for management of all cases of fetal hydrocephalus is not possible because of the varied etiologies. For example, optimal timing and the need for intervention in hydrocephalus associated with myelomeningocele is probably different from that associated with a Dandy-Walker cyst or aqueductal stenosis. A call for a moratorium on further intrauterine procedures for CSF diversion was issued as early as 1 year after the first reported human case. This was on the basis of lack of knowledge of the natural history of fetal hydrocephalus, the reported lack of correlation between extent of hydrocephalus and psychomotor performance, and the paucity of follow-up data after the first few procedures (47). Pringle (40) has observed that this situation bears similarities to that with fetal transfusions 3 years after that technique was introduced. Then, as now, significant problems include patient selection, optimal timing of treatment, and the debate over the choice of approach, i.e., open versus closed technique. These issues provide a framework for discussing present therapeutic controversies.

Patient Selection

The most likely group of patients to benefit from intrauterine shunting are those with documented progressive cortical thinning without associated anomalies that alter prognosis, e.g., holoprosencephaly. In 1982, guidelines were established for selection of such patients (21,41). These included (a) the presence of a multispecialty team and the availability of high resolution ultrasonography, tertiary level obstetric and neonatal units, and ready access to pediatric surgery and other pediatric subspecialties; (b) a singleton pregnancy; (c) absence of other significant anomalies; (d) progressive ventricular dilatation and increasing ventricular width relative to hemispheric width, and decreasing thickness of the cortical mantle; (e) a normal karyotype; (f) viral studies; (g) willingness on the part of the patient to be treated by the team and to return for follow-up studies; (h) evidence of immature lungs or gestational age less than 32 weeks gestation; and (i) a general consensus by the team to proceed with treatment.

These guidelines have not been changed in three consecutive meetings of the Fetal Medicine and Surgery Society, the group that evolved from the original participants. Moreover, it is clear that the ability to detect other anomalies by ultrasound, karyotyping, and viral studies has improved with experience (8,12,27).

Timing of Intervention

Although it is clear that intrauterine shunting may restore ventricular size toward normal in both animal and human studies, both the natural history of the ventriculomegaly and its correlation with long-term psychomotor outcome remain poorly defined. The combined results of three recent reports on the natural history of fetal ventriculomegaly have shown that 27 of 87 fetuses (31%) survived and 17 infants (19.5%) were normal (9,11,19,27). These data cannot be compared to the data from patients treated by ventriculoamniotic shunting. However, the relative survival and data on neurologic outcome are interesting. Thus, the rate of survival in the treated group was higher (83%) than the combined untreated groups (31%) (27). Normal development was low (34%) in treated fetuses as well as untreated fetuses (19.5%) compared to treated neonates (66%). Treated neonates are, of course, already strongly selected because of survival and probably other less readily defined factors.

Conversely, it may be argued that fetal treatment was "too little, too late." It is clear that fetal hydrocephalus may, like hydrocephalus in the premature newborn, evolve significantly before an increase in head circumference, full fontanel, and signs of intracranial hypertension become obvious (48). In Lorber's (25) series of newborns with isolated hydrocephalus, the best rates of survival and intellectual development were in infants who were shunted early. The most important factor contributing to a poor prognosis for neonatal idiopathic isolated hydrocephalus may be delayed treatment (48). However, in the group of fetuses with aqueductal stenosis who were treated with ventriculoamniotic shunting, 28 of 32 (87.5%) survived, but only 12 of the survivors (37.5%) were normal, suggesting that fetal intervention may only have improved survival without improving outcome (27).

Nonprogressive ventriculomegaly during the fetal period may progress and require treatment after birth in many patients. In the report on the natural history of untreated fetal ventriculomegaly by Glick et al. (19), 11 of 24 fetuses had enlarged ventricles without other identified anomalies. Ventricular size remained stable throughout gestation. However, three of the group required shunting at birth and an additional two by 5 months of age.

Open Versus Closed Technique

Several fetuses treated by ventriculoamniotic shunting had complications of shunt obstruction or dislodgement of the catheter, often requiring reinstrumentation of the brain or early delivery. The ventriculoperitoneal shunt has been shown to be very reliable compared to other catheters in the management of neonatal hydrocephalus (18). It is reasonable to conjecture that results in the fetal series to date would have been improved with more reliable catheters. However, placement of a ventriculoperitoneal shunt in the fetus requires open hysterotomy and would almost certainly be associated with a higher risk of premature labor. In this regard, Harrison et al. (40) were able to maintain a human pregnancy for 14 weeks after hysterotomy for treatment of congenital hydronephrosis. This is the longest period of time that a pregnancy has been maintained after an open procedure.

In view of the additional data since the first fetal CSF diversion procedure was undertaken in 1982, it is probable that the outcome for the next 40 fetal shunting procedures will be more encouraging. When a moratorium on this procedure was again suggested at the annual meeting of the Fetal Medicine and Surgery Society in 1985, there was only minimal support (40). A strong consensus urged that carefully selected cases of hydrocephalus should continue to be considered for intrauterine shunting, both in an effort to refine the criteria for patient selection and to develop more effective shunting techniques. Furthermore, it was emphasized that some of the infants in whom the outcome was disappointing in the initial series of patients most probably would have progressed to require cephalocentesis for delivery and subsequent death. As with the introduction of most potentially promising surgical techniques, e.g., cardiac transplantation, the initial results have been characterized by numerous complications, morbidity, difficulties of selection, and controversy, all of which should be rectified by additional experience. Furthermore, in order for fetal shunting to evolve from its present experimental status to an accepted position in the armamentarium of the pediatric neurosurgeon and perinatologist, it must compare favorably in a prospectively controlled trial (27). If such a point is reached, the ethical dilemma facing the expectant mother and the health care team will be greatly simplified.

REFERENCES

1. Adamsons, K., Freda, V.J., James, L.S., and Towell, M.E. (1965): Prenatal treatment of erythroblastosis fetalis following hysterotomy. *Pediatrics,* 35:848–855.
2. Barron, D.H. (1950): An experimental analysis of some factors involved in the development of the fissure patterns of cerebral cortex. *J. Exp. Zool.,* 113:553–581.
3. Birnholz, J.C., and Frigoletto, F.D. (1981): Antenatal treatment of hydrocephalus. *N. Engl. J. Med.,* 304:1021–1023.
4. Bland, R.S., Nelson, L.H., Meis, P.J., et al. (1983): Gonococcal ventriculitis associated with ventriculoamniotic shunt placement. *Am. J. Obstet. Gynecol.,* 147:781–784.
5. Bors, E. (1925): Die Methodik der Interuterinen Operation am Uberlebenden Saugetierfoetus. *Arch. Entwickl.-Mech. Org.,* 105:655–666.
6. Brunelli, M.D., and Brunelli, F. (1984): Experimental fetal microsurgery as related to myelomeningocele. *Microsurgery,* 5:24–29.
7. Cambria, S., Gambardella, G., Cardia, E., and Cambria, M. (1984): Experimental endo-uterine hydrocephalus in fetal sheep and surgical treatment by ventriculo-amniotic shunt. *Acta Neurochir.,* 72:235–240.
8. Chervenak, F.A., Berkowitz, R.L., Tortora, M., and Hobbins, J.C. (1985): The management of fetal hydrocephalus. *Am. J. Obstet. Gynecol.,* 151:933–942.
9. Chervenak, F.A., Duncan, C., Ment, L.R., et al. (1984): Outcome of fetal ventriculomegaly. *Lancet,* 2:179–181.
10. Clewell, W.H., Johnson, M.L., Meier, P.R., et al. (1982): A surgical approach to the treatment of fetal hydrocephalus. *N. Engl. J. Med.,* 306:1320–1325.
11. Clewell, W.H., Meier, P.R., Manchester, D.K., Manco-Johnson, M.L., Pretorius, D.H., and Hendee, R.W., Jr. (1985): Ventriculomegaly: Evaluation and management. *Semin. Perinatol.,* 9:98–102.
12. Daffos, F., Capella-Pavlosvsky, M., and Forestier, F. (1983): A new procedure for fetal blood sampling *in utero:* Preliminary results in fifty three cases. *Am. J. Obstet. Gynecol.,* 146:985–987.
13. Denton, P. (1981): Selective pregnancy termination in thalassemia. *Med. J. Aust.,* 13:654–656.
14. Dutta, D.C. (1979): Destructive operation in obstructed labor. *J. Indian Med. Assoc.,* 72:204–206.
15. Fleischer, A.C., Kirchner, S.G., and Thieme, G.A. (1985): Prenatal detection of fetal anomalies with sonography. *Pediatr. Clin. North Am.,* 32:1523–1536.
16. Foote, C.L., and Foote, F.M. (1949): Changes in the thyroid gland of hamster embryos hyphosectomized by decapitation. *Anat. Rec.,* 105:163–164.
17. Freda, V.J., and Adamsons, K. (1964): Exchange transfusion *in utero.* Report of a case. *Am. J. Obstet. Gynecol.,* 89:817–821.
18. Glick, P.L., Harrison, M.R., Halks-Miller, M., et al. (1984): Correction of congenital hydrocephalus *in utero.* II. Efficacy of *in utero* shunting. *J. Pediatr. Surg.,* 19:870–881.
19. Glick, P.L., Harrison, M.R., and Nakayama, D.K. (1984): Management of ventriculomegaly in the fetus. *J. Pediatr.,* 105:97–105.
20. Goldman, P.S., and Galkin, T.W. (1978): Prenatal removal of frontal association cortex in the Rhesus monkey: Anatomical and functional consequences in postnatal life. *Brain Res.,* 52:451–485.
21. Harrison, M.R., Filly, R.A., Golbus, M.S., et al. (1982): Fetal treatment. *N. Engl. J. Med.,* 307:1651–1652.

22. Hodgen, G.D. (1981): Antenatal diagnosis and treatment of fetal skeletal malformations with emphasis on *in utero* surgery for neural tube defects and limb bud regeneration. *JAMA,* 246:1079–1083.

23. Hooker, D., and Nicholas, J.S. (1930): Spinal cord section in rat fetuses. *J. Comp. Neurol.,* 50:413–467.

24. Liley, A.W. (1963): Intrauterine transfusion of fetus in hemolytic disease. *Br. Med. J.,* 2:1107–1109.

25. Lorber, J. (1970): Medical and surgical aspects in the treatment of congenital hydrocephalus. *Neuropediatrie,* 2:239–246.

26. Lorber, J., and Grainger, R.G. (1983): Cerebral cavities following ventricular puncture in infants. *Clin. Radiol.,* 14:98–109.

27. Manning, F.A., Harrison, M.R., Rodeck, C., et al. (1986): Catheter shunts for fetal hydronephrosis and hydrocephalus. Report of the International Fetal Surgery Registry. *N. Engl. J. Med.,* 315:336–340.

28. Michejda, M. (1983): Correction of spina bifida and encephaloceles in the fetal monkey. Presented at Management of a Fetus with a Correctable Congenital Defect, Aspen, Colorado, June 4–7.

29. Michejda, M. (1984): Intrauterine treatment of spina bifida: Primate model. *Z. Kinderchir.,* 39:259–261.

30. Michejda, M., and Hodgen, G.D. (1981): *In utero* diagnosis and treatment of non-human primate fetal skeletal anomalies. I. Hydrocephalus. *JAMA,* 246:1093–1097.

31. Michejda, M., and Hodgen, G. (1982): Induction of neural tube defects in non-human primates. In: *Proceedings of the World Conference on Prevention of Physical and Mental Congenital Defects,* Strasbourg.

32. Michejda, M., Patronas, N., DiChiro, G., et al. (1984): Fetal hydrocephalus. II. Amelioration of fetal porencephaly by *in utero* therapy in nonhuman primates. *JAMA,* 251:2548–2552.

33. Michejda, M., and Pringle, K. (1986): Editorial. *Fetal Therapy,* 1:3–7.

34. Kerr, J.M., and Munro, J.M. (1971): Destructive operations of the foetus. In: *Operative Obstetrics,* 8th ed., edited by J.C. Moir and P.R. Myerscough, p. 713. Bailliere, Tindall and Cassell, London.

35. Myers, R.E. (1969): Brain pathology following fetal vascular occlusion: An experimental study. *Invest. Ophthalmol.,* 8:41–50.

36. Myers, R.E. (1972): Two patterns of perinatal brain damage and their conditions of occurrence. *Am. J. Obstet. Gynecol.,* 112:246–276.

37. Nakayama, D.K., Harrison, M.R., Berger, M.S., et al. (1983): Correction of congenital hydrocephalus *in utero.* I. The mode: Intracisternal kaolin produces hydrocephalus in fetal lambs and Rhesus monkeys. *J. Pediatr. Surg.,* 18:331–338.

38. Nicholas, J.S. (1925): Notes on the application of experimental methods upon mammalian embryos. *Anat. Rec.,* 31:385–394.

39. Pretorius, D.H., Russ, P.D., Rumack, C.M., and Manco-Johnson, M.L. (1986): Diagnosis of brain neuropathology *in utero. Neuroradiology,* 28:386–397.

40. Pringle, K.C. (1986): Fetal surgery: It has a past, has it a future? *Fetal Therapy,* 1:23–31.

41. Pringle, K.C. (1986): *In utero* surgery. *Adv. Surg.,* 19:101–138.

42. Rakic, P., and Goldman-Rakic, P.S. (1985): Use of fetal neurosurgery for experimental studies of structural and functional brain development in non-human primates. In: *Perinatal Neurology and Neurosurgery,* edited by R.A. Thompson, J.R. Green, and S.D. Johnsen. Spectrum Publications, New York.

43. Rodeck, C.H., Mibashan, R.S., Abramovicz, J., and Campbell, S. (1982): Selective fetocide of the affected twin by fetoscopic air embolism. *Prenat. Diagn.,* 2:189–194.

44. Soper, R.T. (1983): The Pandora's box of antenatal surgery, *Am. Surg.,* 49:285–289.

45. Stephenson, S.R., and Waever, D.D. (1981): Prenatal diagnosis—A compilation of diagnosed conditions. *Am. J. Obstet. Gynecol.,* 141:319–343.

46. Taub, E., Barro, G., Miller, E., et al. (1974): Feasibility of spinal cord or brain surgery in fetal Rhesus monkeys. *Soc. Neurosci.,* Fourth Annual Meeting.

47. Venes, J.L. (1983): Management of intrauterine hydrocephalus (Letter to the editor). *J. Neurosurg.,* 58:793–794.

48. Vintzileos, A.M., Ingardia, C.J., and Nochimson, D.J. (1983): Congenital hydrocephalus: A review and protocol for perinatal management. *Obstet. Gynecol.,* 62:539–549.

49. Wilberger, J.E., and Baghai, P. (1983): Fetal neurosurgery. *Neurosurgery,* 13:596–600.

Fetal Neurology, edited by
A. Hill and J.J. Volpe.
Raven Press, New York © 1989.

11

Current Perspectives on the Diagnosis, Prognosis, and Management of Fetal Hydrocephalus

Frank A. Chervenak

*Department of Obstetrics and Gynecology, The New York Hospital–
Cornell Medical Center, New York, New York 10021*

Ventriculomegaly refers to an abnormal increase in the volume of the cerebral ventricles and has many causes. Although the term *hydrocephalus* is sometimes reserved for those cases of ventriculomegaly resulting from increased cerebrospinal fluid pressure, in this chapter the term *hydrocephalus* will be used interchangeably with *ventriculomegaly* because *hydrocephalus* has been the more common term in the obstetrical literature.

Hydrocephalus may be due to intraventricular or extraventricular obstruction of cerebrospinal fluid, an increase in cerebrospinal fluid production, or a relative decrease in the amount of brain substance. Table 1 lists the more common examples of these various types of hydrocephalus.

The incidence of fetal hydrocephalus ranges from 0.12 to 2.5 per 1,000 total births (27). The subsequent diagnosis and management of this condition represents a common challenge for obstetricians. This chapter will review the current understanding of diagnosis and prognosis of fetal hydrocephalus and associated anomalies, and the options for obstetrical management.

DIAGNOSIS

Before the advent of sonography, the diagnosis of fetal hydrocephalus was based on the radiologic demonstration of an enlarged fetal head. With the introduction of A-mode and early B-mode ultrasound, a transverse diameter of the fetal head could be measured and severe hydrocephalus with macrocephaly could be diagnosed antenatally without the use of ionizing radiation.

Recent advances in diagnostic imaging now permit examination of the ventricles

TABLE 1. *Common etiologies of fetal hydrocephalus*

Obstruction to cerebrospinal fluid flow at the	
Aqueduct fo Sylvius	X-linked aqueductal stenosis
	Aqueductal stenosis caused by viral etiology
Foramen of Luska and Magendie	Dandy-Walker malformation
Foramen magnum[a]	Arnold-Chiari malformation
Arachnoid granulations	Infection
	Hemorrhage
Excessive cerebrospinal fluid production	Choroid plexus papilloma
Ventriculomegaly relative to decreased	
brain substance	Impaired cortical development

[a]Obstruction to cerebrospinal flow in the Arnold-Chiari malformation may also occur at the Aqueduct of Sylvius.

themselves. This is an important development because ventricular dilatation often precedes cranial enlargement. When evaluating a fetus for hydrocephalus, it is best to measure the size of the bodies of the lateral ventricles because they display less anatomic variation than other components of the ventricular system (Fig. 1).

Because it is not always possible to visualize the medial wall of the lateral ventricle, the ratio of lateral ventricle width to hemispheric width (LV/HW), as defined by Jeanty et al. (13) and Johnson et al. (14), has proven most useful (Fig. 2). The LV width is measured from the midline echo to the first echo of the lateral wall of the LV at the point where the ventricular wall runs parallel to the midline. The HW is measured on the same side and in the same plane as the LV width and

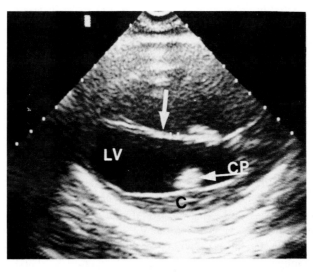

FIG. 1. Transverse cranial sonogram demonstrating enlarged lateral ventricle (LV), compressed cerebral cortex (C), and choroid plexus (CP). (*Arrow* points to midline echo.)

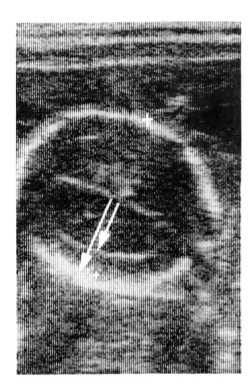

FIG. 2. Transverse cranial sonogram with arrows pointing to the lateral wall of the lateral ventricle and the inner edge of the distal skull. Lateral ventricle/hemispheric width ratio of 69% is abnormally increased for gestational age of 24 weeks. (From ref. 2.)

is the largest distance between the midline and the inner edge of the skull, measured perpendicular to the midline. Because the LV/HW decreases with gestational age, utilization of a nomogram relating LV/HW and gestational age is necessary (Figs. 3 and 4).

The LV/HW has been demonstrated to be an accurate predictor of fetal hydrocephalus over a wide range of gestational ages (1), including those less than 24 weeks (2). However, it should be noted that the absence of ventriculomegaly at a single time in gestation does not preclude its later development, and serial examinations are indicated for any high-risk pregnancy.

Certain pitfalls in the detection of fetal hydrocephalus must be considered to avoid false positive diagnoses. Because artifactual echoes often obscure accurate readings on the proximal side of the head, ventriculomegaly is best assessed in the distal hemisphere (Fig. 5). Another potential source for misinterpretation is a crescent-shaped hypoechoic area, which may be visualized in the distal hemisphere (Fig. 6). In such cases, following the lateral wall of the LV from the area of the frontal horns to the body is useful in the assessment of LV width. In addition, in true hydrocephalus, lateral displacement of the choroid plexus should be observed (Fig. 1). Although dilatation of the occipital, temporal, or frontal horns may be early signs of hydrocephalus (Figs. 7 and 8), the diagnosis of hydrocephalus should not be based solely on these criteria because there is marked variation in

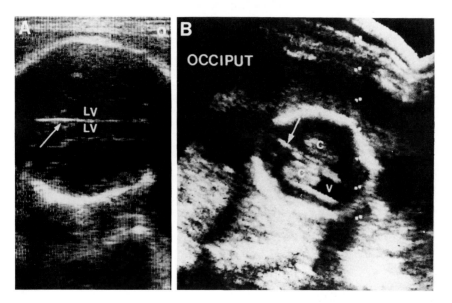

FIG. 3. A: Sonogram through the fetal cranium at the lateral ventricular level demonstrating intracranial anatomy at 32 weeks of gestation. The ratio of lateral ventricle to hemispheric width (LV/HW) is 21%, normal for this gestation. *Arrows* point to midline, lateral wall of LV and inner skull table. **B:** Ultrasonic section through the level of the LV demonstrating intracranial anatomy at 18 weeks of gestation. The LV/HW of 47% and the prominent choroid plexuses are normal for this gestational age. C, choroid plexus. *Arrow* points to midline. (From ref. 1.)

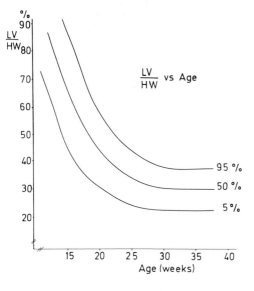

FIG. 4. Nomogram relating lateral ventricle (LV) to hemispheric width (HW) ratio to gestational age. (Modified from ref. 13.)

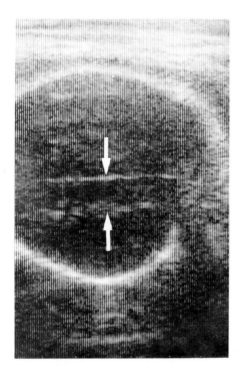

FIG. 5. Cranial sonogram demonstrating reverberation artifact in proximal hemisphere with *arrows* pointing to lateral ventricle in distal hemisphere.

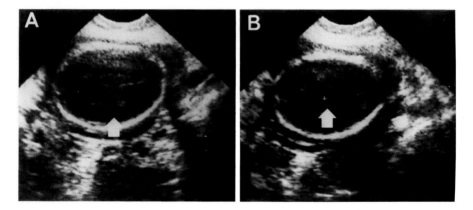

FIG. 6. A: Cranial sonogram with *arrow* pointing to hypoechoic area in normal fetus. B: Cranial sonogram with *arrow* pointing to lateral ventricle. (From ref. 2.)

the ventricular system in normal fetuses. Lastly, it should be remembered that a slightly increased LV/HW may not indicate pathologic ventriculomegaly. Because the natural history of ventricular enlargement in early gestation is uncertain (6,10), the diagnosis of hydrocephalus is most accurate if progressive ventricular enlargement is documented with serial sonography.

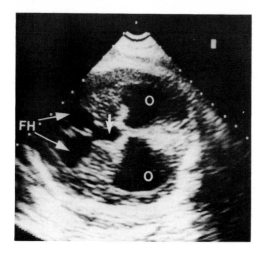

FIG. 7. Cranial sonogram demonstrating dilated frontal horns (FH), occipital horns (O), and third ventricle (*arrow*).

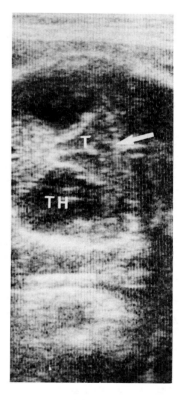

FIG. 8. Cranial sonogram demonstrating dilated temporal horns (TH), thalamus (T), and third ventricle (*arrow*).

When fetal hydrocephalus is identified, careful investigation for associated anomalies is indicated. In a recent study of 53 cases of fetal hydrocephalus, there was isolated hydrocephalus in only 17%, whereas major malformations were present in 83% (3). In addition to a thorough evaluation of the fetus by real-time sonography, M-mode fetal echocardiography and amniocentesis for determination of fetal karyotype should be performed. Figures 9 to 15 illustrate some anomalies found in conjunction with fetal hydrocephalus. Awareness of a severe anomaly in association with fetal hydrocephalus is invaluable in counseling parents regarding management options.

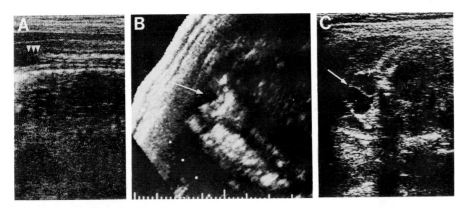

FIG. 9. A: Longitudinal sonogram demonstrating open spina bifida (*arrow*). **B:** Transverse sonogram demonstrating open spina bifida (*arrow*). **C:** Transverse sonogram demonstrating membrane covering meningomyelocele (*arrow*). (From ref. 1.)

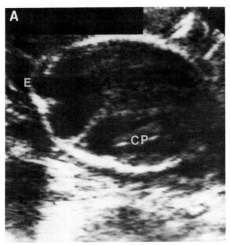

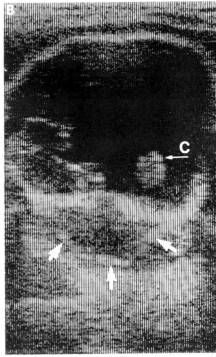

FIG. 10. A: Cranial sonogram demonstrating hydrocephalus. *Arrows* outline encephalocele. CP, choroid plexus. **B:** Cranial sonogram demonstrating hydrocephalus CP, choroid plexus; E, small encephalocele.

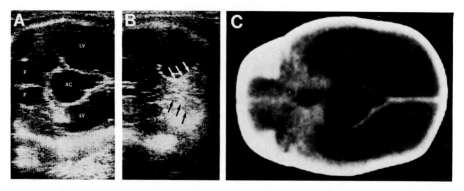

FIG. 11. A: Hydrocephalus with midline arachnoid cyst (AC). F, frontal horns; LV, lateral ventricles. B: Normal posterior fossa demonstrated in same patients is outlined by *arrows*. This finding excludes a Dandy-Walker cyst. C: Neonatal computed axial tomography confirming presence of midline arachnoid cyst. (From ref. 1.)

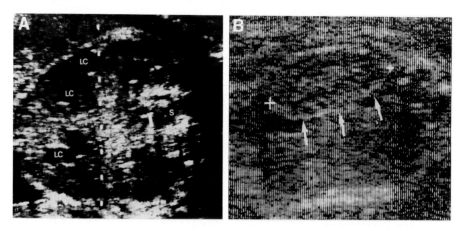

FIG. 12. A: Transverse scan through fetal liver demonstrating liver cysts in fetus with Meckel syndrome. LC, liver cyst; S, spine. B: Transverse scan through fetal abdomen demonstrating polycystic kidney in same fetus as A. Kidney circumference/abdominal circumference = 60%, abnormally increased for gestational age of 30 weeks. (*Arrows* outline kidney.) (From ref. 1.)

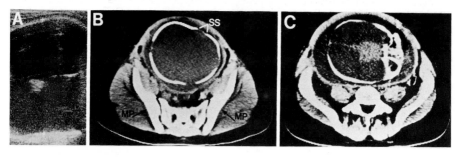

FIG. 13. A: Macrocephaly (biparietal diameter, 11.1 cm) with no visible cortex. B: *In utero* CAT scan showing widening of sutures of fetal calvarium. The skull is filled by homogeneous low-density tissue with no evidence of cortex present. MP, maternal pelvis; SS, separated suture. C: *In utero* CAT scan at lower level demonstrating presence of diencephalon. Autopsy confirmed the antenatal diagnosis of hydranencephaly. (From ref. 1.)

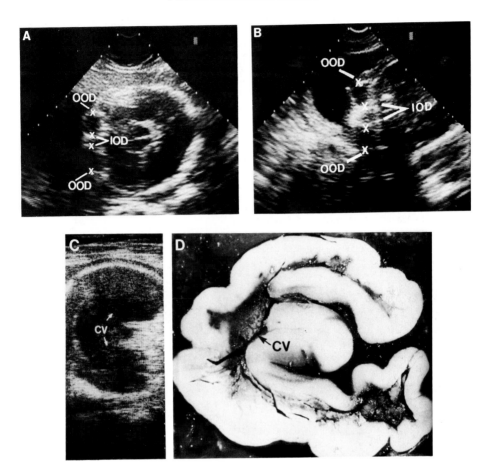

FIG. 14. Antenatal diagnosis of alobar holoprosencephaly based on hypotelorism and absence of midline echo at the level of the cerebral ventricles. **A:** Transverse scan through the orbits of affected fetus demonstrating an inner orbital distance (IOD) of 14 mm and an outer orbital distance (OOD) of 43 mm, both decreased for gestational age of 28 weeks. **B:** Transverse scan through the orbits of normal fetus, for comparison, demonstrating an IOD of 18 mm and an OOD of 49 mm, both normal for gestational age of 28 weeks. **C:** Transverse sonogram through fetal skull and demonstrating common ventricle (CV) and absence of midline structures. **D:** Transverse section of fetal brain at autopsy demonstrating a collapsed CV, failure of separation of cerebral hemispheres, and absence of corpus callosum. (From ref. 7.)

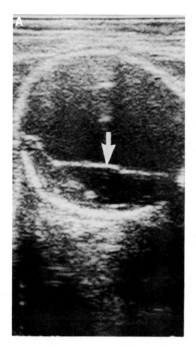

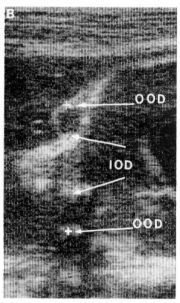

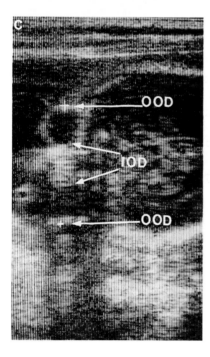

FIG. 15. Antenatal diagnosis of median cleft face syndrome in a fetus with hydrocephalus based on hypertelorism and cleft lip. **A:** Cranial sonogram demonstrating hydrocephalus. *Arrow* points to midline echo. **B:** Transverse scan through the orbits of the affected fetus demonstrating hypertelorism with inner orbital distance (IOD) and outer orbital distance (OOD) that are increased for the gestational age of 31 weeks. **C:** Transverse scan through the orbits of a normal fetus for comparison, at 31 weeks of gestation, demonstrating normal IOD and OOD. **D:** Oblique scan through lower part of fetal face showing intact palate (P), cleft lip (C), and a mass (M) protruding from lip. **E:** Demonstration of scanning plane. **F:** Sagittal scan showing fetal profile and relationship of mass (M) to nose (N) and lip (L). **G:** Demonstration of scanning plane. (From ref. 2a.)

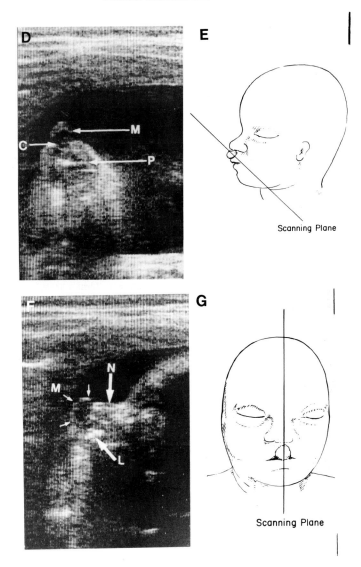

PROGNOSIS

Before the availability of ventriculoperitoneal shunt placement for neonates with hydrocephalus, the prognosis for fetal hydrocephalus was dismal. In 1954, Feeny and Barry (9) reported that only 10 of 93 hydrocephalic infants survived to be discharged from hospital. In 1962, Laurence and Coates (15) reported 182 cases of fetal hydrocephalus in which surgery was not performed. The likelihood of surviving to adulthood was less than 23% (15).

With the development of neonatal neurosurgical shunting of hydrocephalus, the prognosis improved considerably. Lorber and Zachary (17) attempted a prospective randomized trial that compared shunting with conservative management. However, 11 of the 13 infants in the control group needed surgery to correct neurologic deterioration or rapidly increasing head circumference, and the trial was ended.

Raimondi and Soare (24) reported 200 consecutive infants with neonatal hydrocephalus who had shunt procedures performed at Children's Memorial Hospital in Chicago. Only five of these infants died. Intellectual outcome related to the type of hydrocephalus, the age at initial shunt placement, and shunt function but not to the severity of the hydrocephalus or to the total number of shunt revisions. For Caucasians with internal hydrocephalus, the mean IQ was 84.5 ± 25.8, which was not statistically significantly below the mean of the normal population. Infants with hydrocephalus associated with such other problems as porencephaly or Dandy-Walker cyst had significantly lower mean IQ. In this series, infants with congenital hydrocephalus were not clearly differentiated from those who developed hydrocephalus during the neonatal period. However, in other reports, follow-up is given for congenital hydrocephalus. At the University of Washington School of Medicine, 16 of 19 (86%) treated infants with congenital hydrocephalus achieved an IQ of at least 80 (26). Of 37 infants with congenital hydrocephalus and macrocephaly managed at Georgetown University Medical Center, 32 (86%) survived (21). Of the survivors, 17 (53%) had a normal IQ (>80) and 6 (19%) had a borderline IQ (65–80). Furthermore, those with borderline IQ were competitive in educational settings.

Others have corroborated that hydrocephalic infants without associated congenital malformations who are treated surgically in the postnatal period have an excellent chance to achieve normal intelligence, irrespective of the initial severity of the hydrocephalus. At the University of Pennsylvania, 10 neonates with virtual absence of the cerebral substance on computerized tomography (CT) scans were followed (28). Two well-defined clinical entities were identified. Five infants had hydranencephaly with absence of cortical activity on electroencephalograms (EEG) and a picture of minimal occipital brain parenchyma on CT scan. Although these infants were shunted, there was no neurologic or radiologic improvement. On the other hand, the remaining five infants had severe hydrocephalus with minimal frontal cerebral mantle on CT and the presence of electrical activity on EEG. After shunting procedures, a remarkable increase in brain substance was demonstrated in the latter group by serial CT scans, and neurologic development was either normal or only slightly delayed. The reason for the retention of cerebral function despite a markedly thinned cerebral cortex may be that ventricular dilation results in preferential thinning of the white matter, whereas the gray matter on the convoluted surface of the cerebral cortex is relatively spared (25).

Lorber (16) followed 56 infants with severe congenital hydrocephalus (cortex ≤10 mm) over an 8-year period in Sheffield. Of the 46 infants who survived, 4 were of superior intelligence; 29 were of average to good average intelligence; 5 were in the educationally subnormal range; and 6 were profoundly retarded. Intellectual outcome improved if shunting was performed before 6 months of age. Lorber (16) concluded:

> These results suggest that no case of primary congenital hydrocephalus should be considered hopeless and all should have the benefit of the best treatment, irrespective of the degree of hydrocephalus, because the majority will do well if treated in the first few months of life. Even the most extreme degrees of hydrocephalus are compatible with normal physical development, a normal sized head, and superior intelligence, if operative treatment is not delayed.

However, it should be remembered that studies of outcome of neonatal hydrocephalus are subject to selection biases. Three recent obstetrical series on the outcome of fetal hydrocephalus (5,11,23) demonstrate that severe anomalies occur in association with fetal hydrocephalus in a majority. The nature of these anomalies (e.g., alobar holoprosencephaly, thanatophoric dysplasia with cloverleaf skull) rather than the hydrocephalus per se determined a dismal prognosis in most cases.

MANAGEMENT

The obstetric management of fetal hydrocephalus is dependent on gestational age at the time of diagnosis and the presence of associated anomalies. Management options include termination of pregnancy before fetal viability, ventriculoamniotic shunt placement, cephalocentesis before delivery, and/or cesarean section.

The therapeutic value of ventriculoamniotic shunt placement (Figs. 16–18) has not been clearly established. Michejda and Hodgen (22) reported improved outcome when monkeys with steroid-induced hydrocephalus were treated with ventriculoamniotic shunts. Clewell et al. (8) first described the successful placement of a ventriculoamniotic shunt in a human fetus with hydrocephalus. Further experience in human fetuses has not been encouraging (19), in part because of the high frequency of other anomalies in association with hydrocephalus. The recent report by Manning et al. (18) of the International Fetal Surgery Registry describes a 10% procedure-related death rate and a 53% occurrence of serious handicaps for 44 ventriculoamniotic shunt placements.

Clearly, further investigation is necessary to assess the potential benefits and hazards of ventriculoamniotic shunt placement in the management of fetal hydrocephalus (11). At the present time, ventriculoamniotic shunt placement should be

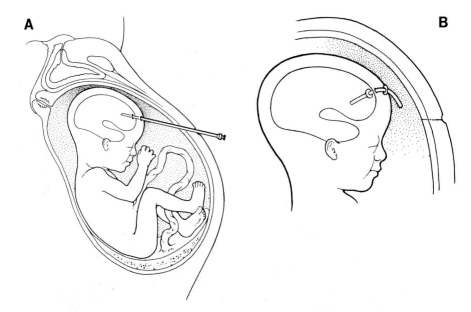

FIG. 16. A, B: Method of ventriculoamniotic shunt placement. A trocar is inserted through a 12-gauge needle into the dilated ventricular system. The trocar is then removed and the shunt system passed through the needle. The overlying needle is then removed leaving the shunt system in place, which connects the ventricular system with the amniotic fluid.

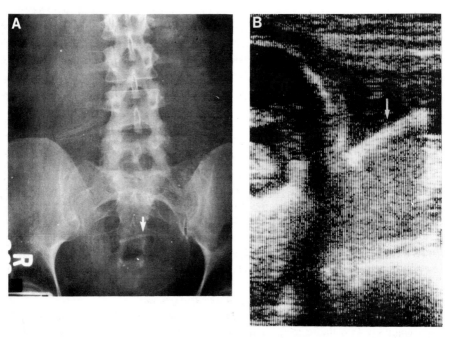

FIG. 17. A: Radiograph demonstrating ventriculoamniotic shunt entering fetal skull (*arrow*). B: Cranial sonogram demonstrating ventriculoamniotic shunt protruding from fetal skull (*arrow*). (From ref. 3.)

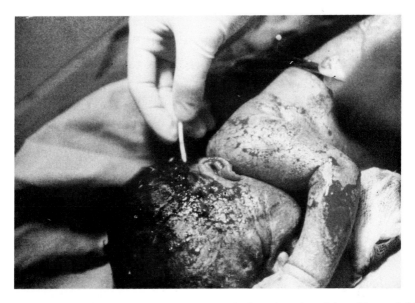

FIG. 18. Ventriculoamniotic shunt protruding from skull of newborn infant. (From ref. 3.)

limited to cases of isolated progressive ventriculomegaly when the fetus is too immature to be delivered for postnatal shunting. A multidisciplinary team consisting of a perinatologist, ultrasonographer, neurosurgeon, neonatologist, geneticist, and social worker is necessary to provide integrated care (12). In addition, full parental disclosure of currently known benefits and risks of the procedure is mandatory, so that consent is fully informed concerning this therapeutic intervention of uncertain efficacy.

As soon as pulmonary maturity is demonstrated, delivery of the fetus with hydrocephalus is recommended to permit optimal neurosurgical management of the neonate. Thus, amniocentesis is performed weekly from 36 weeks of gestation. This recommendation is based on the potential ill effects of prolonged compression of the cerebral cortex. At the present time, there are no clear guidelines as to when preterm delivery for progressive hydrocephalus is indicated before fetal lung maturity. The risks of respiratory distress syndrome with subsequent delay in ventriculoperitoneal shunt placement must be balanced against the potential hazards of progressive ventriculomegaly. Serial sonography may be helpful in this management decision. If delivery before fetal lung maturity is decided on, maternal corticosteroid administration is recommended to reduce the risk of occurrence and the severity of respiratory distress syndrome in the neonate.

Cephalocentesis is a technique in which a needle is passed transabdominally or transvaginally into the dilated ventricular system of the fetus and sufficient cerebrospinal fluid is aspirated to permit vaginal delivery. Figure 19 illustrates how an 18-gauge needle can be guided into the fetal skull through the maternal abdomen

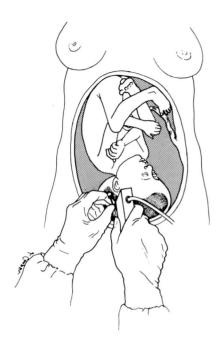

FIG. 19. Method of cephalocentesis. An 18-gauge needle is placed into fetal skull through the maternal abdomen with real-time sonographic guidance. (From ref. 3.)

under local anesthesia (Figs. 20 and 21). The potential morbidity associated with this procedure is well documented by pathologic and sonographic evidence of associated intracranial hemorrhage (Figs. 22–25) (3), the high perinatal mortality associated with the procedure (3), and the occurrence of fetal heart rate deterioration after cephalocentesis (20).

The author believes that in view of the potential for normal and even superior intelligence for those infants with hydrocephalus provided optimum neonatal neurosurgical care, fetuses with isolated hydrocephalus and macrocephaly are best delivered by cesarean section. Because cortical mantle thickness correlates poorly with subsequent intelligence, cephalocentesis cannot be advocated even in cases of severe isolated hydrocephalus. However, if there is no demonstrable cortex, hydranencephaly is most probably present. Because this condition has a dismal prognosis, cephalocentesis might be appropriate. In instances where hydrocephalus is associated with anomalies indicative of a very poor prognosis [e.g., alobar holoprosencephaly (7) or thanatophoric dysplasia with cloverleaf skull (4)], cephalocentesis and subsequent vaginal delivery may be the most appropriate form of management.

In conclusion, this chapter has attempted to review the current status of the diagnosis, prognosis, and management of fetal hydrocephalus. Uncertainties remain in each of these three areas and include the accuracy of antenatal diagnoses in the prediction of anomalies in association with fetal hydrocephalus, the understanding of prognosis for the various types of fetal hydrocephalus, the role of ventriculoam-

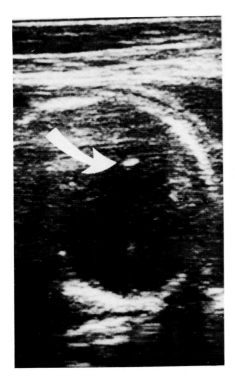

FIG. 20. Sonogram of fetal head with *arrow* pointing to tips of 18-gauge needle in dilated ventricle. (From ref. 3.)

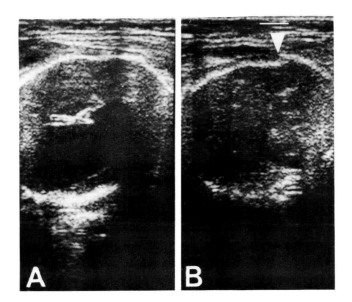

FIG. 21. **A:** Sonogram of fetal head before cephalocentesis. **B:** Sonogram of fetal head after cephalocentesis with *arrow* pointing to overlapping cranial sutures. (From ref. 3.)

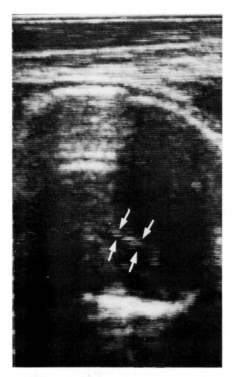

FIG. 22. Sonogram of fetal head after cephalocentesis, with *arrows* outlining stream of blood. (From ref. 3.)

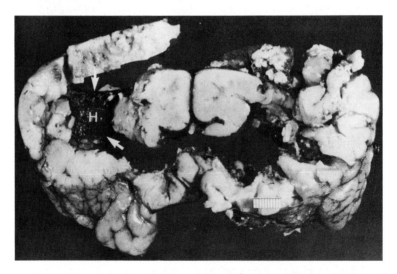

FIG. 23. Section of brain demonstrating intraventricular hemorrhage (H) resulting from cephalocentesis. (From ref. 3.)

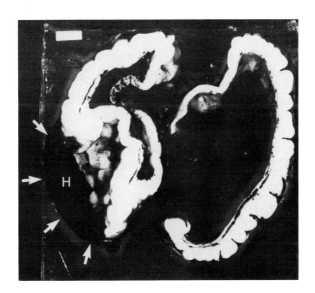

FIG. 24. Coronal section of brain demonstrating a large subarachnoid hemorrhage (H) resulting from cephalocentesis. (From refs. 3 and 12a.)

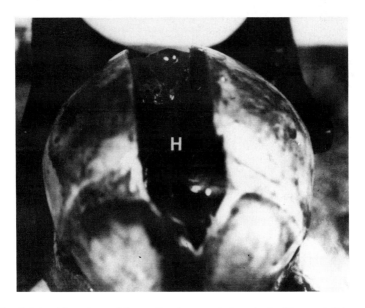

FIG. 25. Subdural hematoma (H) resulting from cephalocentesis. (From ref. 3.)

niotic shunt placement and the selection of appropriate candidates for this procedure, the place of elective delivery before fetal lung maturity when there is rapidly progressive hydrocephalus, the possibility of transabdominal cephalocentesis with removal of a limited amount of cerebrospinal fluid without worsening of fetal prognosis, and the safety of vaginal delivery for the infant with hydrocephalus without macrocephaly.

REFERENCES

1. Chervenak, F.A., Berkowitz, R.L., Romero, A., et al. (1983): The diagnosis of fetal hydrocephalus. *Am. J. Obstet. Gynecol.*, 147:703–716.
2. Chervenak, F.A., Berkowitz, R.L., Tortora, M., et al. (1984): Diagnosis of ventriculomegaly before fetal viability. *Obstet. Gynecol.*, 64:652–656.
2a. Chervenak, F.A., Blakemore, J.K., Isaacson, G., et al. (1983): Antenatal sonographic findings of thanatophoric dysplasia with cloverleaf skull. *Am. J. Obstet. Gynecol.*, 146:984–988.
   fetal hydrocephalus. *Am. J. Obstet. Gynecol.*, 151:933–942.
4. Chervenak, F.A., Blakemore, K.J., Isaacson, G., et al. (1983): Antenatal sonographic findings of thanatophoric dysplasia with cloverleaf skull. *Am. J. Obstet. Gynecol.*, 146:984–985.
5. Chervenak, F.A., Duncan, C., Ment, L.R., et al. (1984): Outcome of fetal ventriculomegaly. *Lancet*, 2:179–181.
6. Chervenak, F.A., Hobbins, J.C., Wertheimer, I., et al. (1985): The natural history of ventriculomegaly in a fetus without obstructive hydrocephalus. *Am. J. Obstet. Gynecol.*, 152:574–575.
7. Chervenak, F.A., Isaacson, G., Mahoney, M.J., et al. (1984): The obstetrical significance of holoprosencephaly. *Obstet. Gynecol.*, 63:115–121.
8. Clewell, W.H., Johnson, M.L., Meier, P.R., et al. (1982): A surgical approach to the treatment of fetal hydrocephalus. *N. Engl. J. Med.*, 306:1320–1325.
9. Feeny, J.K., and Barry, A.P. (1954): Hydrocephaly as a cause of maternal mortality and morbidity. *J. Obstet. Gynecol. Br. Emp.*, 61:652–656.
10. Glick, P.L., Harrison, M.R., Halks-Miller, M., et al. (1984): Correction of congenital hydrocephalus *in utero*. I. Efficacy of *in utero* shunting. *J. Pediatr. Surg.*, 19:870–881.
11. Glick, P.L., Harrison, M.R., Nakayama, D.K., et al. (1984): Management of ventriculomegaly in the fetus. *J. Pediatr.*, 105:97–105.
12. Harrison, M.R., Filly, R.A., and Golbus, M.S. (1982): Fetal treatment. *N. Engl. J. Med.*, 307:1651–1652.
12a. Isaacson, G. (1984): Postmortem examination of infant brains. *Arch. Pathol. Lab. Med.*, 108:80–82.
13. Jeanty, P., Dramaix-Wilmet, M., Delbeke, D., et al. (1981): Ultrasonic evaluation of fetal ventricular growth. *Neuroradiology*, 21:127–131.
14. Johnson, M.L., Dunne, M.G., Mack, L.A., et al. (1980): Evaluation of fetal intracranial anatomy by static and real-time ultrasound. *J. Clin. Ultrasound*, 8:311–318.
15. Laurence, K.M., Coates, S. (1962): The natural history of hydrocephalus. *Arch. Dis. Child.*, 37:345–362.
16. Lorber, J. (1968): The results of early treatment of extreme hydrocephalus. *Dev. Med. Child. Neurol. (Suppl.)*, 16:21–29.
17. Lorber, J., and Zachary, R.B. (1968): Primary congenital hydrocephalus: Long-term results of controlled therapeutic trial. *Arch. Dis. Child.*, 43:516–527.
18. Manning, F.A., Harrison, M.R., Rodek, C., et al (1986): Catheter shunts for fetal hydronephrosis and hydrocephalus: Report of the international fetal surgery registry. *N. Engl. J. Med.*, 315:336–340.
19. Manning, F.A., Lange, I.R., Morrison, I., et al. (1984): Treatment of the fetus *in utero:* Evolving concepts. *Clin. Obstet. Gynecol.*, 27:378–390.
20. McCrann, D.J., and Schifrin, B.S. (1973): Heart rate patterns of the hydrocephalic fetus. *Am. J. Obstet. Gynecol.*, 117:69–74.
21. McCullough, D.C., and Balzer-Martin, L.A. (1982): Current prognosis in overt neonatal hydrocephalus. *J. Neurosurg.*, 57:378–383.
22. Michejda, M., and Hodgen, G.D. (1981): *In utero* diagnosis and treatment of nonhuman primate fetal skeletal anomalies. I. Hydrocephalus. *JAMA*, 246:1093–1097.
23. Pretorius, D.H., Davis, K., Manco-Johnson, M.L., et al. (1985): Clinical course of fetal hydrocephalus: 40 cases. *AJR*, 144:827–831.

24. Raimondi, A.J., and Soare, P. (1974): Intellectual development in shunted hydrocephalic children. *Am. J. Dis. Child.,* 127:664–671.
25. Rubin, R.C., Hochwald, G., Liwnicz, B., et al. (1972): The effect of severe hydrocephalus on size and number of brain cells. *Dev. Med. Child. Neurol.,* 27:117–120.
26. Shurtleff, D.B., Folz, E.L., and Loeser, J.D. (1973): Hydrocephalus: A definition of its progression and relationship to intellectual function, diagnosis, and complications. *Am. J. Dis. Child.,* 125:688–693.
27. Stein, S.C., Feldman, J.G., Apfel, S., et al. (1981): The epidemiology of congenital hydrocephalus. A study in Brooklyn, NY, 1968–1976. *Childs Brain,* 8:253–262.
28. Sutton, L.N., Bruce, D.A., and Schut, L. (1980): Hydranencephaly versus maximal hydrocephalus: An important clinical distinction. *Neurosurgery,* 6:34–38.

Fetal Neurology, edited by
A. Hill and J.J. Volpe.
Raven Press, New York © 1989.

Commentary on Chapters 10 and 11

*Alan Hill and **Joseph J. Volpe

*Division of Neurology, Department of Paediatrics, University of British Columbia,
British Columbia's Children's Hospital, Vancouver, British Columbia, Canada V6H 3V4;
and **Division of Pediatric Neurology, Washington University School of Medicine,
St. Louis, Missouri 63110*

The preceding two chapters provided the reader with two somewhat different perspectives of fetal hydrocephalus. Thus, Dr. Manwaring, a neurosurgeon with an interest in intrauterine intervention, discussed fetal surgery with some enthusiasm, albeit tempered, and Dr. Chervenak, an obstetric-perinatal specialist, exhibited less enthusiasm for such an approach. Both investigators emphasized the importance of careful intrauterine assessment before decision making.

The major etiologies of fetal hydrocephalus are relatively few (10). Those cases identified *at birth* include approximately one-third with aqueductal stenosis, one-third with myelomeningocele and the Arnold-Chiari malformation, and the remainder with primarily communicating hydrocephalus or the Dandy-Walker malformation. The etiologies of those cases identified *in utero* differ in the larger proportion of cases with associated anomalies. Indeed, in the obstetric series approximately 70% to 85% of cases exhibited major associated neural and/or extraneural anomalies by ultrasonographic examination and, importantly, an additional 20% of cases exhibited such anomalies at birth that were not detected by intrauterine ultrasound examination. Indeed, less than 10% of cases identified *in utero* were "pure" or "isolated" hydrocephalus. Herein then lies the problem with intrauterine therapy, i.e., there are very few cases that can be considered potential candidates. In addition, even in the presence of isolated hydrocephalus, it is unlikely that intrauterine intervention favorably alters the outcome relative to prompt postnatal treatment.

The prognosis for congenital hydrocephalus thus depends presumably on the etiology and the presence of associated congenital abnormalities. Consideration of these factors underscores the importance of establishing a specific etiology, whenever possible, in each individual case (7,9).

In this context, recent advances in radiologic techniques play a major role in the investigation of fetal hydrocephalus. Thus, antenatal *ultrasonography* is a valuable technique for the assessment of the size and shape of the ventricular system in the fetus and provides a good correlation with measurements of ventricular size obtained by postnatal computed tomography (5,8). Although ultrasound examination of the ventricles has become the method of choice for the diagnosis of fetal hydrocephalus, it is important to recognize that a single assessment of ventricular size may be inconclusive. This may be owing to technical error or to both the relatively large variation of normal ventricular size and rate of growth of the fetal brain during the second trimester. In some instances, severe fetal hydrocephalus may be detected before the 20th week of gestation, which may allow termination of pregnancy as a management option. However, because of the large variation of normal ventricular size, it has been demonstrated that ventricles that appear abnormally large between 15 to 18 weeks of gestation may subsequently appear normal on follow-up studies, and in fact, the infant may be normal at birth. Thus, during this period (i.e., 15–18 weeks of gestation), normal ventricular size may overlap with the ventriculomegaly of early fetal hydrocephalus, and this overlap makes serial ultrasound studies necessary in order to distinguish abnormal from normal ventricular size. Of course, this reliance on serial imaging to establish an unequivocal diagnosis of hydrocephalus may preclude a sufficiently early diagnosis to allow for termination of the pregnancy as a management option. Consequently, major research efforts in the future should be directed toward the identification of measurements that will distinguish reliably between normal and clearly abnormal ventricular size. None of the parameters of ventricular size that are currently available, e.g., ventricular ratio (4), are entirely satisfactory. To confound this issue further, it is clear that in some instances unequivocal intrauterine ventriculomegaly may be nonprogressive. However, the implications of nonprogressive ventriculomegaly for neurological development remain largely unknown.

Recent data that deal with the outcome of congenital hydrocephalus suggest that there is only limited correlation between ventricular size or cortical thickness at birth and long-term neurological sequelae (10). An obvious exception is the encephaloclastic process that results in hydranencephaly, in which the complete absence of cortex clearly determines the severely abnormal neurological outcome. However, hydranencephaly may be difficult to distinguish *in utero* from severe congenital hydrocephalus in which there is an extremely thin cortical mantle. The use of newer ultrasound transducers (10 MHz) that permit detailed imaging of the near-field of the cranium in infants may help to distinguish between the two entities.

The coexistence of other fetal anomalies with hydrocephalus plays the dominant role in determining outcome. In many but unfortunately not all instances, these associated congenital anomalies may be identified also by ultrasonography (8), provided that the entire fetus is visualized. Preliminary data suggest a contributory role for magnetic resonance imaging (MRI) for the identification of such abnormalities. A major advantage of this technique in pregnancy is the lack of ionizing radiation. Thus, MRI has been used to demonstrate renal anomalies and holoprosencephaly in the fetus and is considered to be particularly useful in patients with oligohydramnios (6). Because of the implications of such coexisting abnormalities for adverse outcome, decision making may be simplified, especially during early pregnancy, when the diagnosis of hydrocephalus is equivocal.

Recent technical advances from both human experience and experimental studies in intrauterine shunting have been encouraging. However, the limited experience in the human fetus does not allow final conclusions to be drawn. Preliminary data suggest that intrauterine shunting may decrease ventricular size and prevent progression of the ventricular enlargement (1). If ventriculomegaly is associated with increased intracranial pressure, fetal shunting may restore normal anatomy, i.e., both the ventricular size and head size may return to normal. However, the duration of such benefit has been limited by the mechanical and technical problems of shunt dislodgment and obstruction. It is also clear that in many infants, neurological outcome is abnormal despite effective ventricular drainage. This relates to the fact that developmental prognosis depends as much on the etiology of the hydrocephalus as on the severity and the stage of pregnancy when the shunting is performed. For example, in X-linked hydrocephalus with its high frequency of associated anomalies, prenatal shunting of the hydrocephalus is of doubtful benefit.

The current approach to management of prenatal hydrocephalus may be summarized as follows: if serial antenatal ultrasound examinations demonstrate hydrocephalus and there are no coexisting congenital anomalies, delivery by elective cesarean section (provided that the lungs are mature) would permit early postnatal ventricular shunting. Such an approach would minimize the possible occurrence of cerebral injury from the hydrocephalus per se or from the delivery of an enlarged head in those infants who may have potential for reasonable neurological outcome. However, if antenatal studies demonstrate coexisting cerebral or systemic anomalies, standard obstetrical management, including vaginal delivery with or without cephalocentesis, may be considered (2,3). At the present time, a third option is to perform intrauterine shunting. However, this remains an experimental procedure. The criteria for patient selection, choice of operative technique, and equipment will no doubt continue to evolve. The existence of the International Registry for Fetal Surgery should maximize the accumulation of information derived from the experience to date. However, it will be several years before meaningful follow-up data are available to assess the value of the procedure.

REFERENCES

1. Birnholz, J.C., and Frigoletto, F.D. (1981): Antenatal treatment of hydrocephalus. *N. Engl. J. Med.*, 303:1021–1023.
2. Clewell, W.H., Johnson, M.L., Meier, P.R., et al. (1982): A surgical approach to the treatment of fetal hydrocephalus. *N. Engl. J. Med.*, 306:1320–1325.
3. Cochrane, D.D., and Myles, T. (1982): Management of intrauterine hydrocephalus. *J. Neurosurg.*, 57:590–596.
4. Denkhaus, H., and Winsberg, F. (1979): Ultrasonic measurement of the fetal ventricular system. *Radiology*, 131:781–787.
5. Hadlock, F.P., Deter, R.L., and Park, S.K. (1981): Real-time sonography: Ventricular and vascular anatomy of the fetal brain *in utero*. *A.J.R.*, 136:133–137.
6. McCarthy, S.M., Filly, R.A., Stark, D.D., Callen, P.W., Golbus, M.S., and Hricak, H. (1985): Magnetic resonance imaging of fetal anomalies *in utero:* Early experience. *A.J.R.*, 145:677–682.

7. McCullough, D.C., and Balzer-Martin, L.A. (1982): Current prognosis in overt neonatal hydrocephalus. *J. Neurosurg.*, 57:378–383.
8. Nyberg, D.A., Mack, L.A., Hirsch, J., Pagon, R.O., and Shepard, T.H. (1987): Fetal hydrocephalus: Sonographic detection and clinical significance of associated anomalies. *Radiology,* 163:187–191.
9. Serlo, W., Kirkinen, P., Jouppila, P., and Herva, R. (1986): Prognostic signs in fetal hydrocephalus. *Child's Nerv. Syst.*, 2:93–97.
10. Volpe, J.J. (1987): *Neurology of the Newborn,* pp. 25–28, W.B. Saunders, Philadelphia.

Fetal Neurology, edited by
A. Hill and J.J. Volpe.
Raven Press, New York © 1989.

12

Current Perspectives on the Diagnosis, Prognosis, and Management of Fetal Spina Bifida

Frank A. Chervenak and Glenn Isaacson

*Department of Obstetrics and Gynecology, The New York Hospital–
Cornell Medical Center, New York, New York 10021*

Spina bifida refers to a defect in the spine resulting from failure of fusion of the vertebral arches. However, this constitutes only a minor part of the overall problem. In fact, the associated maldevelopment of the spinal cord and hydrocephalus represents much more important issues. The most severe form of spinal dysraphism, meningomyelocele, is one of the most devastating congenital disorders and ultimately affects multiple organ systems (Fig. 1). A meningomyelocele, by definition, contains abnormal central nervous tissue (i.e., malformed, maldeveloped spinal cord). The lesions are typically single and large and are composed of a "neural plaque," i.e., the dysraphic spinal cord, which is covered by a membrane of meningeal origin and malformed spine. Meningomyeloceles are usually located in the lower thoracolumbar, lumbar, and lumbosacral areas.

Spina bifida is the most common *major* congenital malformation in the Western world. However, there is significant geographic variation in the occurrence of this lesion. The highest reported incidences are in Ireland and Wales. Spina bifida occurs more often in infants of women of lower socioeconomic classes and those at the extremes of their childbearing age. However, the incidence of open spina bifida has decreased greatly in the last 10 to 15 years. This relates in part to improvements in antenatal diagnosis, which allows more knowledgeable choice of management. However, obstetrical intervention accounts for only half of the reduction in incidence, and there remains no clear explanation for the substantial reduction in incidence. For example, in Ireland the birth incidence of spina bifida decreased by 50% over 4 years in the early 1980s, despite the fact that termination of pregnancy was illegal. Even at the present time, the incidence of spina bifida remains subject to considerable regional and temporal fluctuation. Thus, in 1984

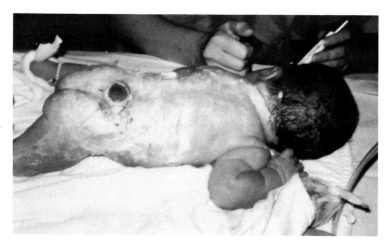

FIG. 1.   Intact lumbosacral meningomyelocele in a neonate.

the incidence of this disorder ranged from 1.8 per 10,000 births in Finland to 17.2 per 10,000 in Northern Ireland. In the United States the incidence was 4.9 per 10,000, and in Great Britain 6 per 10,000 (10,16,18,25).

DIAGNOSIS

Ultrasound is the principal technique available for the diagnosis of neural tube defects *in utero*. On ultrasound scans, spina bifida is manifested by a splaying of the posterior ossification centers of the spine, which produces a U-shaped appearance of the vertebra (7,8,19) (Figs. 2 and 3). In addition, the posterior ossification centers in defective vertebrae are spaced more widely than those in vertebrae above and below the defect. In this context, it should be remembered that there is a normal progressive widening of the spinal canal in the cervical region. Although spina bifida may be visualized on longitudinal scanning, meticulous transverse examinations along the entire vertebral column are necessary to detect smaller defects. In the third trimester, the posterior vertebral elements, including the laminae and spinous processes, are normally visible sonographically. Absence of these structures further supports the diagnosis of spina bifida.

The plane produced by oblique angulation of the ultrasound transducer allows visualization of the anterior vertebral elements; however, the posterior elements may not be demonstrated, and the appearance thus may simulate spina bifida (4). To avoid such errors, careful attention must be directed toward maintenance of a true transverse orientation along the normal curvature of the spine. The ischial tuberosities, iliac crests, and ribs may be used to aid in orientation.

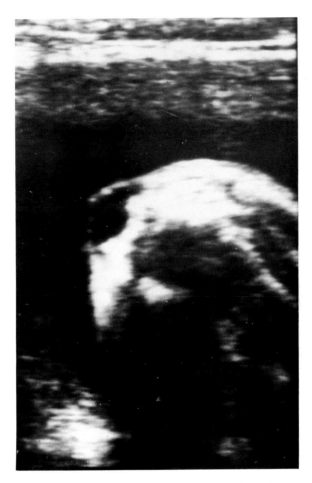

FIG. 2. Transverse sonogram of fetal spina bifida demonstrating splaying of the posterior ossification centers producing a U-shaped appearance and an intact protruding sac.

A recent report by Nicolaides et al. (17) suggests that examination of the fetal head may permit the diagnosis of the Arnold-Chiari malformation, which is associated nearly invariably with spina bifida (Fig. 4). The Arnold-Chiari malformation is an anomaly of the hindbrain, consisting principally of (a) variable displacement of the inferior cerebellar vermis into the upper cervical canal, and (b) similar caudal displacement of the medulla and fourth ventricle. Almost all cases of spina bifida are complicated by the Arnold-Chiari malformation, and 90% to 95% of these patients have evidence of hydrocephalus (1).

Thus, in addition to the specific importance of the Arnold-Chiari malformation, the abnormality may serve as an important marker for spina bifida. Two characteristic sonographic signs (the "lemon" and the "banana") of the Arnold-Chiari

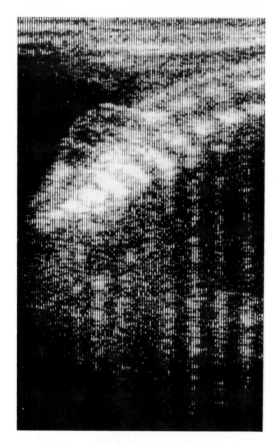

FIG. 3. Sagittal sonogram of lumbosacral spina bifida demonstrating absent posterior elements and protruding sac.

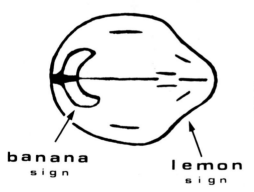

banana
sign

lemon
sign

FIG. 4. Diagrammatic representation of "banana" and "lemon" signs in a fetus with spina bifida. (From ref. 17.)

malformation have been recently described. Thus, scalloping of the frontal bones may produce a lemon-like configuration to the skull of an affected fetus in axial section during the second trimester. The caudal displacement of the cranial contents within the pliable fetal skull is thought to produce this scalloping effect. In addition, as the cerebellar hemispheres are displaced into the cervical canal, they are flattened rostro-caudally and the cisterna magna is obliterated; these changes result in flattened, sonographic appearance with a central curvature, thus simulating a banana. In severe cases, it may be impossible to visualize the cerebellar hemispheres by scanning of the fetal head. These characteristic cranial ultrasonographic appearances should alert the sonographer to examine further for the presence of spina bifida and may reveal this diagnosis in previously unsuspected cases (2,17) (Figs. 5 and 6).

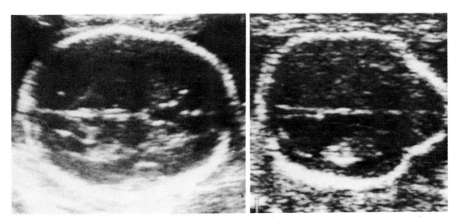

FIG. 5. Left: Transverse section of the normal fetal head in an 18-week fetus at the level of the cavum septi pellucidi. **Right:** Transverse section of the fetal head at the level of the cavum septi pellucidi in an 18-week fetus with open spina bifida showing the "lemon" sign. (From ref 17.)

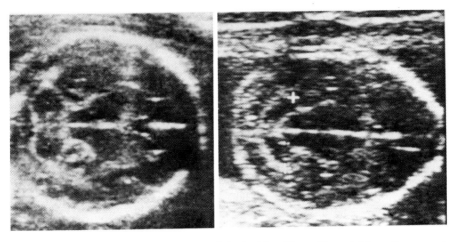

FIG. 6. Left: Suboccipital bregmatic view of the fetal head in an 18-week fetus with a normal cerebellum and cisterna magna. **Right:** Suboccipital bregmatic view of the fetal head in an 18-week fetus with open spina bifida demonstrates the "banana" sign (+). (From ref. 17.)

PROGNOSIS

The prognosis for any individual case of spina bifida is dependent on several factors. The most important of these are the presence or absence of nerve tissue in the meningeal sac and the spinal level and extent of the lesion. Paralysis of the lower extremities and incontinence of bowel and bladder functions are the most common neurological sequelae. In addition, intelligence is often affected (9,13,22,23). With the advent of routine serum alpha-fetoprotein screening and the subsequent option of abortion of fetuses with open neural tube defects, the relative proportion of the less severe lesion, meningocele, among liveborn infants with spina bifida has increased.

The optimal management for the neonate with meningomyelocele has been the subject of much debate. Before 1960, nonsurgical treatment of the infant with meningomyelocele was the rule because of the excessive risks of operation during the neonatal period. Closure of the defect was considered at 12 to 18 months of age, when the hydrocephalus had stabilized and epithelization of the sac had occurred, thus decreasing the operative risk (9). With the introduction of shunt systems with valves for treatment of hydrocephalus as well as other improvements in neonatal neurosurgery, more aggressive management became possible. In the 1960s, Sharrard and associates (22) conducted a controlled study of immediate versus delayed closure of spina bifida at the Sheffield Children's Hospital. The study was discontinued when it was realized that mortality, infectious morbidity, and muscle function appeared to be decreased in the group treated with early operative closure. Subsequently, Lorber (13,15) reviewed the experience at the same institution and established criteria for nonsurgical treatment of the newborn based on the presence of gross paralysis of legs, thoracolumbar lesion, kyphosis or scoliosis, very advanced hydrocephalus, intracerebral birth injury, and other gross congenital defects. In a subsequent prospective study (14), two-thirds of neonates did not meet the selection criteria for active treatment and were allowed to die. The possibility of active euthanasia in order to alleviate pain and suffering was considered by Freeman (5).

The prognosis for spina bifida has changed in recent years. Currently more than 90% of infants have long-term survival; some of these grow to be productive adults with normal or superior intelligence. Early closure of defects, as well as ventriculoperitoneal or ventriculoarterial shunting of hydrocephalus, and management of urinary and fecal incontinence by surgery, dietary management, and biofeedback techniques are responsible in part for these relative improvements (11,12), although the prognosis for severely affected infants generally remains poor because of a high incidence of severe and permanent multisystem defects.

MANAGEMENT

If meningomyelocele is diagnosed late in the third trimester or if termination of pregnancy is declined when a meningomyelocele is diagnosed earlier, a team approach involving the obstetrician, pediatric neurosurgeon, pediatric neurologist,

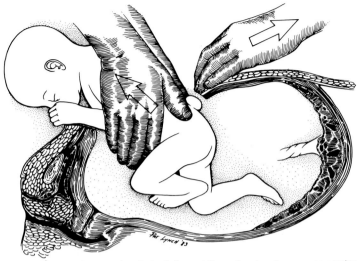

FIG. 7. Fetus with meningomyelocele is delivered through a low transverse uterine incision. Both fetal flanks are grasped, and gentle traction is applied in an outward direction. The assistant retracts the edge of the uterine incision as the body is delivered. (From ref. 3.)

and neonatologist is advisable for optimum planning of management. In addition, a perinatal social worker may provide invaluable support for the family both before and following delivery. Fetal surveillance, including bioelectric fetal heart rate monitoring and serial sonography, is essential to assess fetal growth, head size, and severity of hydrocephalus. Unless an obstetric indication takes precedence, delivery should be considered after documentation of fetal lung maturity.

Unfortunately, there is a paucity of clinical information with regard to the optimal route of delivery for infants with meningomyelocele. In a retrospective study (published in 1970) of the deliveries of 130 infants with meningomyelocele (24), 14% had evidence of cerebral birth injury. The authors suggested that the spinal neurologic deficit in many newborns increased during delivery (24). In another retrospective series (6), an increased incidence of intrapartum distress was reported in the fetus with a meningomyelocele. In the latter study, the diagnosis of fetal distress was based on the presence of thick meconium or persistent bradycardia and was associated with cephalic presentation (6). Furthermore, autopsy studies of Ralis and Ralis (20,21) suggested that labor and delivery may have a detrimental effect on the infant with meningomyelocele, especially with breech presentation.

In view of the potential risks of vaginal delivery and the lack of evidence that vaginal delivery is nontraumatic for the infant with a meningomyelocele, cesarean section should be offered to the parents as a potentially beneficial procedure. The following technique is generally recommended. If the lower uterine segment is well developed, the section may be performed by means of a low transverse incision. After the head is delivered, the biacromial diameter is positioned horizontally. Both fetal flanks are grasped, and gentle traction is applied in an outward direction away from the uterine wall near the meningomyelocele. The assistant retracts the edge of the uterine incision as the body of the infant is delivered (3)

(Fig. 7). Further clinical studies are necessary, especially with smaller lesions, to determine whether atraumatic abdominal delivery may improve long-term neurologic function.

REFERENCES

1. Bell, J.E., Gordon, A., and Maloney, A.F.J. (1980): The association of hydrocephalus and Arnold-Chiari malformation with spina bifida in the fetus. *Neuropathol. Appl. Neurobiol.,* 6:29–39.
2. Campbell, J., Gilbert, W.M., Nicolaides, K.M., and Campbell, S. (1987): Ultrasound screening for spina bifida: Cranial and cerebellar signs in a high risk population. *Obstet. Gynecol.,* 70:247–250.
3. Chervenak, F.A., Duncan, C., Ment, L.R., et al. (1984): Perinatal management of meningomyelocele. *Obstet. Gynecol.,* 63:376–380.
4. Dennis, M.A., Drose, J.A., Pretorius, D.H., and Manco-Johnson, M.L. (1985): Normal fetal sacrum simulating spina bifida: "Pseudodysraphism." *Radiology,* 155:751–754.
5. Freeman, J.M. (1972): Is there a right to die quickly? *J. Pediatr.,* 80:904.
6. Guha-ray, D.K. (1977): Open spina bifida (OSB) and intrapartum fetal distress. *J. Reprod. Med.,* 19:277–279.
7. Hobbins, J.C., Grannum, P.A.T., Berkowitz, R.L., et al. (1979): Ultrasound in the diagnosis of congenital anomalies. *Am. J. Obstet. Gynecol.,* 134:331–345.
8. Hobbins, J.C., Venus, I., Tortora, M., et al. (1982): Stage II ultrasound examination for the diagnosis of fetal abnormalities with an elevated amniotic fluid alpha-fetoprotein concentration. *Am. J. Obstet. Gynecol.,* 142:1026–1029.
9. Ingraham, F.D., and Hamlin, H. (1943): Spina bifida and cranium bifidum. II. Surgical treatment. *N. Engl. J. Med.,* 228:631.
10. International Clearinghouse for Birth Defects Monitoring Systems (1983): *Annual Report.* ISSN 0743-5703:14.
11. Leonard, C.O., and Freeman, J.M. (1981): Spina bifida: A new disease. *Pediatrics,* 68:136–137.
12. Lorber, J. (1969): Ventriculo-cardiac shunts in the first week of life. Results of a controlled trial in the treatment of hydrocephalus in infants born with spina bifida cystica or cranium bifidum. *Dev. Med. Child Neurol. [Suppl.],* 20:13–22.
13. Lorber, J. (1971): Results of treatment of myelomeningocele: An analysis of 524 unselected cases, with special reference to possible selection for treatment. *Dev. Med. Child Neurol.,* 13:279–303.
14. Lorber, J. (1973): Early results of selective treatment of spina bifida cystica. *Br. Med. J.,* 4:201–204.
15. Lorber, J. (1974): Selective treatment of myelomeningocele: To treat or not to treat? *Pediatrics,* 53:307–308.
16. Lorber, J., and Ward, A.M. (1985): Spina bifida—A vanishing nightmare? *Arch. Dis. Child.,* 60:1086–1091.
17. Nicolaides, K.M., Campbell, S., Gabbe, S.G., and Guidetti, R. (1986): Ultrasound screening for spina bifida: Cranial and cerebellar signs. *Lancet,* 2:72–74.
18. Office of Population Censuses and Survey (1986): *OPCS Monitor,* MB31862.
19. Pearce, J.M., Little, D., and Campbell, S. (1985): The diagnosis of abnormalities of the fetal central nervous system. In: *The Principle and Practice of Ultrasonography in Obstetrics and Gynecology,* 3d ed., edited by R.C. Saunders and A.E. James, pp. 246–248, Appleton-Century-Crofts, Norwalk.
20. Ralis, A.Z. (1975): Traumatizing effect of breech delivery on infants with spina bifida. *J. Pediatr.,* 87:613–616.
21. Ralis, A.Z., and Ralis, H.M. (1972): Morphology of peripheral nerves in children with spina bifida. *Dev. Med. Child Neurol. [Suppl.],* 27:109–116.
22. Sharrard, W.J., Zachary, R.B., Lorber, J., et al. (1963): A controlled trial of immediate and delayed closure of spina bifida cystica. *Arch. Dis. Child.,* 38:18–22.
23. Shurtleff, D.B. (1980): Myelodysplasia: Management and treatment. *Curr. Probl. Pediatr.,* 10:1–98.
24. Stark, G., and Drummond, M. (1970): Spina bifida as an obstetrics problem. *Dev. Med. Child Neurol. [Suppl.],* 12:157.
25. Stein, S.C., Feldman, J.G., Friedlander, M., et al. (1982): Is myelomeningocele a disappearing disease? *Pediatrics,* 69:511–514.

Fetal Neurology, edited by
A. Hill and J.J. Volpe.
Raven Press, New York © 1989.

Commentary on Chapter 12

*Alan Hill and **Joseph J. Volpe

*Division of Neurology, Department of Paediatrics, University of British Columbia,
British Columbia's Children's Hospital, Vancouver, British Columbia, Canada 6VH 3V4;
and **Division of Pediatric Neurology, Washington University School of Medicine,
St. Louis, Missouri 63110

Drs. Chervenak and Isaacson in Chapter 12 discussed the diagnosis, prognosis, and management of fetal spina bifida, which represents only one type of neural tube defect. Other neural tube defects listed in order of decreasing severity include craniorachischisis totalis, anencephaly, myeloschisis, encephalocele, and meningomyelocele/Arnold-Chiari malformation (20). Because the first three conditions are incompatible with survival beyond the newborn period and their diagnostic features differ principally only in severity from the milder forms of neural tube defects, this discussion focuses on the restricted forms of neural tube defects, i.e., encephalocele and meningomyelocele.

Encephalocele is considered a restricted disorder of anterior neural tube closure that occurs in the occipital region in approximately 80% of cases but may be located rarely in the frontal, temporal, or parietal regions. Spina bifida is an associated finding in approximately 30% of cases.

Diagnosis by intrauterine ultrasonography has been reported and may permit elective termination of the pregnancy before fetal viability (6,7). Ultrasonography of a fetus with an encephalocele may reveal a sac-like structure adjacent to the head and neck region with an associated bony defect (8,16,18). The differential diagnosis of this lesion must include cystic lymphangioma and iniencephaly. The fetal kidneys must be assessed because polycystic kidneys and encephalocele are features of Meckel's syndrome, which is inherited in an autosomal recessive fashion with a 25% risk of recurrence in subsequent pregnancies (21).

Although the outcome of encephaloceles is difficult to predict accurately from the available data, the possibility of reasonable intellectual outcome does exist. However, more than half of all cases are associated with hydrocephalus and/or impaired intellect and motor deficits (1,14). Nevertheless, similar to current concepts in the treatment of meningomyelocele, neurosurgical intervention is now recommended for most encephaloceles except for massive lesions and those associated with severe microcephaly (12).

In contrast to encephalocele, which results from restricted failure of closure of the anterior neural tube, myelomeningocele implies restricted failure of posterior neural tube closure. A prenatal diagnosis may be made either biochemically by alpha-fetoprotein or acetylcholinesterase determinations in amniotic fluid (10) or by fetal ultrasonography. There is some indication that quantification of acetyl-cholinesterase in amniotic fluid may ultimately replace the alpha-fetoprotein test on the basis of its greater accuracy and reliability (2). Determination of maternal serum alpha-fetoprotein levels has been suggested for large-scale screening for neural tube defects (15). The fetal spine may be outlined by ultrasonography before 14 weeks gestation (4), and the spinal abnormalities are discussed by Drs. Chervenak and Isaacson. It should be remembered that occasionally the sac may not be ultrasonically visualized when the intrauterine pressure equals that of the cerebrospinal fluid. In addition, compression of the fetal vertebral column by the uterine wall can obscure the sac. Scanning may be helpful in distinguishing meningoceles from meningomyeloceles by the finding of echogenic material within the sac. The degree of fetal lower limb movement ultrasonically visualized has not been prognostically helpful and may be seen in the presence of a higher level lesion. In these instances, further herniation of the cord through the defect may have occurred with the intrauterine pressure at delivery and resulted in further damage (3,9). It must also be remembered that until late in pregnancy, fetuses with spina bifida characteristically have smaller biparietal diameters. Thus, ultrasonic dating should be validated by other ultrasonic criteria (femur length, abdominal circumference) when a spinal deformity is suspected (17).

The functional outcome of myelomeningocele correlates principally with the spinal level of the lesion (20). Thus, patients with lesions below S1 may be expected to learn to walk unassisted, whereas those with lesions above L2 are usually ultimately wheelchair bound; patients with L4/L5 lesions may be ambulatory with crutches. Young children with lesions as high as the thoracolumbar level may ambulate by utilizing standing braces. Lesions above an L2 level are generally associated with significant scoliosis (11,13). The site of the lesion is also important in the prediction of hydrocephalus from the Arnold-Chiari malformation. Thus, with occipital, thoracic, or sacral lesions, the incidence of hydrocephalus is approximately 60%, compared to at least a 90% incidence with thoracolumbar, lumbar, or lumbosacral lesions. It should be remembered that overt clinical signs of hydrocephalus may not be evident at birth but usually develop within 2 or 3 weeks of age. Eighty percent of infants who develop hydrocephalus with myelomeningocele develop clinical signs within 6 weeks of age (19). In addition to the site of the lesion, the severity of orthopedic and urinary tract complications, as well as major hypoxic-ischemic cerebral insult or associated congenital cerebral malformation, may affect outcome significantly. Hydrocephalus per se does not appear to affect outcome to a major degree. However, infection after shunt placement does correlate with intellectual outcome.

It is clear that all management decisions must be made on the basis of optimal understanding of the prognosis of the lesion. For example, there is a prevalent notion that early closure of the back lesion within 24 or 48 hr is desirable to minimize infection and loss of motor function. However, in a recent study of 110 infants, the incidence of ventriculitis was 10% in those infants whose lesions were closed within the first 48 hr versus 12% in infants whose lesions were closed in 3 to 7 days and 8% if lesions were closed after 7 days. Prophylactic antibiotic use reduced this incidence further. Furthermore, the severity of lower extremity paralysis was not influenced by the timing of surgery (5). Thus, it appears that closure of the back lesion is not as urgent as was previously thought and that time is available for rational decision making, which involves the family as well as a team that includes the obstetrician, neonatologist, neurologist, and neurosurgeon.

REFERENCES

1. Brandensky, G. von, and Klick, A. (1969): Encephalocele and hydrocephalus. *Z. Kinderchir.*, 7:583.
2. Brook, D.J.H., Barron, L., and Van Heyningen, V. (1985): Prenatal diagnosis of neural tube defects with a monoclonal antibody specific for acetylcholinesterase. *Lancet*, 1:5.
3. Campbell, S. (1977): Early prenatal diagnosis of neural tube defects by ultrasound. *Clin. Obstet. Gynecol.*, 20:351–359.
4. Campbell, S., Pryse-Davies, J., Coltart, T.M., Seller, M.J., and Singer, J.D. (1975): Ultrasound in the diagnosis of spina bifida. *Lancet*, 1:1065–1068.
5. Charney, E.B., Weller, S.C., Sutton, L.N., et al. (1985): Myelomeningocele newborn management: Time for a decision making process. *Pediatrics*, 75:58–64.
6. Chervenak, F.A., Berkowitz, R.L., Tortora, M., and Hobbins, J.C. (1985): The management of fetal hydrocephalus. *Am. J. Obstet. Gynecol.*, 151:933–942.
7. Chervenak, F.A., Isaacson, G., Mahoney, M.J., et al. (1984): The obstetric significance of holoprosencephaly. *Obstet. Gynecol.*, 63:115–121.
8. Graham, D., Johnson, T.R.B., Jr., Winn, K., and Sanders, R.C. (1982): The role of sonography in the prenatal diagnosis and management of encephalocele. *J. Ultrasound Med.*, 1:111–115.
9. Hobbins, J.C., Grannum, P.A.T., Berkowitz, R.L., Silverman, R., and Mahoney, M.S. (1979): Ultrasound in the diagnosis of congenital anomalies. *Am. J. Obstet. Gynecol.*, 134:331–345.
10. Kimball, M.E., Milunsky, A., and Alpert, E. (1977): Prenatal diagnosis of neural tube defects. III. A re-evaluation of the alpha-fetoprotein assay. *Obstet. Gynecol.*, 49:532.
11. Liptak, G.S., and Masiulis, B.S. (1984): Letter. *Pediatrics*, 74:165.
12. Matson, D. (1969): *Neurosurgery of Infancy and Childhood.* Charles C. Thomas, Springfield, IL.
13. McLaughlin, J.F., and Shurtleff, D.B. (1979): Management of the newborn with myelodysplasia. *Clin. Pediatr.*, 18:463–476.
14. Mealy, J., Jr., Dzenitis, A.J., and Hockey, A.A. (1970): The prognosis of encephaloceles. *J. Neurosurg.*, 32:209–218.
15. Milunsky, A., Elliot, A., Neff, R.K., and Frigoletto, F.D., Jr. (1980): Prenatal diagnosis of neural tube defects. IV. Maternal serum alpha-fetoprotein screening. *Obstet. Gynecol.*, 55:60.
16. Miskin, M., Rudd, N.L., Dische, M.R., Benzie, R., and Pirani, B.B.K. (1978): Prenatal ultrasonic diagnosis of occipital encephalocele. *Am. J. Obstet. Gynecol.*, 130:585–587.
17. Roberts, A.B., and Campbell, S. (1980): Letter to the editor. *Br. J. Obstet. Gynaecol.*, 87:927–928.
18. Shaff, M.I., Blumenthal, B., and Coetzee, M. (1977): Meningo-encephalocele: Prepartum ultrasonic and feto-amniographic findings. *Br. J. Radiol.*, 50:754–757.
19. Stein, S.C., and Schut, L. (1979): Hydrocephalus in myelomeningocele. *Childs Brain*, 4:413–419.
20. Volpe, J.J. (1987): *Neurology of the Newborn*, 2nd ed., W.B. Saunders, Philadelphia.
21. Wapner, R.J., Kurtz, A.B., Ross, R.D., and Jackson, L.G. (1981): Ultrasonographic parameters in the prenatal diagnosis of Meckel syndrome. *Obstet. Gynecol.*, 57:388–392.

Fetal Neurology, edited by
A. Hill and J.J. Volpe.
Raven Press, New York © 1989.

13

Influences of the Brain on Normal and Abnormal Muscle Development

*Pierre Jacob and **Harvey B. Sarnat

*University of Ottawa Faculty of Medicine and The Children's Hospital of Eastern Ontario, Ottawa, Ontario, Canada K1H 8L1; and **University of Calgary Faculty of Medicine and Alberta Children's Hospital, Calgary, Alberta, Canada T2T 5C7*

Many factors influence muscle development in muscular dystrophies, congenital myopathies, and other neuromuscular disorders. Abnormalities of suprasegmental or upper motor neuron function in the fetus must be included among the factors that alter the development of motor units and thereby play a role in pathogenesis of these disorders by altering the physiological discharge pattern of lower motor neurons. Such cerebral influences affect development of muscle in terms of histochemical differentiation as well as growth and morphology of myofibers. These cerebral influences, in association with degeneration or other intrinsic muscle factors, may contribute to the composite of abnormalities recognizable in muscle biopsies of many genetically determined diseases.

A review of normal fetal development of muscle fibers and its relation to the development of the central nervous system is a prerequisite to an understanding of the evolving histopathological changes observed in the different varieties of dystrophies and congenital myopathies. The association of certain cerebral dysgenesis with aberrations in muscle fiber maturation suggests a uniform pathophysiological process to which developmental myopathies might be linked.

EMBRYONIC MUSCLE DEVELOPMENT

Several studies provide direct data on the microscopic characteristics of human myogenesis (27,28,38,60). In view of the relative paucity of complete and adequate human material, attempts to provide information on muscle growth and development have been based on information from studies of muscle development in other mammalian species or from the study of myogenesis *in vitro*. Such animal data fill some of the gaps in the studies of human embryos, particularly during the early stages of myogenesis.

All somatic striated muscles of vertebrates originate from the mesodermal layer in the embryo. Neurulation, i.e., the formation of the neural tube, occurs during the 3rd and 4th weeks of gestation. The nervous system differentiates on the dorsal aspect of the embryo as a plate of tissue in the middle of the ectoderm. The underlying notochord and chordal mesoderm induce formation of the neural plate at approximately 18 days of gestation. Under influence of the chordal mesoderm, the lateral margins of the neural plate are induced to invaginate and close dorsally to form the neural tube. After closure of the neural tube, neural crest cells differentiate into dorsal root ganglia, sensory ganglia of cranial nerves, autonomic ganglia, Schwann cells, and cells of the pia and arachnoid. Furthermore, nerve cells of the adrenal medulla and certain skeletal elements of the head and face are derived from the neural crest.

The neural tube is the origin of the central nervous system. Beneath the neural plate, mesenchymal cells migrate laterally and anteriorly to form a continuous layer, which subdivides further as development continues. The myotomal plates appear as a pair of thickened bands of mesoderm located on either side of the neural tube. A strip of intermediate mesoderm (6) lies between the myotomal plate and the lateral mesoderm.

Elongation of the embryo and formation of recognizable subdivisions of the body are accompanied by additional changes in the myotomal plate and lateral mesoderm. Elongation of the embryo is associated with regression of the node and the primitive streak in the caudal direction. As this regression occurs, paired blocks separate sequentially from the strips of undifferentiated lateral mesoderm to form paired somites on either side of the neural tube. Table 1 presents the major stages of human brain development. The body wall, mesenteries, and internal organs also originate from the lateral mesoderm. Subsequently, the somites divide into dermatome and scleratome. Myotomes develop from the dermatome to form limb and trunk muscles. Cervical and cranial bulbar muscles are derived from the specialized somites of the branchial arches.

Although animal experiments offer some insight, the mechanisms that regulate the differentiation of various limb muscles are poorly understood. The mechanical role of insinuating nerves has been studied (52). Thus, in limbs deprived of innervation, subsequent muscle patterning occurs normally (82). Furthermore, normal muscle differentiation occurs when investing nerves are destroyed before the initiation of muscle splitting. Muscles and tendinous insertions develop independently and connect subsequently (46). Neither physical continuity with the tendon nor the generation of tension plays a role in this mechanism, but tendons that fail to establish a muscular connection dedifferentiate eventually into mesenchyme (64).

Connective tissue cells guide the migration of myogenic cells. Myoblasts originate from mesenchymal cells. Although myoblasts have few histological features to distinguish them from other mesodermal cells, their programmed commitment to myogenesis is demonstrated in cell culture. When these mitotic mesenchymal cells develop myofilament proteins, synthesize creatine kinase, and acquire membrane sensitivity to acetylcholine, they become recognizable as myoblasts, both *in*

TABLE 1. *The major stages of human brain development*

Time of occurrence (weeks)	Stages of human development		Major events	
3–4	Neurulation	Notochord	Neural plate	Neural tube
				Neural crest cells
			Neural tube	Brain differentiation of prosencephalon, mesencephalon and rhombencephalon at 20 days
				Spinal cord
				Dura
				Cranium and vertebra
			Neural crest cells	Dorsal root ganglia
				Pia and arachnoid
				Schwann cells
				Autonomic ganglia, etc.
4–7	Caudal neural tube formation	Canalization followed by regressive differentiation		
5–6	Ventral induction	Precordal mesoderm	Face and forebrain	
		Prosencephalon	Cleavage of prosencephalon into cerebral vesicles to form the 2 cerebral hemispheres at 33 days	
8–16	Neuronal proliferation	Cellular proliferation in the ventricular and subventricular zones	Differentiation of hypothalamus	
			Optic vesicles	
			Olfactory bulbs and tracts	
		Proliferation of vascular tree, particularly venous	First fibers in internal capsule at 41 days	
		Interkynetic nuclear migration	Thalamus and basal ganglia	
		Neuroblasts		
		Glioblasts		
12–20	Migration	Radial migration in cerebrum	Cortical lamination	
			Neuronal migration is completed in the cerebral cortex at about 5 months postnatally	
		Radial tangential migration in the cerebellum	Completed at about 1 year postnatally	
24 to postnatal	Organization	Late neuronal migration in cerebrum and cerebellum		
		Alignment, orientation and layering of cortical neurons		
		Synaptic contacts		
		Proliferation of glia and differentiation		
Peak at birth to years postnatal	Myelination	Bulbospinal tracts	24 to postnatal	
		Motor roots	24 to postnatal	
		Medial lemniscus	24 to postnatal	
		Pyramidal tract	38 to 2 years postnatally	
		Frontopontine tract	7–8 months to postnatal to 2 years	
		Corpus callosum	4 months postnatal to 16 years	

vivo and *in vitro*. Myoblast proliferation is extensive by 7 weeks gestation, and at that time, these cells begin to form primary myotubes. Myotubes are nonmitotic, multinucleated, elongated cells that occur in clusters of 4 to 12. Intervening spaces between clusters of myotubes contain other mesodermal cells, such as fibroblasts and probably angioblasts as well as additional myoblasts.

The nuclei of myotubes are arranged in a linear fashion in the center of the fiber. The space between nuclei is occupied by mitochondria and other organelles; contractile filaments form a peripheral cylinder and align themselves in parallel. Thus, sarcomeres with distinct Z-bands are formed. Primary myotubes continue to develop until their numbers correspond to the preprogrammed number of muscle fibers for a specific muscle. By 15 weeks of gestation, primary myotubes approach a more mature state, and often, undifferentiated mononuclear cells are enclosed within the same basal lamina, as "satellite cells."

As maturation proceeds, myofibrils increase in number and size. Nuclei migrate to the periphery of the myofiber, which is surrounded by its own basal lamina, termed the *sarcolemma*. Numerous individual undifferentiated satellite cells continue to divide and fuse beneath the basal lamina of these immature muscle fibers until the 30th week of embryonic development. Some remain separated even during postnatal development and constitute the satellite cell population seen in neonatal muscle biopsies.

It is not until the 18th or 19th gestational week that histochemical fiber types may be first recognized. Before that time all fibers react as subtype 2C with calcium-mediated myofibrillar adenosine triphosphatase (ATPase) stains. Subsequently, small numbers of type 1 fibers (slow twitch, oxidative) appear, followed by subtype 2B (fast twitch, glycolytic) and finally type 2A (fast twitch, oxidative, glycolytic). As type 1 fibers develop, they grow more rapidly and are larger in size than type 2 fibers. They always remain uniformly distributed and are never grouped in normal fetal muscle. By 24 weeks of gestation, about 10% of fetal fibers are type 1 and/or larger fibers (i.e., Wohlfart b fibers). By 28 weeks gestation, types 1 and 2 fibers are present in mature proportions, and differences in size of the two myofibers types are no longer easily detectable. At term, 10% of type 2C fibers persist (19,28), whereas in the adult, 2C fibers represent only 5% of type 2 fibers or about 2.5% of the total myofibers.

Table 2 summarizes the major stages of human muscle development. The time of initial formation of neuromuscular contact during structural maturation of the neuromuscular junction has not been defined precisely. Intramuscular nerves may be recognized during the 8th week of gestation. Primitive neuromuscular contacts appear during the 9th or 10th gestational week (37).

Although myoblast differentiation, fusion, and subsequent myotube formation occur independently of neural influence in tissue culture, long-term motor neuronal inductive inputs are required for further development and maintenance of muscle fibers. Afferent nerves are known to have a greater inductive effect than motor innervation on differentiation of intrafustal muscle fibers and muscle spindle formation (49,50,80). Thus, mesodermal cells initiate the formation of myotubes in-

TABLE 2. *The major stages of human muscle development*

Time of occurrence gestational age (weeks)	Stages of human muscle development	Major events
<5	Premyoblastic	Mesenchymal cells not differentiated
5–8	Myoblastic	Active mitosis and fusion of mesenchymal cells
		Synthesis of actin and myosin
8–9		Intramuscular nerves
9–10		Primitive neuromuscular contact (Motor end-plates)
8–15	Myotubular	Mitosis ended
		Alignment of myofilaments
		Formation of sarcomeres
		Connective tissue septae divide muscle into fascicles
15–20	Immature myocytic	Migration of nuclei toward periphery
18–24	Early histochemical	Appearance of type I
		Wolfhart b (large size, more differentiated)
		Later appearance of type 2B then 2A
24–28	Late histochemical	Mature proportion of type 1 and type 2 fibers
		Fibers equal in size
28+	Mature myocytic	Maturation (morphological and histological)

dependently of neuronal stimulation, but neuronal influence is crucial for further maturation of muscle fibers.

Several studies have demonstrated the importance of trophic nerves on development, maturation, and differentiation of muscle fibers (9,10). If denervation occurs before 20 weeks gestation, there is failure of differentiation into fiber subtypes. This phenomenon also occurs, albeit less pronounced, following the administration of curare. The period that is most sensitive to denervation occurs during the 9th or 10th week of gestation and corresponds to the time during which spinal motor axons enter the limb and extend to the periphery. In the chick, the first neuromuscular junctions form at the same time that the first myotubes are detected in the limb (52,59).

Motor neurons and muscles differentiate in parallel fashion. Thus, motor axons reach their target at the same time that myoblasts form myotubes and muscle cell nuclei migrate to the subsarcolemmal region (45). It is often thought that the neuromuscular interaction occurs only in the direction of nerve to muscle. However, these interactions should be considered bidirectional. Thus, during development, muscle also exerts a powerful regulatory influence on the nerve that innervates it. The regulation of motor neuron function by muscles involves three major aspects:

1. Muscles determine the specificity of connections of nerve fibers to individual muscles.
2. Muscles help to determine the number of motor neuroblasts surviving to maturity.
3. Finally, muscles are involved in the refinement of connection during periods of synapse elimination. Polysynaptic innervation of muscle fibers is transient.

During the period immediately following motor neuron proliferation, a large fraction of immature motor neurons die. This phenomenon has been studied most extensively in mice and chicks (4,36,62) but occurs in all species with nervous systems, including simple nematode worms and insects. One hypothesis proposes that spinal muscular atrophy results from failure of the mechanism that arrests the physiological death of surplus motor neuroblasts in the embryo (76). Thus, a normal developmental process may become pathological by persistence into late fetal and postnatal life.

Abnormal suprasegmental influences from a dysplastic brainstem, cerebellum, and/or cerebrum on the developing motor unit may potentially alter the rate of maturation of striated muscles or cause abnormal proportions and sizes of histochemical fiber types. In order to alter the histochemical profile of muscle, the cerebral disorder must exert its influence between the 18th and 28th weeks of gestation. Thus, birth trauma or asphyxia in full-term and in most premature infants would not contribute significantly to these developmental abnormalities of muscle.

The association of cerebral abnormalities with progressive muscular dystrophy has been recognized for many years (29). These conditions are generally termed the *congenital muscular dystrophies*. Although the term congenital muscular dystrophy has become widely accepted, it is a poor label because by definition all muscular dystrophies are genetically determined and hence could be considered congenital diseases. It would be more accurate to refer to such conditions as symptomatic at birth or in early infancy. Other conditions with involvement of both brain and muscle include certain congenital myopathies and cerebral dysgeneses, notably cerebellar hypoplasia.

Thus, these disorders with involvement of both muscle and brain may be classified as (a) muscular dystrophies of early onset and associated with central nervous system abnormalities; (b) congenital myopathies; and (c) delayed muscle maturation with cerebellar hypoplasia and other cerebral dysgeneses.

MUSCULAR DYSTROPHIES OF EARLY ONSET

The muscular dystrophies of early onset, i.e., which are clinically symptomatic at birth or during early infancy, may be classified further into several subcategories:

1. Fukuyama muscular dystrophy;
2. cerebro-ocular dysplasia-muscular dystrophy syndrome;

3. heterogeneous muscular dystrophies associated with possible intellectual problems, other central nervous system abnormalities, and/or hypodensity of cerebral white matter on CT scan;
4. Duchenne (and Becker) muscular dystrophy;
5. neonatal myotonic dystrophy.

Fukuyama Muscular Dystrophy

The combination of muscular dystrophy evident at birth and central nervous system abnormalities was first described in Japan by Fukuyama (31). This autosomal
recessive disease is characterized by clinical abnormalities suggestive of both myopathy and encephalopathy during the first few months of life (30). This type of
congenital muscular dystrophy was thought to be confined to Japan, but cases have
been reported recently from Australia (29), Holland (48), Canada (57), and in non-
Japanese Americans (61).

In Japan, the ratio of Duchenne dystrophy to the Fukuyama form of muscular
dystrophy is 2.8:1 (86). The incidence of Duchenne muscular dystrophy in Japan
is similar to that in the United States, i.e., 13 to 33 per 100,000 liveborn males
(90). Prevalence in the population is approximately 2.8 per 100,000. A high percentage of mothers of patients with Fukuyama muscular dystrophy have spontaneous abortions, and mothers often report decreased fetal movements (31). At birth,
the affected infants are hypotonic with poor suck and weak cry. The face is ex-
pressionless and weakness is generalized, although proximal muscles are more severely affected than distal muscles. Contractures, principally of the knees and
elbows, are frequently present at birth or may develop subsequently. Fifty percent
of patients present with pseudohypertrophy of muscles, most often the gastroc-
nemii, and 30% of affected infants exhibit a funnel-shaped chest deformity.

Both afebrile and febrile convulsions are observed in more than 50% of cases of
Fukuyama muscular dystrophy. Myopia occurs frequently but more severe ocular
abnormalities are observed only rarely. Motor and intellectual development is retarded. Only a small percentage of affected children are able to stand by 4 years
of age and independent walking is achieved rarely because of weakness and
progressive contractures. Death occurs usually around 10 years of age. Muscle
biopsies demonstrate nonspecific dystrophic changes and extensive endomysial
connective tissue proliferation. Fifty percent of cases of Fukuyama muscular dystrophy show abnormalities on CT scan, which usually consist of a reduction of
white matter and, in some cases, moderate ventricular dilatation (23).

The major pathological change observed in the central nervous system is polymicrogyria of the cerebral cortex and cerebellum, associated with neuronal hetero-
topias. Restricted areas of pachygyria or agyria have also been reported (31).
Partial fusion of the cerebral hemispheres, as well as aberrant formation of the
pyramidal tracts, also has been described.

Cerebro-ocular Dysplasia with Muscular Dystrophy

The central nervous system involvement associated with the syndrome of cere-bro-ocular dysplasia with muscular dystrophy varies from ocular anomalies to severe central nervous system abnormalities. Congenital hypotonia, joint contrac-tures affecting multiple joints, as well as mental retardation and hydrocephalus, are common findings (16,87).

The cerebral malformations consist of agyria, varying degrees of polymicrogy-ria, hypomyelination of cerebral white matter, diffuse leptomeningeal gliodermal proliferation with neuronal heterotopia, cerebellar polymicrogyria and hypoplasia, and absence of the pyramidal tracts. Partial fusion of the frontal lobes occurs fre-quently.

Ocular pathology includes corneal abnormalities, congenital cataracts, anterior chamber angle abnormalities, retinal dysplasia with or without retinal detachment, and hypoplasia of optic nerves (87). The muscle biopsies demonstrate nonspecific dystrophic changes as well as foci of inflammation that are more frequent than in Fukuyama muscular dystrophy. Death occurs frequently before 2 years of age. Santavuori et al. (70) have described a similar syndrome with longer survival. A more heterogeneous group of patients may be identified with muscular dystrophy of early onset, normal or decreased intelligence, macrocephaly, and epilepsy. Hy-podensity of subcortical white matter is evident on the cerebral CT scans of these children, and white matter spongiosis is found histologically (20,88).

Duchenne Muscular Dystrophy

Microscopic examinations of the brain have demonstrated minor morphological abnormalities in boys with Duchenne muscular dystrophy (21,66). In this type of dystrophy, walking is often delayed, but this delay in gross motor development is probably owing to the myopathy rather than the CNS factors. Subsequently, proxi-mal weakness, lumbar lordosis, and neck flexor weakness become manifest be-tween ages 3 and 5 years. Scoliosis and contractures develop later and cardiac involvement is common. At least one-third of patients have evidence of mental subnormality, and only 10% of the children have above average intelligence. The muscle biopsy is diagnostic. Death usually occurs late in the second decade.

Myotonic Dystrophy

Myotonic dystrophy is an autosomal dominant disease with great variability in expression and penetrance (34). Clinical abnormalities occur in many organ sys-tems, including eyes, gonads, and other endocrine organs, as well as brain and pituitary. Patients have weakness of facial and jaw muscles, ptosis of eyelids, and distal limb weakness. Myotonia appears generally after 5 years of age. Mental re-tardation is a frequent finding, and minor morphological abnormalities have been described in the brains of affected children (67).

The muscle biopsies demonstrate atrophy or hypoplasia of histochemical type 1 fibers (13), which may be so marked that they appear as nuclear clumps. Generally, there is an increase in the number of myofibers with internal nuclei. The features described above are characteristic of the mature form of the disease and differ from those observed in the neonatal form of myotonic dystrophy (22).

Infants who are symptomatic during the newborn period are usually born to affected mothers, and pregnancy is often complicated by polyhydramnios, poor fetal movements (77), and an increased rate of spontaneous abortion. Other maternal complications include prolonged first stage of labor, diminished uterine contraction during the second stage, retained placenta, postpartum hemorrhage, and sensitivity to anesthetic agents (35).

The clinical features of congenital myotonic dystrophy include characteristic facial weakness with a tented upper lip (carp mouth appearance) (1,77). Jaw weakness is also pronounced. This combination of facial and jaw weakness is largely responsible for the feeding problems as well as the respiratory difficulties encountered in these infants. Newborns are severely hypotonic and often areflexic at birth. Delayed motor development, mental retardation, and ankle contractures are observed frequently. Decreased peristalsis, abdominal distension, and constipation result from involvement of smooth muscle of the bowel wall (77).

The muscle pathology in affected infants demonstrates several unusual features (43,79) that evolve into more typical changes of myotonic dystrophy with maturation. In early infancy, there is marked hypoplasia of muscles, particularly affecting respiratory muscles. Muscle fibers are reduced in diameter and number. The muscle biopsy demonstrates delayed or arrested maturation of fibers in all stages of development. The fibers appear round in cross section, and the presence of central nuclei in association with histochemical and ultrastructural features of myotubes denotes the immaturity of the fiber (Fig. 1).

Although myotubes are recognized most frequently, more detailed analysis with electron microscopy discloses scattered primitive myoblasts and an excessive number of satellite cells. Muscle fibers with peripheral sarcolemmal nuclei but lacking histochemical differentiation may also be noted. Occasional fibers appear mature with complete differentiation. The involvement is variable in different muscles in the same infant. The largest number of immature fibers is observed in the muscles associated with joint contractures, as well as in the diaphragm and the pharyngeal muscles. In contrast to findings in the muscle biopsies of older children or adults with this disease, active degenerative changes are absent. Endomysial fibrosis, split fibers, and striated annulets also are not common. Atrophy of predominantly type 1 muscle fibers may be observed in early infancy in muscles that are not severely affected by maturational delay (2). Occasional infants with myotonic dystrophy have presented with congenital muscle fiber-type disproportion (CMFTD) or decreased size of type 1 myofibers (2). Immaturity of striated muscle in neonatal myotonic dystrophy may be accompanied by features of dysmaturity of other organs, especially the lungs. These observations support the concept of arrest or abnormal development of muscle at specific stages of development, rather than active degeneration (79).

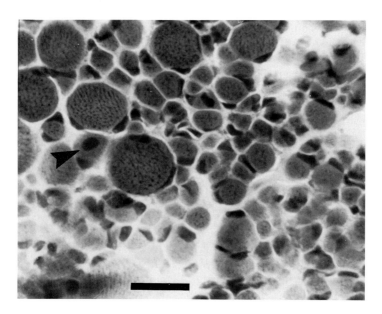

FIG. 1. Vastus lateralis muscle biopsy of neonate with myotonic dystrophy, already symptomatic at birth with weakness, hypotonia, areflexia, fascial wasting, and contractures. All stages of muscle fiber development are seen, including small immature myocytes lacking histochemical differentiation, large mature myofibers, scattered centronuclear myotubes (*arrowhead*), and primitive myoblasts (seen with EM). Modified Gomori trichrome stain. Bar = 15 μm.

The muscular dystrophies, including Duchenne and myotonic dystrophies, are genetic diseases. The expression of the genetic abnormality is not limited to striated muscle but in fact affects every cell in the body. On the other hand, factors other than the primary genetic defect and degeneration of muscle fibers may influence muscle development in the muscular dystrophies. Thus, type 1 fiber predominance is common in Duchenne muscular dystrophy as well as in Fukuyama muscular dystrophy, and selective type 1 myofiber atrophy is prominent in myotonic dystrophy.

Investigation of hereditary muscular dystrophy in hamsters shows that muscle fiber maturation may be altered either by selective denervation of specific muscles or by hypophysectomy (39,40,42,44). Similarly, growth hormone deficiency in human Duchenne muscular dystrophy alters the expression of the mutant gene. Although the muscle biopsy of patients with growth hormone deficiency still demonstrates features of dystrophy with necrosis, inflammation, and fibrosis, there is modification of the clinical expression of the gene such that the weakness appears less marked (91). Thus, it appears that influences other than those of peripheral nerve or genetically determined factors may play a role in the expression of dystrophy and in the maturation of muscle fibers.

Upper motor neuron lesions during embryonic life may also explain histochemical alterations in other muscle diseases, i.e., the congenital myopathies. CMFTD and fiber-type predominance, in particular, are associated with cerebellar hypoplasia and developmental anomalies of the brainstem (73).

CONGENITAL MYOPATHIES

Because many congenital myopathies present clinically with hypotonia in the newborn period, they may be difficult to distinguish on clinical grounds alone. Electromyography may demonstrate normal or nonspecific mild myopathic features. In these situations, the muscle biopsy often provides the definitive diagnosis.

Congenital Muscle Fiber-type Disproportion

CMFTD is characterized by disproportion in sizes and ratios of fiber-types (26,71,72). Type 1 fibers are uniformly smaller in size and more numerous than type 2 fibers, often constituting 80% of total fibers. Autosomal dominant and recessive forms have been reported, but most cases are sporadic and probably not genetically determined. Affected children often have delayed motor milestones but normal intellectual development (11,53). Muscle weakness is disproportionately mild compared to the hypotonia, and tendon stretch reflexes may be diminished or even absent (26). Skeletal abnormalities, including contractures, congenital hip dislocation, kyphoscoliosis, clubfeet, high-arched palate, dolichocephaly, and small stature are characteristic findings (14). The hypotonia and weakness may appear to progress clinically during the first 2 years of life. Subsequently, improvement usually becomes evident, concomitant with natural growth and development. Although contractures may lead to significant disability in some patients, many children do not become functionally disabled.

There is considerable support for the hypothesis that CMFTD is not a primary disease of muscle. The normal morphological appearance of motor neurons and the myopathic motor unit profile by electromyography suggests that this is a developmental disease of skeletal muscle cells. No specific cellular or molecular abnormality has been identified. The hypertrophy of the type 2 fibers is probably compensatory (12).

There is increasing recognition of the fact that abnormal suprasegmental innervation of muscle in the fetus may alter fiber-type differentiation. Thus, midthoracic spinal cord transection in neonatal rats causes developmental arrest in the soleus muscles in the stage of late histochemical differentiation (55). Cerebral control of motor neurons is involved in the differentiation of slow myosin isoenzyme (54). However, the muscle of neonatal rats is much less mature at birth than human muscle. Human infants with cerebral dysgenesis or lacking corticospinal tracts at birth but with normal brainstem and cerebellum do not demonstrate abnormalities or changes in the skeletal muscle maturation or the histochemical differentiation of muscle. If the brain influences the differentiation of fiber types in the human fetus, suprasegmental pathways arising in the brainstem and cerebellum appear to be more important than those originating in the cerebral cortex (73).

CMFTD is a syndrome of diverse etiologies that has been reported in infants with myotonic dystrophy (2), Krabbe's globoid cell leukodystrophy with neuropathy (17,56), fetal alcohol syndrome (56), glycogenoses II and III (56), and rigid spine syndrome (17) and may be associated also with central nuclei in muscle (81).

The characteristic clinical pattern associated with nemaline rod disease is similar to that of CMFTD. In addition to nemaline rods, type 1 fiber predominance and smallness of type 1 fibers are found in the muscle biopsy. This association suggests a common pathogenesis for these conditions. Thus, CMFTD may represent the primary developmental disorder, whereas nemaline rods represent a secondary reaction of muscle. Figures 2 and 3 illustrate these two entities.

Some studies suggest that CMFTD is a developmental disorder of muscle that arises secondary to neurogenic influences (71). It has been postulated that an abnormally high rate of embryonic cell death early in gestation may result in abnormally large permanent motor units supplied by surviving motor neurons. A continuous rapid rate of discharge of these motor neurons may represent an attempt to induce growth of muscle fibers. The result would be maturation of muscle fibers and induction of histochemical type 1 fibers, but the large size of the motor units would prevent individual fibers from achieving a normal diameter.

The consistent occurrence of CMFTD in Krabbe's disease supports a neurogenic

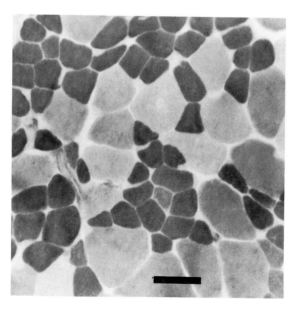

FIG. 2. Congenital muscle fiber-type disproportion. Histochemical type I myofibers (dark) are uniformly smaller and more numerous than type II fibers (light). Myofibrillar adenosine triphosphatase (ATPase), preincubated at pH 4.6. Bar = 20 μm.

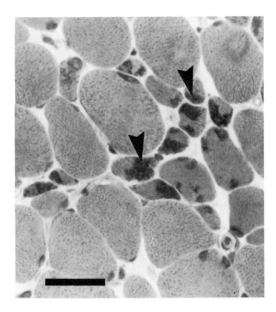

FIG. 3. Muscle biopsy of 2-year-old child with nemaline rod disease. The rod structures (*arrowheads*) aggregate selectively in the small myofibers that stain histochemically at type I uniformly. The large fibers free of rods are type II. Modified Gomori trichrome stain. Bar = 15 μm.

etiology (17). Segmental demyelination, as well as axonal degeneration of peripheral nerves, occurs in this disease, but these neuropathic changes are not usually evident in early infancy, whereas CMFTD and involvement of central brainstem tracts are already prominent at birth.

Fully mature motor neurons are able to sustain abnormally large motor units, and this fact provides the basis of histochemical type grouping in muscles of adult patients with neuropathy and reinnervation of denervated motor units. Nevertheless, even if the individual muscle fibers of these large adult motor units are not uniformly small as in CMFTD, often a greater than normal variability of muscle fiber diameter persists within the group, and many fibers remain atrophic. Consequently, if the mature motor neuron cannot exert a uniform trophic control over an excessively large motor unit, an immature one would be expected to exert even less uniform control. Thus a minority of motor neurons in CMFTD may innervate a relatively small number of muscle fibers, and these may represent the motor units capable of differentiating into type 2 fibers. The large size of the type 2 muscle fibers in CMFTD is more pronounced in older infants and children than in neonates and probably represents compensatory hypertrophy in motor units of nearly normal size.

In some nonprogressive congenital neuromuscular diseases of developmental origin, most muscle fibers are differentiated histochemically as type 1 fibers, whereas type 2 fibers are sparse or fail to develop (18,63). Perinatal neuropathies or infantile anterior horn cell diseases are distinguished from conditions with hypoplasia of type 1 muscle fibers by the presence of hypertrophic type 1 muscle fibers that are mostly grouped. The giant fibers observed in infantile spinal muscular atrophy (Werdnig-Hoffmann disease) are probably related to small motor units that are not affected and undergo compensatory hypertrophy. The fact that they are mainly type 1 fibers supports the concept that a continuous rapid rate of discharge of motor neurons induces growth of immature muscle fibers.

Thus, perinatal muscle undergoing a high rate of neural stimulation is characterized by muscle fiber hypertrophy if the motor unit is small and in fiber hypoplasia if the motor unit is large. However, in both situations, the neural stimulation induces histochemical type 1 muscle fibers (51,69).

Centronuclear Myopathies

Central nuclei in muscle fibers represent a nonspecific myopathic finding. Internal nuclei may be a secondary phenomenon resulting from migration of the nucleus from the normal subsarcolemmal position, e.g., polymyositis, or may reflect retention of the primitive embryonic position in the myofiber caused by delayed maturation. In addition to central nuclei, the criteria for true myotubes include lack of histochemical differentiation and confinement of oxidative enzymatic activity to mitochondria and glycogen to central zones between nuclei rather than interspersed throughout the intermyofibrillar spaces (Fig. 4). Furthermore, ultrastructural findings of delayed maturation of the sarcotubular system and triad formation may be present (72). Neonatal myopathies that demonstrate large numbers of fetal myotubes may be regarded as true myotubular myopathies. However, older children with centronuclear myopathies, who lack the accompanying criteria of myotubes, have been described erroneously as "myotubular myopathy." The lack of precision in the use of this term has led to considerable confusion in the literature.

The centronuclear myopathies are a group of diseases characterized by the internal position of nuclei in many muscle fibers observed on muscle biopsy. The muscle fibers are usually abnormally small in caliber. The central area of increased activity of oxidative enzymes and decreased activity of ATPase within fibers suggests persistence of fetal myotubes (84). Three major categories have been identified and are described below.

The clinical features of neonatal X-linked centronuclear myopathy include severe hypotonia and weakness (5). Pregnancy is often complicated by decreased fetal movements and polyhydramnios. Hypotonia, diminished or absent cry, suck, cough, and swallow reflexes, as well as respiratory distress, are evident immediately after birth. Assisted ventilation is often needed and severe dysphagia may necessitate feeding by nasogastric tube. Although there is often a fatal outcome during infancy, progression of muscle weakness does not occur if the patient survives beyond this time. Muscle tissue studied many months after birth demonstrates no further maturation, with persistence of 90% predominance of myotubes (78).

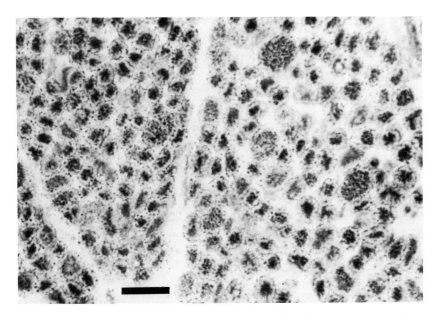

FIG. 4. Muscle biopsy of neonate with myotubular myopathy. More than 90% of total myofibers are small centronuclear fibers showing mitochondrial oxidative enzymatic activity in the center of the fiber between nuclei and in the subsarcolemmal region. Note the few large, more mature fibers with a mature trabeculated network of activity in the intermyofibrillar sarcoplasm. NADH-TR. Bar = 20 μm.

In the second type, clinical abnormalities become apparent in early childhood. At birth, these children may demonstrate generalized hypotonia and ptosis without external ophthalmoplegia. Affected children have delayed motor milestones during infancy with slowly progressive ophthalmoplegia, facial and proximal muscle weakness, and loss of deep tendon reflexes. Autosomal dominant inheritance has been suggested but has not been confirmed. Among these patients, there is a relatively high frequency of convulsions, mental deficiency, and abnormal electroencephalograms. These features support the hypothesis that the observed muscle changes may be secondary to a primary defect in the developing central nervous system.

In the third type, the onset of clinical abnormalities is more insidious and may remain unnoticed during the first and second decades (33). Clinical presentation is usually one of progressive limb girdle weakness, affecting mainly the legs. Autosomal dominant inheritance is the rule.

It is unknown whether the central nucleation in these conditions is a result of failure of migration of nuclei from the primitive myotubular position or whether the nuclei return to a central position from the periphery. In centronuclear myopathies, studies of spinal cord, motor end plates, and intramuscular nerves have all been normal (25).

Nemaline Rod Myopathy

The distinguishing feature of this congenital myopathy is the presence within muscle fibers of multiple small rod-like inclusions that represent structural proteins derived from the Z-band. This myopathy is associated with predominance of type 1 muscle fibers, frank CMFTD, or almost complete failure of differentiation of type 2 fibers.

Clinically, muscular hypotonia that may be mild or severe is evident in all cases during the first year of life. There may be respiratory or feeding difficulties. Motor development is delayed. However, severe cases have been reported at birth with immediate respiratory difficulties and neonatal death (41,83).

In milder cases, motor skills improve slowly during childhood, associated with growth. Thus, the condition is often considered benign. However, muscles of proximal and distal limbs, trunk, and neck are small and weak, and this involvement may be associated with considerable lumbar lordosis. In addition, there may be weakness of facial, pharyngeal, and laryngeal muscles. Weakness of extraocular muscles is not a feature of this disease.

The inheritance pattern has been the subject of great interest. It appears that only an autosomal dominant mode of inheritance with reduced penetrance could explain the findings (3). Asymptomatic family members may demonstrate rods in muscle fibers (7). Other changes include smallness and predominance of type 1 muscle fibers, internal nuclei, and nonspecific myopathic changes (3,7).

A disease of late onset with nemaline rods is manifest by a limb-girdle syndrome, affecting predominantly the lower extremities (24). Onset is usually during the 5th or 6th decade, and this disease is probably not related to congenital nemaline rod disease or other developmental disorders. In nemaline myopathy of childhood onset, abundant rods are present within a majority of type 1 fibers with marked reduction or complete absence of histochemical type 2 fibers. Persisting type 2 fibers also contain sparse rods.

Rods are composed principally of actin and alpha-actinin and originate in the Z-bands. Rods do not occur in intrafusal muscle fibers or in smooth muscles (41). These observations, in addition to the fact that type 1 fibers are affected principally, has raised the possibility that a neural abnormality may be responsible for rod formation. Failure of differentiation of the type 2 lower motor neuron has been postulated. Studies of the spinal cord in nemaline myopathy have been inconclusive. One report described a quantitative reduction in the number of lower motor neuron cell bodies in lumbar cord (15,47), whereas another (65) concluded that the number of motor neurons is normal but that their size is reduced.

Because nemaline rods originate in the Z-bands, a lesion that might precede the formation of nemaline rods is Z-band streaming. Z-band streaming is a phenomenon observed both in normal and abnormal muscles (58). Cases with nemaline rods as well as central cores and focal loss of cross-striations within the same muscle and even within the same muscle fibers have been reported (8). These observations suggest a common origin for all three lesions.

Another hypothesis suggests that nemaline rods in human muscle result from longitudinal splitting and disruption of muscle fibers secondary to deficient regeneration of myofibrils associated with neurotrophic abnormality (32).

A third hypothesis proposes that nemaline rod formation in the congenital disorder may be associated with the persistence of a fetal type of myosin (85). The type 1 fiber predominance in congenital nemaline rod disease is associated with the substitution of a hybrid slow myosin light-chain electrophoretic pattern for the mixed pattern of myosin found in normal muscle (89).

CEREBELLAR HYPOPLASIA ASSOCIATED WITH MATURATION ABNORMALITY OF MUSCLE FIBERS

Recent studies report the association of altered histochemical profiles in muscle of children with cerebellar hypoplasia (73). These children have variable causes for their cerebellar abnormality, and the latter is not necessarily associated with cerebral malformations (75).

The muscle abnormality associated most frequently with cerebellar hypoplasia appears to be a lack of maturation of muscle or a numerical predominance of a specific fiber type, either type 1 or type 2 (Fig. 5). Delayed maturation and/or de-

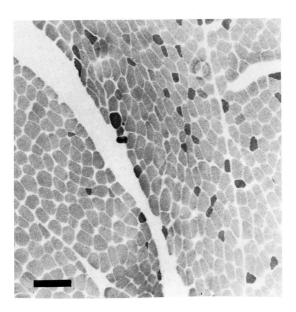

FIG. 5. Vastus lateralis muscle biopsy of a 6-year-old boy with cerebellar hypoplasia but no primary neuromuscular disease. More than 90% of total myofibers are type I (light), whereas only a few scattered type II fibers (dark) are differentiated. Fiber type-predominance is common in the presence of suprasegmental disease influencing fetal muscle development *in utero*. Myofibrillar adenosine triphosphatase (ATPase), preincubated at pH 9.8. Bar = 50 μm.

creased size of either type 1 or type 2 muscle fibers are other known abnormalities associated with these conditions. The only consistent clinical finding in affected children is moderate or severe hypotonia, which may be associated with mild weakness, ataxia, nystagmus, and depressed tendon stretch reflexes (73).

In summary, changes in muscle fibers associated with cerebellar hypoplasia may be classified into three categories:

1. Maturational delay or arrest with incomplete histochemical differentiation;
2. Fiber-type predominance of more than 80% of either type 1 or type 2 muscle fibers;
3. CMFTD involving selective hypotrophy of type 1 fibers as well as type 1 fiber predominance.

Infants with a dysplastic brainstem and almost complete absence of descending motor fibers to the spinal cord have demonstrated normal muscle development and maturation of histochemical profiles, indicating that motor units are capable of developing normally at the segmental spinal level (73,74). However, abnormal suprasegmental impulses during the stage of histochemical differentiation between the 18th and 28th week of gestation may alter development. The cerebellum has no direct efferent pathway to the spinal cord but exerts inhibitory influences by means of the Purkinje cells. Thus, the influence of the cerebellum on motor function affects the thalamus and subsequently the motor cortex to modify corticospinal tract function. In addition, there are direct Purkinje cell projections to the vestibular nuclei and brainstem reticular formation.

The corticospinal tract is the only direct pathway from the forebrain to the spinal cord. Between 18 and 28 weeks of gestation, the corticospinal tract is small and unmyelinated and its influence on muscle control and muscle development is probably insignificant. However, small descending bulbospinal pathways (also called subcorticospinal pathways) mature at precisely the same time as histochemical differentiation of muscle occurs and may play an important role in muscle development. These pathways include the vestibulospinal, reticulospinal, olivospinal, tectospinal, and rubrospinal tracts. Many of these descending tracts have medial and lateral divisions within the brainstem, often with antagonistic function. At the time of birth, the myelination of the subcorticospinal pathways is much more advanced than that of the corticospinal tracts. The subcorticospinal pathways may play a significant role during the neonatal period and early infancy, as is evident from the normal postural changes observed in premature infants as well as the abnormal postures observed in infants with neurological disease (63). However, opisthotonic posturing, strong adduction of the thumbs, and the flexion of the fingers and toes in term infants may result from injury of the cerebral cortex without significant impairment of brainstem function.

In summary, selective type 1 myofiber atrophy is a prominent feature of congenital myotonic dystrophy, whereas type 1 fiber predominance is common in Duchenne and Fukuyama muscular dystrophies. Congenital myopathies demonstrate changes compatible with developmental arrest or abnormality of development of muscle fibers. Infants with cerebellar hypoplasia demonstrate altered histochemical profiles of muscle fibers. Although recent studies support the concept of a close relationship between muscle fibers and upper motor neurons, more detailed correlation of muscle development in relation to specific central tracts is needed. Whether suprasegmental effects modulate, stimulate, or inhibit muscle maturation is an important unresolved question.

REFERENCES

1. Aicardi, J., Conti, D., and Goutieres, F. (1974): Les formes neo-natales de la dystrophie myotonique de Steinert. *J. Neurol. Sci.,* 22:149–164.
2. Argov, Z., Gardner Medwin, D., Johnson, M.A., and Mastaglia, F.L. (1980): Congenital myotonic dystrophy. Fibre-type abnormalities in two cases. *Arch. Neurol.,* 37:693–696.
3. Arts, W.F., Bethlem, J., Dingemans, K.P., et al. (1978): Investigations on the inheritance of nemaline myopathy. *Arch. Neurol.,* 35:72–77.
4. Banker, B.Q. (1981): Physiologic death of neuron in the developing anterior horn of the mouse. In: *Human Motor Neuron Diseases,* edited by L.P. Rowland, pp. 473–491. Raven Press, New York.
5. Barth, P.G., Van Wijngaarden, G.K., and Bethlem, J. (1975): X-linked myotubular myopathy with fatal neonatal asphyxia. *Neurology,* 25:531–536.
6. Bellairs, R., and Portch, P.A. (1977): Somite formation in the chick. In: *Vertebrate Limb and Somite Morphogenesis,* edited by D.A. Ede, J.R. Hinchliffe, Jr., and M. Balls, pp. 449–463. Cambridge University Press, Cambridge, England.
7. Bender, A.N., and Willner, J.P. (1978): Nemaline (rod) myopathy: The need for histochemical evaluation of affected families. *Ann. Neurol.,* 4:37–42.
8. Bethlem, J., Arts, W.F., and Dingemans, K.P. (1978): Common origin of rods, cores, miniature cores, and focal loss of cross-striation. *Arch. Neurol.,* 35:555–556.
9. Bonner, P.H. (1978): Nerve dependent changes in clonable myoblast populations. *Dev. Biol.,* 66:207–219.
10. Bonner, P.H., and Hauschka, S.D. (1978): Clonal analysis of vertebrate morphogenesis. 1. Early developmental events in the chick limb. *Dev. Biol.,* 37:317–328.
11. Brooke, M.H., Carroll, J.E., and Ringel, S.P. (1979): Congenital hypotonia revisited. *Muscle Nerve,* 2:84–100.
12. Carpenter, S., and Karpati, G. (1984): Congenital fibre-type disproportion. In: *Pathology of Skeletal Muscle,* edited by S. Carpenter and G. Karpati, pp. 449–453. Churchill Livingston, Edinburgh.
13. Casanova, G., and Jerusalem, F. (1979): Myopathology of myotonic dystrophy: A morphometric study. *Acta Neuropathol., (Berl.),* 45:231–240.
14. Clancy, R.R., Kelts, K.A., and Oehlert, J.W. (1980): Clinical variability in congenital fibre-type disproportion. *J. Neurol. Sci.,* 46:257–266.
15. Dahl, D.S., and Klutxow, F.W. (1974): Congenital rod disease: Further evidence of innervational abnormalities as the basis for the clinicopathologic features. *J. Neurol. Sci.,* 23:371–385.
16. Dambska, M., Wisniewski Sher, J.H., and Solish, G. (1982): Cerebrooculo-muscular syndrome. A variant of Fukuyama congenital cerebromuscular dystrophy. *Clin. Neuropathol.,* 1:93–98.
17. Dehkharghani, F., Sarnat, H.B., Brewster, M.A., and Roth, S.I. (1981): Congenital muscle fibre type disproportion in Krabbe's leukodystrophy. *Arch. Neurol.,* 38:585–591.
18. Dinn, J.J., and O'Doherty, N. (1980): Congenital type 2 fibre deficient myopathy. *Ir. J. Med. Sci.,* 149:53–58.
19. Dubowitz, V. (1963): Enzymatic maturation of skeletal muscle. *Nature,* 197:1215.
20. Dubowitz, V. (1979): Involvement of the nervous system in muscular dystrophies in man. *Ann. NY Acad. Sci.,* 317:431–439.
21. Dubowitz, V., and Crome, L. (1969): The central nervous system in Duchenne muscular dystrophy. *Brain,* 92:805–808.
22. Dyken, P.R., and Harper, D.S. (1973): Congenital dystrophia myotonica. *Neurology,* 23:465–473.

23. Echenne, B., Arthuis, M., Billard, C., et al. (1986): Congenital muscular dystrophy and cerebral CT scan anomalies. *J. Neurol. Sci.*, 75:7–22.
24. Engel, A.G. (1986): Late onset rod myopathy (A new syndrome?). Light and electron microscopic observation in two cases. *Mayo Clin. Proc.*, 41:713–741.
25. Engel, W.K., Gold, G.N., and Karpati, G. (1968): Type 1 fibre hypotrophy and central nuclei: A rare congenital abnormality with a possible experimental model. *Arch. Neurol.*, 18:435–444.
26. Fardeau, M., Harpey, J.P., Caille, B., and Lafourcade, J. (1975): Hypotonies neo-natales avec disproportion congenitale des differents types de fibre musculaire et petitesse relative des fibres de Type 1. *Arch. Fr. Pediatr.*, 32:901–914.
27. Farkas-Bargeton, E., Diebler, M.F., Arsenio-Nunes, M.L., et al. (1977): Etude de la maturation histochimique, quantitative et ultrastructurale du muscle foetal humain. *J. Neurol. Sci.*, 31:245–259.
28. Fenichel, G.M. (1966): A histochemical study of developing human skeletal muscle. *Neurology*, 16:741–745.
29. Fowler, M., and Manson, J.I. (1973): Congenital muscular dystrophy with malformation of the central nervous system. In: *Clinical Studies in Myology. Part 2*, edited by B.A. Kakulas, pp. 192–197. Excerpta Medica, Amsterdam.
30. Fukuhara, N., Yuasa, T., Tsubaki, T., et al. (1978): Nemaline myopathy: Histological, histochemical and ultrastructural studies. *Acta Neuropathol.*, 42:33–41.
31. Fukuyama, Y., and Osawa, M. (1984): A genetic study of the Fukuyama type congenital muscular dystrophy. *Brain Dev.*, 6:373–380.
32. Fukuyama, Y., Osawa, M., and Suzuki, H. (1981): Congenital progressive muscular dystrophy of the Fukuyama type. Clinical, genetic and pathological considerations. *Brain Dev.*, 3:1–29.
33. Haninan, D.G.F., and Haleema, M.A. (1972): Centronuclear myopathy in old age. *J. Pathol.*, 108:237–248.
34. Harper, P.S. (1979): *Myotonic Dystrophy. Major Problems in Neurology*, vol. 9. W.B. Saunders, Philadelphia.
35. Harper, P.S. (1986): Myotonic disorders. In: *Myology*, edited by A.G. Engel and B.Q. Banker, pp. 1274–1276. McGraw-Hill, New York.
36. Hollyday, M., and Hamburger, V. (1976): Reduction of the naturally occurring motor neuron loss by enlargement of the periphery. *J. Comp. Neurol.*, 170:316–320.
37. Juntunen, J., and Teravainen, H. (1972): Structural development of myoneural junctions in the human embryo. *Histochemie*, 32:107–112.
38. Kamieniecka, Z. (1968): The stages of development of human fetal muscles with reference to some muscular diseases. *J. Neurol. Sci.*, 7:319–329.
39. Karpati, G. (1979): General discussion on hamster dystrophy. *Ann. NY Acad. Sci.*, 317:89–91.
40. Karpati, G., Armann, M., Carpenter, S., and Prescott, S. (1983): Reinnervation is followed by necrosis by denervated skeletal muscles of dystrophic hamsters. *Exp. Neurol.*, 82:358–365.
41. Karpati, G., Carpenter, S., and Anderman, F. (1971): A new concept of childhood nemaline myopathy. *Arch. Neurol.*, 24:291–304.
42. Karpati, G., Carpenter, S., and Prescott, S. (1982): Prevention of skeletal muscle fibre necrosis in hamster dystrophy. *Muscle Nerve*, 5:369–372.
43. Karpati, G., Carpenter, S., Watters, G.V., et al. (1973): Infantile myotonic dystrophy: Histochemical and electron microscopic features in skeletal muscle. *Neurology*, 23:1066–1077.
44. Karpati, G., Jacob, P., Carpenter, S., and Prescott, S. (1985): Hypophysectomy mitigates skeletal muscle fibre. Damage in hamster dystrophy. *Ann. Neurol.*, 17:60–64.
45. Kelly, A.M., and Zacks, S.I. (1969): The fine structure of motor end plate myogenesis. *J. Cell Biol.*, 42:154–169.
46. Kieny, M., and Chevalier, A. (1979): Autonomy of tendon development in the embryonic chick wing. *J. Embryol. Exp. Morphol.*, 49:153–165.
47. Konno, H., Iuasaki, Y., Yamamoto, T., and Inosaka, T. (1987): Nemaline bodies in spinal muscular atrophy. An autopsy case. *Acta Neuropathol.*, 74:84–88.
48. Krijgsman, J.B., Barth, P.G., Stam, F.C., Slooff, J.L., and Jaspar, H.H.J. (1980): Congenital muscular dystrophy and cerebral dysgenesis in a Dutch family. *Neuropadiatrie*, 11:108–120.
49. Kucera, J. (1981): Histochemical profile of cat intrafusal muscle fibres and their motor innervation. *Histochemistry*, 73:397–418.
50. Kucera, J. (1982): Histological study of an unusual cat muscle spindle deficient in motor innervation. *Anat. Embryol.*, 165:39–49.

51. Kugelburg, E. (1976): Adaptive transformation of rate soleus motor units during growth: Histochemistry and contraction speed. *J. Neurol. Sci.,* 27:269–289.
52. Landmesser, L., and Morris, D.G. (1975): The development of functional innervation in the hind limb of the chick, *J. Physiol.,* 249:301–326.
53. Lenard, H.G., and Goebel, H.H. (1975): Congenital fibre-type disproportion. *Neuropadiatrie,* 6:220–231.
54. Margreth, A., and Dalla Sibera, L. (1980): Postnatal changes in myosin composition of slow muscle in relation to the differentiation of motoneurons. *Muscle Nerve,* 3:273. (Abstract)
55. Margreth, A., Dalla Sibera, L., Salviati, G., and Ischia, N. (1980): Spinal transection and the postnatal differentiation of slow myosine isoenzymes. *Muscle Nerve,* 3:483–486.
56. Martin, J.J., Clara, R., Ceuterick, C., and Joris, C. (1976): Is congenital fibre-type disproportion a true myopathy? *Acta Neurol. Belg.,* 76:335–344.
57. McMenamin, J.B., Becker, L.E., and Murphy, E.G. (1982): Fukuyama type congenital muscular dystrophy. *J. Pediatr.,* 101:580–582.
58. Meltzer, H.Y., Kuncl, R.W., Click, J., and Yang, V. (1976): Incidence of Z-band streaming and myofibrillar disruptions in skeletal muscle from healthy young people. *Neurology,* 26:853–857.
59. Milfer, S.F., Searls, R.L., and Fonte, V.G. (1973): An ultrastructural study of early myogenesis in the chick wing bud. *Dev. Biol.,* 30:374–391.
60. Minquetti, G., and Mair, W.G.P. (1981): Ultrastructure of developing human muscles. *Biol. Neonate,* 40:276–294.
61. Nonaka, I., and Chou, S.M. (1979): Congenital muscular dystrophy. In: *Handbook of Clinical Neurology,* vol. 41, edited by P.J. Vinken and G.W. Bruyn, pp. 27–50. North Holland, Amsterdam.
62. Nurcombe, V., McGrath, P.A., and Bennet, M.R. (1981): Postnatal death of motor neurons during the development of the brachial spinal cord of the rat. *Neurosci. Lett.,* 27:249–254.
63. Oh, S.J., and Danon, M.J. (1983): Nonprogressive congenital neuromuscular disease with uniform type 2 fibres. *Arch. Neurol.,* 40:147–150.
64. Pantou, M.P., Hedayat, I., and Kieny, M. (1982): The pattern of muscle development in the chick leg. *Arch. Anat. Microsc. Morphol. Exp.,* 71:194–206.
65. Robertson, W.C., Kawamura, Y., and Dyck, P.J. (1978): Morphometric study of motor neurons in congenital nemaline myopathy and Werdnig-Hoffmann disease. *Neurology,* 28:1057–1061.
66. Rosman, N.P. (1970): The cerebral defect and myopathy in Duchenne muscular dystrophy. *Neurology,* 20:329–335.
67. Rosman, N.P., and Rebeiz, J.J. (1967): The cerebral defect and myopathy in myotonic dystrophy. *Neurology,* 17:1106–1112.
68. Saint-Anne Dargassies, S. (1974): *Le Developpement Neurologiqué du Nouveau-né à Terme et Premature.* Masson et cie Editeurs, Paris.
69. Salmons, S., and Sreter, F.A. (1976): Significance of impulse activity in the transformation of skeletal muscle type. *Nature,* 263:30–34.
70. Santavuori, P., Leisti, J., and Krurs, S. (1977): Muscle, eye and brain disease—A new syndrome. *Neuropadiatrie,* 8:550.
71. Sarnat, H.B. (1982): Developmental disorders of muscle. In: *Skeletal Muscle Pathology,* edited by J.N. Walton and F.L. Mastaglia. Churchill Livingstone, Edinburgh.
72. Sarnat, H.B. (1983): *Muscle Pathology and Histochemistry,* pp. 45–66. American Society of Clinical Pathologists Press, Chicago.
73. Sarnat, H.B. (1985): Le cerveau influence-t-il le developpement musculaire du foetus humain? *Can. J. Neurol. Sci.,* 12:111–120.
74. Sarnat, H.B. (1986): Cerebral dysgeneses and their influence on fetal muscle development. *Brain Dev.,* 8:495–499.
75. Sarnat, H.B., and Alcala, H. (1980): Human cerebellar hypoplasia. A syndrome of diverse causes. *Arch. Neurol.,* 37:300–305.
76. Sarnat, H.B., Jacob, P., and Jimenez, C. (1988): L'atrophie spinale musculaire: La disparition de la fluorescence a l'A.R.N. des neurones moteurs en degenerescence: Une etude a l'acridine-orange. *Rev. Neurol. (in press).*
77. Sarnat, H.B., O'Connor, T., and Byrne, P.A. (1976): Clinical effects of myotonic dystrophy on pregnancy and the neonate. *Arch. Neurol.,* 33:459–465.
78. Sarnat, H.B., Roth, S.I., and Jimenez, J.F. (1981): Neonatal myotubular myopathy: Neuropathy and failure of postnatal maturation of fetal muscle. *Can. J. Neurol. Sci.,* 8:313–320.

79. Sarnat, H.B., and Silbert, S.W. (1976): Maturation arrest of fetal muscle in neonatal myotonic dystrophy: A pathological study of four cases. *Arch. Neurol.,* 33:466–474.
80. Schroeder, S.M., Kemme, P. T., and Scholz, L. (1979): The fibre structure of denervated and reinervated muscle spindles: Morphometric study of intraspinal muscle fibres. *Acta Neuropathol.,* 46:96–106.
81. Seay, A. R., Ziter, F.A., and Petajan, J.H. (1977): Rigid spine syndrome: A type 1 fibre myopathy. *Arch. Neurol.,* 34:119–122.
82. Sengel, T., and Kieny, M. (1963): Sur le role des organes axiaux dans la differentiation de la pteryle spinale de l'embryon de poulet. *CR Seances Acad. Sci. [D],* 256:774–777.
83. Shafiq, S.A., Dubowitz, V., Peterson, H., et al. (1967): Nemaline myopathy. Report of a fatal case with histochemical and electron microscopic studies. *Brain,* 90:817–828.
84. Spiro, A.J., Shy, G.M., and Gonatas, N.K. (1966): Myotubular myopathy. Persistence of fetal muscle in an adolescent boy. *Arch. Neurol.,* 14:1–14.
85. Sreter, F.A., Astrom, K.E., Romanul, F.C., et al. (1976): Characteristics of myosin in nemaline myopathy. *J. Neurol. Sci.,* 27:99–116.
86. Takeshita, K., Yoshina, K., Kitahara, T., Nakashima, T., and Kato, N. (1977): Survey of Duchenne type and congenital type of muscular dystrophy in Shimane, Japan. *Jpn. J. Hum. Genet.,* 22:43–47.
87. Toufighi, J. Sanani, J.W., Suzaki, L., and Sadda, R.L. (1984): Cerebro-ocular dysplasia muscular dystrophy syndrome. *Acta Neuropathol.,* 65:110–123.
88. Turner, J.W.A. (1949): On amyotoia congenita. *Brain,* 72:25–34.
89. Volpe, P., Damiani, E., Margreth, A., et al. (1982): Fast to slow change of myosin in nemaline myopathy: Electrophoretic and immunologic evidence. *Neurology,* 32:37–41.
90. Walton, J.N., and Gardner-Medwin, D. (1981): Progressive muscular dystrophy and the myotonic disorders. In: *Disorders of Voluntary Muscle,* 4th ed., edited by J.N. Walton, pp. 486–487. Churchill Livingstone, Edinburgh.
91. Zatz, M., Betti, R.T.D., and Levy, G.A. (1981): Benign Duchenne muscular dystrophy in a patient with growth hormone deficiency. *Am. J. Med. Genet.,* 10:301–304.

Fetal Neurology, edited by
A. Hill and J.J. Volpe.
Raven Press, New York © 1989.

Commentary on Chapter 13

*Alan Hill and **Joseph J. Volpe

*Division of Neurology, Department of Paediatrics, University of British Columbia,
British Columbia's Children's Hospital, Vancouver, British Columbia, Canada V6H 3V4;
and **Division of Pediatric Neurology, Washington University School of Medicine,
St. Louis, Missouri 63110

Drs. Jacob and Sarnat raised the important possibility that the developmental neuromuscular disorders should be regarded more correctly as disorders that involve predominantly the motor system from its origins in the cerebral cortex to its termination in muscle. The presence of neuromuscular disease in the fetus may significantly influence the evaluation of fetal movement as a parameter for assessment of fetal well-being. Recent data suggest that factors other than primary genetic defects and/or degeneration of muscle fibers may influence muscle development in the muscular dystrophies and other developmental neuromuscular disorders. Thus, the embryonic development of muscle should be considered in the light of corresponding development in the central and peripheral nervous system. Although the factors responsible for myogenesis are not entirely understood, there is experimental evidence to suggest that motor innervation plays a major role. Thus, denervation of the soleus muscle in the rat, when myogenesis is in the myotubular stage, results in maturational delay with persistence of myoblasts and failure of histochemical differentiation (1). Similarly, the role of the motor neuron in the determination of muscle fiber type has been demonstrated by cross-innervation and reinnervation after denervation experiments (2,4). It appears that motor innervation influences both muscle fiber differentiation and growth of individual muscle fibers.

The effects of upper motor neuron disease on the developing motor unit are not well understood. It may be speculated that such disorders may alter the physiological discharge pattern of lower motor neurons during the histochemical stage of muscle development, i.e., 20 to 28 weeks gestation, which in turn may result in maturational delay and/or abnormal proportions and relative sizes of histochemical fiber types. Because the corticospinal tracts are small and unmyelinated at midgestation, they are unlikely to play a major role in muscle development. Thus, the muscle biopsies of children with spastic diplegia caused by corticospinal abnormalities demonstrate only atrophy of type II fibers, resembling disuse atrophy of normal, mature muscle. In contrast, the multiple small bulbospinal tracts, including the vestibulospinal, reticulospinal, olivospinal, tectospinal, and rubrospinal tracts are relatively well myelinated during this stage of embryogenesis and may influence the developing motor unit. Neuropathological studies have demonstrated characteristic pathological findings in muscle of patients with infratentorial malformations involving the cerebellum or brainstem, which cannot be explained on the basis of primary myopathy or denervation of muscle alone. These abnormalities may be classified as (a) maturational arrest or delay of histochemical differentiation; (b) predominance of more than 80% of either type I or II fibers; (c) congenital muscle fiber-type disproportion with type I fiber predominance and hypotrophy (6). These abnormalities of muscle may contribute to the clinical alterations in muscle tone often observed in children with such malformations.

Similar abnormalities of muscle, i.e., selective type I fiber atrophy or type I fiber predominance, may be observed in the muscular dystrophies, including Duchenne muscular dystrophy, Fukuyama-type congenital muscular dystrophy, Emery-Driefuss dystrophy, and facio-scapulo-humeral dystrophies. Thus, suprasegmental influences may contribute to some aspects of the muscle pathology in the muscular dystrophies. Furthermore, upper motor neuron abnormalities may explain the type I fiber predominance observed in some nonprogressive "congenital myopathies" such as congenital fiber-type disproportion, nemaline rod disease (5), and central core disease (3). Because these diseases are not generally fatal, pathological studies of the brain generally are not available and the hypothesis that the congenital myopathies may represent an expression of underlying central nervous system disease has not been proven. The situation may be further complicated in that the abnormal suprasegmental influence may be physiological and transitory, rather than morphological in nature.

REFERENCES

1. Engel, W.K., and Karpati, G. (1968): Impaired skeletal muscle maturation following neonatal neurectomy. *Dev. Biol.*, 17:713–723.
2. Karpati, G., and Engel, W.K. (1968): "Type grouping" in skeletal muscles after experimental reinnervation. *Neurology*, 18:447–455.
3. Morgan-Hughes, J.A., Brett, E.M., Lake, B.D., et al. (1973): Central core disease or not? *Brain*, 96:527–536.
4. Romanul, I.C.A., and Van der Meulen, J.P. (1967): Slow and fast muscle fibres after cross innervation. Enzymatic and physiologic changes. *Arch. Neurol.*, 17:387–402.
5. Sarnat, H.B. (1983): *Muscle Pathology and Histochemistry*. American Society of Clinical Pathologists Press, Chicago.
6. Sarnat, H.B. (1986): Cerebral dysgeneses and their influence on fetal muscle development. *Brain Dev.*, 8:495–499.

Subject Index

$$225$$
$$\times 14$$
$$\overline{}$$
$$100$$
$$25$$
$$\overline{350}$$
$$-1.25$$
$$\overline{7.5}$$